Chinese Perspectives on Cultural Psychiatry

Wei Wang

Editor

Chinese Perspectives on Cultural Psychiatry

Psychological Disorders in "A Dream of Red Mansions" and Contemporary Society

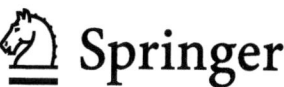 Springer

Editor
Wei Wang
Department of Clinical Psychology
and Psychiatry/School of Public Health
Zhejiang University College of Medicine
Hangzhou, China

ISBN 978-981-13-3536-5   ISBN 978-981-13-3537-2   (eBook)
https://doi.org/10.1007/978-981-13-3537-2

Library of Congress Control Number: 2018964941

This Springer imprint is published by the registered company Springer Nature Singapore Pte Ltd.
The registered company address is: 152 Beach Road, #21-01/04 Gateway East, Singapore 189721, Singapore

Preface

Cultural psychiatry is an important area in psychological medicine and in social science, and many problems in the field remain unclear. The cultural influence on psychological (psychiatric or mental) disorders has been a topic for a long time, and previous studies in this regard have taken primarily a comparative perspective, looking for differences between cultures such as those between Eastern and Western cultures. Nevertheless, few works have focused on the cultural origin and even fewer on the core of a culture and the relationship with psychological problems, especially in Chinese context. This book is proposed to fill the gap by inspecting the elements of Chinese culture and their fitness with Maslow's Hierarchy of Needs Theory (the biological and physiological needs, safety needs, social needs, esteem needs, self-actualization needs, and self-transcendence needs) and their involvements in the psychological disorders. We will propose a link between cultural influence and psychological disorders and present both literature and lab evidence conducted in contemporary China to support it. We will explore the narrative sources in a very influential and realistic novel – *A Dream of Red Mansions* (DRM, a famous Chinese fiction of the seventeenth to eighteenth century) – to study the elements of Chinese culture in ancient China, which provides evidence of the cultural contribution, through its emic part, to some psychiatric symptoms. Admittedly, the positive impact that Chinese culture has on mental health has been recognized and investigated, such as on the personality development, emotion stability, treatment and therapy, and family solidarity. One of our current purposes is to look for the negative impact of Chinese culture on the psychological disorders, which might offer some suggestions for the prevention and management of these disorders worldwide.

Inside the book, we will discuss the Chinese personality structure and personality disorders, bipolar disorders, and other issues related to Chinese culture, with an emphasis on the cultural elements in late imperial and contemporary China, such as Confucianism, Collectivism, family factors, etc., contributing to these disorders. But firstly, we will introduce previous research on some important and distinctive elements of Chinese culture and their relationships with psychological disorders within the framework of Maslow's Hierarchy of Needs Theory. Specifically, the first chapter is set to provide a working hypothesis, a framework for the whole book, and trains of ideas to future studies in this area. In order to look into the core of culture, we will open our discussion with the traditional culture in China, and the materials we used will be from DRM (Chapter "Societal Culture from Late Imperial to contemporary China: As Indirectly Reflected in A Dream of Red Mansions"). The discussion about the cultural continuity in China from earliest times to the present day will be presented as well. Using adjectives chosen from text in DRM, a study looking for the structure of personality will be carried out using the psycho-lexical methodology, so that we might have an idea of what the structure of personality looked like back in time when the novel was written (Chapter "Personality Traits Characterized by the Adjectives in A Dream of Red Mansions"). The personality disorders in the novel affected by Chinese culture will also be discussed (Chapter "Narrations of Personality Disorders in A Dream of Red Mansions"), which will bring implications of the negative influence of Chinese culture on personality pathology.

On the basis of these personality studies, we will then turn to the literature study on the cultural contribution to personality disorder in contemporary China (Chapter "Cultural Contribution to Personality Disorders in China"), and thereafter the structure of personality will be acquired through the development of a questionnaire – the Chinese Adjective Descriptors of Personality (Chapter "Personality Traits in Contemporary China: A Lexical Approach"). Using this questionnaire, we will investigate whether the personality-related Chinese adjectives could predict personality disorder functioning styles well (Chapter "Personality Disorders Predicted by the Chinese Adjective Descriptors of Personality"). Similarly, we will characterize the structure of antisocial personality disorder in the contemporary Chinese culture (Chapter "Adjectival Descriptors for Antisocial Personality Trait in Chinese Culture").

As for the cultural influence on emotion, we will discuss its contribution to bipolar disorder, especially in the Chinese context (Chapter "Bipolar Disorders in Chinese Culture: From a Perspective of Harmony"). We will then apply the Chinese Adjective Descriptors of Personality questionnaire to correlate the affective states of bipolar disorder patients (Chapter "Predicting Affective States of Bipolar Disorder by the Chinese Adjective Descriptors of Personality"). In addition, concerning that family plays an important role in people's life and mental status, we will discuss specifically the relationship between psychiatric/psychological disorders and family factors in the context of Chinese culture (Chapter "Chinese Family Contributions to Psychological Disorders"). Finally, we will continue to consummate the framework which addressing the link between psychological disorders and Chinese culture (Chapter "A Theoretical Framework Explaining Chinese Cultural Contributions to Psychological Disorders"). Therefore, the whole book points to the significance of Chinese culture in sorts of psychological disorder and offers hints to the understanding, preventing, and treatment of these disorders in a Confucian or collectivistic context, such as in China or other parts of the world.

There are definitely important words which I would like to put forward here. I greatly appreciate the hard work and creativity of my colleagues who have contributed to this book; each colleague has also reviewed the whole book and provided their invaluable feedback. In particular, I thank Drs. Hongying Fan and Guorong Ma for their additional terrific job by intellectual and technical assistance.

Hangzhou, China   Wei Wang
12 October 2018

Contents

Contributors[1]

Hao Chai Department of Psychology, College of Education, Zhejiang University of Technology, Hangzhou, China

Wanzhen Chen Department of Social Work, East China University of Science and Technology, Shanghai, China

Hongying Fan Department of Clinical Psychology and Psychiatry/School of Public Health, Zhejiang University College of Medicine, Hangzhou, China

Yanli Jia Department of Clinical Psychology and Psychiatry/School of Public Health, Zhejiang University College of Medicine, Hangzhou, China

Guorong Ma Department of Clinical Psychology and Psychiatry/School of Public Health, Zhejiang University College of Medicine, Hangzhou, China

Xu Shao Department of Clinical Psychology and Psychiatry/School of Public Health, Zhejiang University College of Medicine, Hangzhou, China

Chanchan Shen Department of Clinical Psychology and Psychiatry/School of Public Health, Zhejiang University College of Medicine, Hangzhou, China

Chu Wang Department of Clinical Psychology and Psychiatry/School of Public Health, Zhejiang University College of Medicine, Hangzhou, China

Jiawei Wang Department of Clinical Psychology and Psychiatry/School of Public Health, Zhejiang University College of Medicine, Hangzhou, China

Mufan Wang Faculty of Psychology, Universidad Complutense de Madrid, Madrid, Spain

Wei Wang Department of Clinical Psychology and Psychiatry/School of Public Health, Zhejiang University College of Medicine, Hangzhou, China

---

[1] Note: For Chinese contributors, the order of their given and family names is that the given name comes first then the family name, while for other Chinese persons mentioned in the text, the order of their given and family names is that the family name comes first then the given name.

You Xu Department of Sleep Medicine, the Seventh Hospital of Hangzhou, and Mental Health Center, Zhejiang University College of Medicine, Hangzhou, China

Shaohua Yu Department of Psychiatry, The Second Affiliated Hospital, Zhejiang University College of Medicine, Hangzhou, China

Bingren Zhang Department of Clinical Psychology and Psychiatry/School of Public Health, Zhejiang University College of Medicine, Hangzhou, China

Junpeng Zhu Department of Psychiatry, Zhejiang Provincial People's Hospital, Hangzhou, China

Department of Psychiatry, People's Hospital of Hangzhou Medical College, Hangzhou, China

Abbreviations

BD I	Bipolar I Disorder
BD II	Bipolar II Disorder
CADAP	Chinese Adjective Descriptors for Antisocial Personality Trait
CADP	Chinese Adjective Descriptors of Personality
CCMD	Chinese Classification of Mental Disorders
DRM	A Dream of Red Mansions
DSM	Diagnostic and Statistical Manual of Mental Disorders
HCL-32	Hypomania Checklist-32
ICD	International Classification of Diseases
MDQ	Mood Disorder Questionnaire
NEO-PI-R	Revised NEO Personality Inventory
PCL	Psychopathy Checklist
PERM	Parker Personality Measure
PVP	Plutchik-van Praag Depression Inventory
TCI	Temperament and Character Inventory
TCM	Traditional Chinese Medicine
ZKPQ	Zuckerman-Kuhlman Personality Questionnaire

Technical Chinese Words

Ai (爱)	Affection or love (first appearance in Chapter "Personality Traits in Contemporary China: A Lexical Approach")
Dao (道)	A core concept in Daoism, which refers to the source of heaven and earth and in between, is elusive and vague, deep and obscure, and soundless and formless and thus cannot be seen or touched (Chapter "Societal Culture from Late Imperial to contemporary China: As Indirectly Reflected in A Dream of Red Mansions")
Dao De Jing (道德经)	The Book of the Way and the Book of Virtue, which is the Daoist Classic (Chapter "Societal Culture from Late Imperial to contemporary China: As Indirectly Reflected in A Dream of Red Mansions")
Guan Xi (关系)	Relationship (Chapter "Societal Culture from Late Imperial to contemporary China: As Indirectly Reflected in A Dream of Red Mansions")
He (和)	Harmony (Chapter "Personality Traits in Contemporary China: A Lexical Approach")
Huang Di Nei Jing (黄帝内经)	Yellow Emperor's Internal Canon of Medicine (Chapter "Bipolar Disorders in Chinese Culture: From a Perspective of Harmony")
Junzi (君子)	Superior man or gentleman (Chapter "Hierarchical Needs and Psychological Disorders in China")
Li Ji (礼记)	Record of Rites (Chapter "Hierarchical Needs and Psychological Disorders in China")

Lun Yu (论语)	Analects (Chapter "Societal Culture from Late Imperial to contemporary China: As Indirectly Reflected in A Dream of Red Mansions")
Mianzi (面子)	Face (Chapter "Societal Culture from Late Imperial to contemporary China: As Indirectly Reflected in A Dream of Red Mansions")
Ping (平)	Peace (Chapter "Personality Traits in Contemporary China: A Lexical Approach")
San Gang (三纲)	Three Cardinal Guides or Three Fundamental Bonds (Chapter "Societal Culture from Late Imperial to contemporary China: As Indirectly Reflected in A Dream of Red Mansions")
Sheng Ren (圣人)	Sages (Chapter "Societal Culture from Late Imperial to contemporary China: As Indirectly Reflected in A Dream of Red Mansions")
Shi Ji (史记)	Records of the Grand Historian (Chapter "Personality Traits Characterized by the Adjectives in A Dream of Red Mansions")
Tai Ji Quan (太极拳)	An internal Chinese martial art practiced for both its defense training and its health benefits (Chapter "Hierarchical Needs and Psychological Disorders in China")
Wu Chang (五常)	Five Constant Virtues, including *Rén* (仁, humanity or benevolence), *Yi* (义, righteousness), *Li* (礼, propriety), *Zhi* (智, wisdom), and *Xin* (信, trust or faithfulness) (Chapter "Hierarchical Needs and Psychological Disorders in China")
Wu Lun (五伦)	Five Cardinal Relationships, including *Zhong* (忠, loyalty and duty), *Xiao* (孝, love and obedience), *Rěn* (忍, obligation and submission), *Ti* (悌, seniority and modeling), and *Xin* (信, trust or faithfulness) (Chapter "Hierarchical Needs and Psychological Disorders in China")
Wu Xing (五行)	Five basic elements, including *Jin* (金, metal), *Mu* (木, wood), *Shui* (水, water), *Huo* (火, fire), and *Tu* (土, earth) (Chapter "Bipolar Disorders in Chinese Culture: From a Perspective of Harmony")
Xiao Ren (小人)	A person with vile character (Chapter "Bipolar Disorders in Chinese Culture: From a Perspective of Harmony")

Xiao Shun (孝顺)	Filial piety (Chapter "Societal Culture from Late Imperial to contemporary China: As Indirectly Reflected in A Dream of Red Mansions")
Yin (隐)	Being a hermit (Chapter "Personality Traits Characterized by the Adjectives in A Dream of Red Mansions")
Yin (阴) – *Yang* (阳)	Two forces of the *Dao*, with *Yin* standing for female force, such as passivity and dark, and *Yang* standing for male force, such as activity and light (Chapter "Societal Culture from Late Imperial to contemporary China: As Indirectly Reflected in A Dream of Red Mansions")
Yong (勇)	Courage (Chapter "Personality Traits Characterized by the Adjectives in A Dream of Red Mansions")
Zhong Yong (中庸)	Doctrine of mean (Chapter "Bipolar Disorders in Chinese Culture: From a Perspective of Harmony")

Hierarchical Needs and Psychological Disorders in China

Hongying Fan and Wei Wang

1 Introduction

The word "culture" has rich connotations. According to a Dutch scholar, Hofstede (1991), culture is "the collective programming of the mind which distinguishes the members of one group or category of people from another." Culture is also defined as "both the means and values which arise among distinctive social groups and classes, on the basis of their given historical conditions and relationship, through which they handle and respond to the conditions of existence" (Hall 1980). Psychiatrists and other scholars have recognized the significance of culture in psychological disorders, such that in the Diagnostic and Statistical Manual of Mental Disorders, Fifth Edition (DSM-5, American Psychiatric Association 2013), a widely-acknowledged diagnostic standard in the international psychiatric arena, has included the Cultural Formulation as a part of its Section III – Emerging Measures and Models. Problems associated with social or cultural environment are also considered as a collection of factors influencing health status in the 11th beta version of the International Classification of Diseases (ICD-11, World Health Organization 2017), another widely-acknowledged diagnostic standard in the international psychiatric field.

Similar to other world cultures, the Chinese culture has its advantages regarding its elements of the indigenous perspective. For the last 10 years, the popular term "Qian Xuesen's Question" has been widely reported in China, and caused a stir and heated discussion in China. Praised as the "Father of Missiles in China", Mr. Qian Xuesen was a rocket scientist educated in USA. He returned China in the 1950s and became a national hero for his defining contribution to China's space program. Once in a meeting with the former Chinese Premier – Mr. Wen Jiabao in 2009 about

H. Fan · W. Wang (✉)
Department of Clinical Psychology and Psychiatry/School of Public Health, Zhejiang University College of Medicine, Hangzhou, China
e-mail: drwangwei@zju.edu.cn

© Springer Nature Singapore Pte Ltd. 2019
W. Wang (ed.), *Chinese Perspectives on Cultural Psychiatry*,
https://doi.org/10.1007/978-981-13-3537-2_1

the education reform in China, Mr. Qian questioned the reasons behind that China had not cultivated great innovative-talents (Zhang et al. 2012). Some scholars believe that "one of the most important reasons that China has not fully developed is that not a single university in China is able to follow a model which enables innovation and creativity in science and technology" (Jin and Qi 2009). Definitely, this statement is a very superficial consideration.

Later, the discussion veered away from education and round to the Chinese cultural criticism. Some scholars believe it is the Chinese culture that leads to the embarrassing situation. For instance, Confucianism has been a representative of the Chinese traditional culture in official context for more than 2000 years; while only for centuries has Capitalism been growing in China. Thus, these two components lead to a cultural confusion, which in turn nudging China towards reflections on the Confucius worldview and cultural value, and exploring ways to integrate Confucianism into modern society. From some perspective of view, culture can be regarded as a means of defense against anxiety, therefore "when people are reminded of their mortality, they are motivated to validate and defend their cultural worldviews and values in order to boost their self-esteem and viability of their own culture" (Leng and Salzman 2016). In this sense, the Confucianism renaissance in recent years might not be that hopeful or optimistic. Some Chinese people then turn to reading Mr. Lu Xun's works again for his critiques of the feudal Chinese culture (Liu 2016; Wang 2016; Gao 2018). Mr. Lu Xun was the pen name of Zhou Shuren (1881–1936), who was a leading figure of modern Chinese literature, the titular head of the League of Left-Wing Writers in Shanghai, China in the 1930s.

In context of Chinese culture, patients with psychological disorders display many clinical or epidemiological differences from those of other contexts. For instance, Chinese depressive outpatients reported more somatic symptoms of depression compared with Euro-Canadians (Ryder et al. 2002, 2008); and the prevalence of personality disorders in China was higher than that in Western Europe but lower than that in America (Huang et al. 2009). It is easier to speculate that culture is a reason accounting for these differences.

Mr. Abraham H. Maslow (1943, 1954, 1970a, b) stated that human motivation was based on people's seeking fulfillment and change through personal growth. His model of the hierarchy of needs is one of the most referenced and discussed psychological theories, which emphasizes human's needs in five to eight levels: Biological and psychological needs, Safety needs, Social needs, Esteem needs, Self-Actualization needs, and Self-transcendence needs. Maslow's Hierarchy of Needs Theory has been believed capable to predict how individuals develop (Wicker et al. 1993), how nations develop, and how people's quality of life improves (Sirgy 1986). However, once any need of an individual is not satisfied, his psychological problems appear. Based on the perspective of human needs and the uniqueness of Chinese culture, we are aiming to explain how the risk factors in the culture contribute to the psychological disorders, as illustrated in Fig. 1. This figure introduces us a working hypothesis of the present book, and presents an outline of our strategy to address the psychological disorders in Chinese culture.

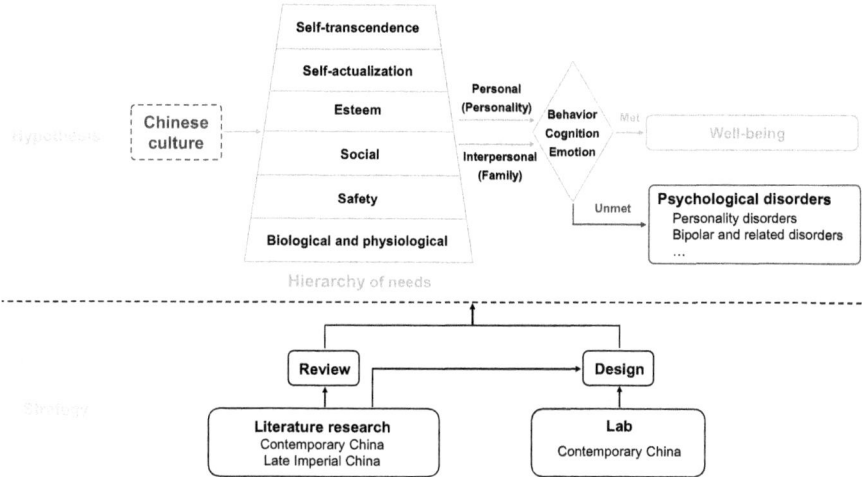

Fig. 1 Working hypothesis (upper part) and testing strategy (lower part) of the relationship between Chinese culture and psychological disorders. The core components of Chinese culture trigger individiduals' psychological processes (behavior, cognition and emotion) to meet their hierarchical needs (Maslow's theory); once the needs are met, they remain well-being; otherwise, they develop psychological disorders. The classical novel text (the late imperial China) and the research literature (in contemporary China) might provide topical reviews and exploring-designs, and the psychological measurements (contemporary China) might offer lab-investigations, both of which help to prove the working hypothesis

2 Involvement of the Biological and Physiological Needs

Human beings are seeking the basic necessities of life, such as air, food, drink, oxygen, shelter, warmth, sex, sleep, etc., namely biological and physiological needs (Maslow 1970a; McLeod 2007). This is definitely the case in China, in addition, for some Chinese people, drinking is the most prominent on the level of needs, which can be traced back to the ancient history. *Li Ji* (礼记, Record of Rites), one of Confucian classics written in more than two thousand years ago, says that "eat and drink, man and woman - the greatest human desires reside in them (饮食男女, 人之大欲存焉)". Throughout the history, drinking has been acting as an essential part in important events of Chinese people, including wedding ceremonies, sacrificial ceremonies, and birthday parties. In modern times, as Chinese business world becoming much highly competitive, drinking is seen as an essential behavior for success, an approach to lessen tensions and to facilitate social exchange among Chinese businessmen (Hao and Young 2000; Cochrane et al. 2003). Hao et al. (1999) also studied Chinese people living in six areas including Hunan Province in Southcentral China, Anhui Province in the East, Jilin Province in the Northeast, Sichuan Province in the Southwest, and Shandong Province in the North, and reported that the male, female and total drinking rates were 84.1%, 29.3% and 59.5% respectively, with more than half of male drinkers and 90.0% of female drinkers used alcohol up to once a week, and more than 16.1% of male drinkers and 2.5% of female drinkers drank once a day or more. Later, Hao et al. (2004) reported that the 1-year drinking rate was 59.0%, and the point prevalence rate of alcohol dependence was 3.8% in 24,992 community residents living in the same five provinces of China mentioned above. There is a phenomenon that in social environment, the more an individual drinks the happier his feeling and the closer his relationship with others, therefore the alcohol related disorders including alcohol dependence are common and high in prevalence. The drinking culture to some extent results in high alcohol use, alcoholism and other related disorders (Cochrane et al. 2003).

Furthermore, the suppressive attitude towards sex in Chinese culture greatly influences the satisfaction of sex needs. However, many psychiatrists, psychologists, trans-culturalists, and anthropologists, who are mostly Chinese and quite deeply experience and understand Chinese culture, share the opinion that Chinese people often take a suppressive attitude toward sex (Tseng and Hsu 1970; Suen 1983). The suppression of sex needs and expression originates from Chinese reverence for Li (礼, propriety), which has strictly moral and social codes, and which is ruled by Confucianism. The Chinese are observed more conservative than people from other cultures generally, and Chinese culture is even described as asexual (Suen 1983). Compared with American people, Chinese were found holding the sex role attitude more conservative (Chia et al. 1994). Similarly, compared with English people, Chinese were found persisting traditional values in mate-selection preferences, implying that Chinese carried out a relatively conservative sexual culture from ancient times to the present day (Higgins et al. 2002). Further, under the influence Chinese culture, Asian college students presented predominantly more conservative views on the interpersonal sexual behavior and sociosexual restrictiveness than non-Asian college students did (Meston et al. 1996).

Unfortunately, the Confucian conservative concept including the suppression of sex needs leads to psychological problems conversely. It has shown that the forced suppression of desire, provided some short-term relief, but often backfired later, leading to the so-called ironic rebound effects (Wegner 1994; Hofmann et al. 2015). As for Maslow's Hierarchy of Needs Theory, the more the desire is suppressed the more psychological disorders occur. In addition, the sexual dysfunction is thought due to anxiety and cognitive interference related to sex needs (Barlow 1986). Investigators have noticed that there is an association between mental health, psychological illness, and sexual functioning well-being (Ace 2007). Laurent and Simons (2009) also found relationships between disorders of sexual desire, arousal, and orgasm comorbid with depression and anxiety. The depression and anxiety levels were increased with conservatism in general population (Crandall 1965).

There are indeed cumulative evidences demonstrating the associations between sexual problems and psychological disorders. Sexual disfunctions were found associated with anxiety and depression: the premature ejaculation was significantly associated with anxiety in men, and the arousal, orgasmic, and enjoyment problems and others were associated with anxiety in women (Dunn et al. 1999). A group of investigators interviewed 4678 Chinese individuals about their perceptions connected with sex and their association with quality of life, and they found that about half participants were disturbed by sexual problems, a rate markedly higher than those in America (Lau et al. 2008). Specifically, it is suggested that at least one sexual problem was significantly associated with the lower overall life satisfaction and worse mental health for both genders. This study also reported prevalences of some sex-related problems: sexual problems ranged from 3.4% (pain) to 29.7% (premature orgasm) for men, and 6.9% (anxiety) to 24.7% (lack of interest) for women, and the erectile and lubrication problems were 9.6 and 23.6% in men and women respectively. These data confirmed the association that the lower satisfaction of sex leads to the higher prevalence of sexual and psychological disorders, and explained that the suppressive attitude to sex needs is associated with the occurrence of psychological disorders in China.

3 Involvement of the Safety Needs

Safety needs are a set of desires to seek security through order and law, including protection from security, order, regulation, limits, stability, etc. (Maslow 1970a; McLeod 2007). Affected by Confucianism, besides the legislative system, moral rules assist in social order under the background of Chinese culture. Individuals were taught to observe the *Wu Chang* (五常, the Five Constant Virtues) of Confucian distillation: *Rén* (仁, Humanity), *Yi* (义, Righteousness), *Li* (礼, Propriety), *Zhi* (智, Wisdom) and *Xin* (信, Faithfulness) (Chen 1986). Chinese people are required to behave and follow these principles in order to have harmony for themselves and the society. The obsession with preserving harmony sets in motion the condition of the excessive power distance and rigid rules, tending to be uniformity in the control of operations (Gray 1988), and to the detriment of flexibility and professionalism (Chan et al. 2001).

The social ideal in the harmonious circumstances is of "every man in his place", in concert with the humanistic idea of "everything in its place" (Lin 1935). Every person is given a definite place or role in the society, i.e., the social status. In the Confucian culture, people are required to admit their own responsibility to support and maintain harmony, then protect the stability of society. According to how well a person serves to enhance the interpersonal standards of the society, his behavior is evaluated, and his relational identity is defined. Compared with Western cultures, where individuality or individual freedoms are highly valued, Chinese culture has a group-oriented behavior within harmonious interaction of group members in priority (Bedford and Hwang 2003). Harmony is a crucial component of relational identity that persons are not permitted to disrupt it, and conversely it impacts on the identity of everyone.

Thus, the objective right and wrong actions in maintaining behavior is taken lightly, and is replaced by maintaining harmony using shame and guilt as more effective methods of social control (Bedford and Hwang 2003). Contrary to people in Individualistic-Occidental culture, an individual in a Collectivistic-Oriental culture would feel unsafe if he fails to fulfill a group requirement or is judged by the group, otherwise he would lose the group status. As Bedford and Hwang (2003) stated, for example, the experience of shame is produced by revelation of a failure or a flaw in one's identity, which is also linked to the fear that one's inadequacies will result in rejection by the group. Shame and guilt could provide energy for and guide the behaviors related to the self-conscious emotions (Tomkins 1970; Weiner 1992; Baumeister et al. 1995; Lindsay-Hartz et al. 1995), and are the prelude to other problems and disorders as well.

The systematic and empirical comparisons of shame and guilt between different cultural backgrounds can reveal the features of one culture. The Chinese are more sensitive to arouse a feeling of shame when other people's actions infringe upon their sense of identity and order, because of their much stronger connectedness with others than Westerners do (Hwang 1999). Stipek (1998) also found that Chinese university students agreed more than Americans did with standpoints, suggesting that individuals should feel ashamed for the negative behavior or outcomes related to family members. The socialization of shame could start on age two-and-a-half in Chinese through the interviews with the primary caregivers and longitudinal observations of spontaneous home interactions (Fung 1999). Shame is a vital factor mediated the linkage from face-lose to relationship deterioration (Kam and Bond 2008). This also happens in other Asian countries, for instance, a cross-cultural study revealed that American children scored highest on pride, whereas Japanese children scored highest on shame, and Korean children scored highest on guilt (Furukawa et al. 2012), confirming the differences between Western and Asian cultures (Bagozzi et al. 1999).

Above all, the Chinese are more sensitive to being personally shamed by actions on the part of others than Westerners are. Bond (1986) claimed that "an individual in Chinese society always belongs to some groups which absorb and reflect that individual's glory or shame". He also pointed out that emotions, including shame and guilt, afflict members of the Chinese family. When the person intends to avoid feelings of guilt, shame, or self-criticism, he feels pressure with a sense of resistance, inner conflict, and anxiety (Deci and Ryan 2000; Soenens and Vansteenkiste 2010).

4   Involvement of the Social Needs

Social needs, also called belongingness and love needs, are the needs to seek affiliation with a group, such as work group, family, affection, relationships, etc. (Maslow 1970a; McLeod 2007). In Sternberg's Triangular Love Theory, there are three components of love: intimacy, passion, and commitment (Sternberg 1986, 1998). Recently scholars have again confirmed the relationship between the three components of love and fundamental motives of humans (Engel et al. 2002). These documentation once again confirm the structure of the social needs.

One of the significant features of Chinese culture regarding the needs for social and love is the family and group orientation (Faure and Fang 2008), or the "high

Collectivism"/"low Individualism" (Hofstede 1984; Hofstede and Bond 1988). The foundation of Chinese culture, the Confucianism, is obviously the primary cause for collectivistic interpersonal relationships (Pye 1972). According to Confucius, human relations and their principles should follow the rules defined by *Wu Lun* (五伦, the Five Cardinal, Relationships): *Zhong* (忠, loyalty and duty) as the principle of the relationship between sovereign and subject; *Xiao* (孝, love and obedience), father and son; *Rĕn* (忍, obligation and submission), husband and wife; *Ti* (悌, seniority and modeling subject), elder and younger brothers; and *Xin* (信, trust), friend and friend. The ethical idea *Rén* (仁, benevolence) was emphasized by Confucius, defined as "goodness in interpersonal relationships", for the sake of interdependence in society (Lin 1939; Tseng and Hsu 1970).

As mentioned above, according to the safety needs, the aspiration of Chinese to keep social harmony leads to Collectivism, with a high degree of interdependence (Hofstede 1980, 1984). Collectivism embraces interdependence, interpersonal harmony, co-operation, and the subordination of personal goals to in-group goals (Triandis et al. 1988). Triandis (1989, 1993, 2001) further characterized Collectivism as emphasizing interdependence, family security, social hierarchies, co-operation, and lower levels of competition, different from independence, freedom, and high levels of competition and pleasure of Individualism. For instance, aiming at fostering harmony and mutual obligation, Collectivism may encourage family members to share responsibilities (Lebra 1976; Markus and Kitayama 1991; Heine 2001).

Investigators have made much effort for a systematic comparison between Collectivism and Individualism (Gao 2001). As expected, strong individualistic values and beliefs in Individualism are harmful to society and the individual psychology; in detail, they are associated with smaller and less satisfying social support networks, less skill in managing both self and others' emotions, lower intentions to seek help from family and friends for personal and suicidal problems, and higher levels of hopelessness and suicide ideation (Scott et al. 2004). Nevertheless, it does not mean that Collectivism is perfect. Regarding personality, people might try very hard to get along with others in order to live a life that coincides with Collectivism, which might result in a dependent trait (Diaz-Guerrero 1979; Triandis and Suh 2002). In Chapter "Narrations of Personality Disorders in A Dream of Red Mansions", we will introduce the proneness to avoidant personality disorder of Chinese females to the Collectivism along with male dominance, which leads to a higher tendency for them to submit to their fate-fatalism.

Indeed, in contrast to the case in Individualistic orientation, where people try to seek control over the fate, Collectivistic orientation is thought to be the reason for the Chinese to submit to their fate-fatalism (Chan 1967). Moreover, the interdependent orientation stunts the expression of negative emotions for fear of disruptive relationships. The Chinese are always more accustomed to controlling and hiding their negative emotions instead of exhibiting them outward (Triandis 2000; Goodwin and Lee 1994; Chen 1995). Other studies have also disclosed the suppression of emotional expression in Chinese people, for instance, the collectivistic context is ruled to less self-disclosure, more expressing indirectly, nonverbally, ambiguously, and contextually, and less expressing in communication styles (Argyle et al. 1986; Gudykunst and Matsumoto 1996).

Fortunately, the self-disclosure is beneficial for interpersonal communication and relationships, because of its positive effects on stress reduction, intimacy building, and social approval increasing for one's ideas (Greenberg and Stone 1992; Posey et al. 2010). Sprecher and Hendrick (2004) examined the connection between self-disclosure and characteristics of individuals and intimate relationship, exposed that self-disclosure had positive association between self-esteem, relationship esteem, responsiveness, and relationship quality including satisfaction, love, and commitment. However, lack of self-disclosure is related to depression (Wei et al. 2005), fear (Bartholomew and Horowitz 1991), anxiety (Hong and Woody 2007), and the feeling of loneliness (Stokes 1987; Wei et al. 2005). On the other hand, the lower score of self-disclosure brings the avoidant attitude toward seeking professional psychological help (Vogel and Wester 2003; Heath et al. 2016). From this point of view, psychologists and psychiatrists might offer assistance to patients with lower self-disclosure, and with the reduction of mental health-related stigma (Henderson et al. 2017).

5 Involvement of the Esteem Needs

An individual needs to seek his esteem through achievement or peer-recognition (Maslow 1970a; McLeod 2007). Based on Maslow's theory, satisfaction of self-esteem needs leads to the feelings of self-confidence, worth, strength, capability, and adequacy, and of being useful and necessary in the world. Hofstede (1980, p. 320) generalized that "relationships among Chinese people are strictly determined by the hierarchy framework", and the workflow is not codified (Yeh 1988). In line with the roles individuals play within society, Chinese people characterize themselves directly according to the needs of self-esteem.

The hierarchy in Chinese society in general depends on the legal and moral rules originating from Confucianism, especially the respect for etiquette, age and social classes (Ho 1985; Faure and Fang 2008), with the dominance of elders and men (Lang 1946; Ho 1987). The principles of *Wu Lun* regarding the relationships between sovereign and subject, father and son, husband and wife, elder and younger brothers, and friend and friend, are fully embodied in the social hierachies of China. Ho et al. (2004) observed that requirements of classic propriety and protocol were rather strict in Confucian societies, stipulating a rigidly hierarchical and authoritarian social-order and allowing authority and role relationships to take the place of individual sentiments, in expressing emotions. The image of *Junzi* (君子, the superior man or gentleman), raised by Confucius as an ideal goal for a man, is asked to maintain tightly controlled to meet the expectation of the strict demands of propriety and protocol.

According to empirical studies, the hierarchy and authoritarian in China might be conductive to social harmony and peace; however, they might contribute to the reduced self-esteem of individuals. Investigators compared the difference of self-esteem between the Chinese and American, and found a positive relationship between self-esteem and self-protection in response to negative feedback in the American, but not in the Chinese (Brockner and Chen 1996). This study indicates a lower self-esteem level in the Chinese, which might fit into that the high self-esteemed persons react to evaluative feedback identified than the low ones do (Taylor and Brown 1988). Tsai et al. (2001) also observed that affiliation with Chinese people was negatively correlated with self-esteem in the Chinese American. In addition, the Chinese and Japanese have lower level of self-esteem than that of North Americans (Heine et al. 1999). Both Chinese and Japanese individuals tend to view and present themselves negatively, whereas North American individuals positively, which might be due to their different cultures. According to Yik et al. (1998), "North American cultures view the self as separate from others, they encourage their members to demonstrate their uniqueness by engaging in self-enhancement strategies (i.e., presentation of the self as superior to others), whereas Chinese and Japanese cultures view the self as connected with others and therefore encourage their members to maintain interpersonal relationships through self-effacement strategies (i.e., presentation of the self as inferior to others)."

The self-esteem has been conceptualized as both a casual factor and an outcome of psychological illnesses, being frequently used as a global indicator of mental health, personal coping resources, and emotional adjustment, either by design or accident (Schwarzer et al. 1997). Rosenberg et al. (1989) conducted a study on self-esteem and adolescent problems, and found a reciprocal effect of between their self-esteem and their school achievement, problem behaviors, and depressive state. In intercultural studies between the Chinese and Western, individuals with lower self-esteem and higher pessimistic thoughts about their accomplishments and personal development were considered to have a lower sense of self-efficacy. The latter was associated with depression, anxiety, helplessness, and physical symptoms, and negatively with optimism (Schwarzer 1993; Schwarzer et al. 1997). Recently, investigators have disclosed the dark-side of the self-esteem, i.e., it is in association with suicide (Zhang et al. 2004), subjective well-being (Cai et al. 2009), body dissatisfaction (Davis and Katzman 1998; Tiggemann 2005), inappropriate use of social media (Andreassen et al. 2017) or internet (Zhao et al. 2017), family dysfunction (Shi et al. 2017), and examination stress (Xiang et al. 2017).

6 Involvement of the Self-Actualization Needs

The self-actualization needs are different from the basic/deficient needs (i.e., biological and physiological, safety, social, and esteem needs), and are motivated to fulfill personal potential, such as self-fulfillment and personal growth seeking. Acquiring knowledge and systematizing the universe have been considered as expressions of self-actualization for an intelligent man. The desire to know and to understand, namely the need of cognition, such as knowledge, meaning interpretation, etc., is a valid approach to self-actualization (Maslow 1970a; McLeod 2007). The cognition need is essential for sharing knowledge (curiosity) and for understanding (the philosophical, theological, value-system-building explanation need). It is also defined as "a need to structure relevant situations in meaningful and integrated ways" or "a need to understand and make reasonable the experiential world" (Cohen et al. 1955). Kruglanski and Webster (1996) defined it as the desire to find an answer to an ambiguous situation, which is widely ramifying consequences for social-cognitive phenomena at the intrapersonal, interpersonal, and group levels of analysis. Of course, there are still other concepts relating to the cognition need that are influenced by culture, for instance, an individual's motivation with respect to information processing and judgment (Webster and Kruglanski 1994).

It is then understandable that the need of cognition is influenced by culture. According to socioemotional selectivity theory (Carstensen et al. 1999), the acquisition of knowledge is a similar concept, which motivates an enormous amount of social behavior including problem-solving approaches, through the pursuit of information. From the perspective of time orientation, the linkage between the need of cognition and culture is concise enough to understand. Implicitly or explicitly in theory, cultural values represent the common ideas, such as what is good, right, and desirable in a society (Williams 1970). Cultural values constitute the fundamental elements of a culture (Kluckhohn 1962) and reflect the essential characteristics of that culture (Hofstede 2001). Cultural values also influence individuals' behavior in a society (Tybout and Artz 1994) by structuring their beliefs and attitudes, which providing them with a whole set of solutions to the problems they encounter (Terpstra and David 1985; Rice 1993; Hofstede 2001).

On the other aspect, the time orientations of a value are divided into three dimensions: past, present, and future (Kluckhohn and Strodbeck 1961). In Chinese culture, the orientation to the past is the core components of the need of cognition (Chinese Culture Connection 1987; Fan 2000). Investigators have compared China with Hindu (Smith 1952), America and Mexico (Spears et al. 2000), and have concluded that the Chinese venerate and respect more for tradition, supporting the past-time orientation feature of the Chinese. The Chinese believe that their interactions with other things or beings are continuous (Yau 1988). Moreover, the tendency towards past-time orientation of the Chinese is linked conceptually with traditionalism, referring greater value on tradition, which is different from the strong future orientation of Australians; thus, the tendency leads less willing of Chinese to initiate changes than of Australians (Lowe and Corkindale 1998). Furthermore, linguistic scholars put more attention to the relationship between languages and cultures, by watching Chinese language as "what is in front of the speaker is in the past, while what is in back of the speaker is in the future" (Ahrens and Huang 2002; Yu 2012).

The activities of Chinese people are regulated by the words and sayings of the witted sages of the distant past in virtue of a high regard for their ancestors (Lam 2002). They historically believe in an old adage: draw lessons from history or take history as a mirror (以史为鉴), which indicates not only a continuity among the past, the present, and the future, but a focus on the past. Yau (1988) has found that when making current consumption choices, Chinese consumers are likely to consider opinions, values and influences of deceased relatives and respected figures.

Unfortunately, the past-time orientations have brought harm to mental health to an individual. Tradition is central of past-time orientations, which holds a belief that no new thing will occur in the present or the future that has not already happened (Kluckhohn and Strodbeck 1961). Many studies have shown that the future-oriented individuals are with higher anxiety (Kendall and Ingram 1989; Getsinger 1978), while the past-oriented individuals are with higher depression (Kendall and Ingram 1989; Eysenck and Fajkowska 2017). In particular, patients with depression were most preoccupied with past events in comparison to healthy participants, meanwhile, the former generally overestimated time, attended to more distant past events and memories, focused less on present and future events, and concentrated on more imminent future events (Wyrick and Wyrick 1977). A high degree of past temporal orientation always gives rise to subsequently elevated levels of distress long after a life trauma had passed, and invokes the temporal disintegration at the time of the trauma (Holman and Silver 1998).

7 Involvement of the Self-Transcendence Needs

In Maslow's Hierarchy of Needs (Maslow 1970b; Baurley 2004; McLeod 2007), other than basic needs of the above-mentioned levels, there are meta-needs (or meta-motivation), where an individual constantly strives to satisfy. The meta-needs include cognitive, aesthetic, self-actualization and self-transcendence needs. Individuals with self-transcendence needs seek further a cause beyond the self and experience a communion beyond the boundaries of the self through peak experience, then help others to achieve self-actualization. As Maslow and other psychologists believe, the individual may be involved in the service to others, devotion to an ideal (e.g., truth or art) or a cause (e.g., social justice, environmentalism, pursuit of science, or religious faith), or a desire to be united with what is perceived as transcendent or divine, or both; or be involved in the mystical experiences and certain experiences with nature, aesthetic experiences, sexual experiences, or other transpersonal experiences, where the individual experiences a sense of identity that transcends or extends beyond the personal self (Maslow 1971; McLeod 2007).

The hierarchy of needs have proposed two paths toward self-transcendence. One is to satisfy all four levels of basic needs and self-actualization needs, the other is to directly transcend the personal self. The self-transcendence touches on the questions such as ultimate concern in spiritual faith or religion. However, scholars have had difficulty applying the sense of religion into the Chinese context, and some of them "even go so far as to say that the dimension of transcendence is itself lacking in the Chinese spiritual universe", because the English word "religion" comes as it does from the Latin "religio", not traditionally existing in the Chinese vocabulary, and it is usually taken to "signify a bond between the human and the divine" (Ching 1993). Religion is different from the spiritual faith (i.e., Christian faith), but it might be understood as the belief in the existence of a god or gods, and the activities that are connected with the worship of them. From this perspective, Daoism can be regarded as a native Chinese religion.

Daoism seems suitable to meet the self-transcendence needs, with its advocacy of integration with the Law of Nature, inaction, and infinite frame of reference, rather than of social attainment, self-development, progressive endeavor, and personal interpretation (Yip 2004). Daoism, along with the psychological theory-schools of Jung, Erikson, and Maslow, shares the common central aspect: "the metamorphosis of one's false (non-genuine) self into one's true (genuine) self", attaining integrity (wholeness) and wisdom (spiritual knowledge) (Rosen and Crouse 2000). In this process, transcendence is a vital step, but not the place to remain, because only continual acts of transformation lead to real personality change. Finally, death completes the cycle of development, returning individuals to the state of wholeness from which they emerged at birth. In agreement with this idea, Daoists set a goal much more than simply to find a means of obviating the death-event, but to attain an exalted state of existence through assimilation to higher realities; therefore, the personal purification and enhanced awareness of reality, i.e., a process of moral, spiritual, and cognitive growth are all included (Kirkland 2008).

By now, the satisfactory observation of Daoism for self-transcendence needs has encouraged some Chinese people. The explanation of distress and the related therapy are included in the Daoist conceptions of personality structure, dynamics, individual differences, and personality development (Hagen 2002). The disconnection between humans and themselves, other human beings, nature, and the universe that supports them, brings distress. Daoist therapy hence pursues translating conceptual theories into real-life practice in order to nurture a healthy human's spirit, through a variety of therapeutic strategies, such as focusing-oriented psychotherapy, reflective therapy, creativity and attachment exercises, meditation, *Tai Ji Quan* (太极拳), cognitive-behavioral, Gestalt, existential, and experiential therapies.

Along these years, Daoism might help some Chinese people to satisfy their self-transcendence needs, and it might be one approach to self-transcendence in the hierarchy of needs. Another way is full of obstacles originating from Chinese future, is centered on Confucianism, and urges people to chase social harmony by a rigidly hierarchical system of reciprocal duties and highly regulated and ritualized behaviors (Scarborough 1998). Therefore, it seems inevitably problematic for the Chinese to satisfy transcendence needs under Chinese culture.

8 Conclusion

Human beings produce culture, which in turn affects them from all aspects. Maslow's Hierarchy of Needs Theory covers all needs of human beings, which are comprehensively exemplified in Chinese culture. The link also helps explain the etiopathology of psychological disorders, through pathways of emotion, cognition, and behavior. Numerous influential elements in Chinese culture were systematically confirmed as risk factors for mental health, such as the unique drink custom, sexual attitude, moral rules, harmony seeking, Collectivism, hierarchal society, legal and moral rules, etiquette, past-time orientation, which more or less are originated from Confucianism or Daoism.

For sure, there are plenty of advantages within Chinese culture, which contribute to maintenance of mental health of Chinese people. Meanwhile, there are intersections within the hierarchy of needs, but these can hardly disturb our observations. Today the Chinese culture has expanded its influence in every corner of the world by economic and political activities, such as migration and trade, which implies much significance in a wider geographic area. Cultural studies therefore have been fruitful in the psychological world. Indeed, these elements in Chinese culture are "emic", and their influences are stable along the traditional and contemporary China. Specifically, the Chinese culture in the late imperial and contemporary China and its influence on the psychological world would be introduced continuously in the following chapters. In Chapter "Societal Culture from Late Imperial to Contemporary China: As Indirectly Reflected in A Dream of Red Mansions", one of the excellent media of Chinese literature, a novel of the seventeenth to eighteenth century, A Dream of Red Mansions, will be under our discussion in this respect.

References

Ace, K. J. (2007). Mental health, mental illness, and sexuality. In M. S. Tepper & A. F. Owens (Eds.), *Sexual health* (Psychological foundations) (Vol. 1, pp. 301–329). Westport: Praeger Publishers/Greenwood Publishing Group.

Ahrens, K., & Huang, C. R. (2002). Time passing is motion. *Language and Linguistics, 3*, 491–519.

American Psychiatric Association. (2013). *Diagnostic and statistical manual of mental disorder* (5th ed.). Washington, DC: American Psychiatric Association.

Andreassen, C. S., Pallesen, S., & Griffiths, M. D. (2017). The relationship between addictive use of social media, narcissism, and self-esteem: Findings from a large national survey. *Addictive Behaviors, 64*, 287–293.

Argyle, M., Henderson, M., Bond, M., Iizuka, Y., & Contarello, A. (1986). Cross-cultural variation in relationship rules. *International Journal of Psychology, 21*, 287–315.

Bagozzi, R. P., Wong, N., & Yi, Y. (1999). The role of culture and gender in the relationship between positive and negative affect. *Cognition and Emotion, 13*, 641–672.

Barlow, D. H. (1986). Causes of sexual dysfunction: The role of anxiety and cognitive interference. *Journal of Consulting and Clinical Psychology, 54*, 140–148.

Bartholomew, K., & Horowitz, L. M. (1991). Attachment styles among young adults: A test of a four category model. *Journal of Personality and Social Psychology, 61*, 226–244.

Baumeister, R., Stillwell, A., & Heatherton, T. (1995). Interpersonal aspects of guilt: Evidence from narrative studies. In J. Tangney & K. Fischer (Eds.), *Self-conscious emotions: The psychology of shame, guilt, embarrassment, and pride* (pp. 255–273). New York: Guilford.

Baurley, S. (2004). Interactive and experiential design in smart textile products and applications. *Personal and Ubiquitous Computing, 8*, 274–281.

Bedford, O., & Hwang, K. K. (2003). Guilt and shame in Chinese culture: A cross-cultural framework from the perspective of morality and identity. *Journal for the Theory of Social Behaviour, 33*, 127–144.

Bond, M. H. (1986). *The psychology of the Chinese people* (p. 247). Hong Kong: Oxford University Press.

Brockner, J., & Chen, Y. R. (1996). The moderating roles of self-esteem and self-construal in reaction to a threat to the self: Evidence from the People's Republic of China and the United States. *Journal of Personality and Social Psychology, 71*, 603–615.

Cai, H., Wu, Q., & Brown, J. D. (2009). Is self-esteem a universal need? Evidence from The People's Republic of China. *Asian Journal of Social Psychology, 12*, 104–120.

Carstensen, L. L., Isaacowitz, D. M., & Charles, S. T. (1999). Taking time seriously: A theory of socioemotional selectivity. *American Psychologist, 54*, 165–181.

Chan, W. (1967). The individual in Chinese religions. In C. A. Moore (Ed.), *The Chinese mind: Essentials of Chinese philosophy and culture*. Honolulu: University of Hawaii Press.

Chan, K. H., Lew, A. Y., & Tong, M. Y. J. W. (2001). Accounting and management controls in the classical Chinese novel: A Dream of the Red Mansions. *International Journal of Accounting, 36*, 311–327.

Chen, C. (1986). *Neo-confucian terms explained*. New York: Columbia University Press.

Chen, G. M. (1995). Differences in self-disclosure patterns among Americans versus Chinese: A comparative study. *Journal of Cross-Cultural Psychology, 26*, 84–91.

Chia, R. C., Moore, J. L., Lam, K. N., Chuang, C. J., & Cheng, B. S. (1994). Cultural differences in gender role attitudes between Chinese and American students. *Sex Roles, 31*, 23–30.

Chinese Culture Connection. (1987). Chinese values and the search for culture-free dimensions of culture. *Journal of Cross-cultural Psychology, 18*, 143–164.

Ching, J. (1993). *Chinese religions*. Maryknoll: Orbis Books.

Cochrane, J., Chen, H. H., Conigrave, K. M., & Hao, W. (2003). Alcohol use in China. *Alcohol and Alcoholism, 38*, 537–542.

Cohen, A. R., Stotland, E., & Wolfe, D. M. (1955). An experimental investigation of need for cognition. *Journal of Abnormal and Social Psychology, 51*, 291–294.

Crandall, J. E. (1965). Some relationships among sex, anxiety, and conservatism of judgment. *Journal of Personality, 33*, 99–107.

Davis, C., & Katzman, M. A. (1998). Chinese men and women in the United States and Hong Kong: Body and self-esteem ratings as a prelude to dieting and exercise. *International Journal of Eating Disorders, 23*, 99–102.

Deci, E. L., & Ryan, R. M. (2000). The "what" and "why" of goal pursuits: Human needs and the self-determination of behavior. *Psychological Inquiry, 11*, 227–268.

Diaz-Guerrero, R. (1979). The development of coping style. *Human Development, 22*, 320–331.

Dunn, K. M., Croft, P. R., & Hackett, G. I. (1999). Association of sexual problems with social, psychological, and physical problems in men and women: A cross sectional population survey. *Journal of Epidemiology and Community Health, 53*, 144–148.

Engel, G., Olson, K. R., & Patrick, C. (2002). The personality of love: Fundamental motives and traits related to components of love. *Personality and Individual Differences, 32*, 839–853.

Eysenck, M. W., & Fajkowska, M. (2017). Anxiety and depression: Toward overlapping and distinctive features. *Cognition and Emotion*. https://doi.org/10.1080/02699931.2017.1330255.

Fan, Y. (2000). A classification of Chinese culture. *Cross Cultural Management, 7*, 3–10.

Faure, G. O., & Fang, T. (2008). Changing Chinese values: Keeping up with paradoxes. *International Business Review, 17*, 194–207.

Fung, H. (1999). Becoming a moral child: The socialization of shame among young Chinese children. *Ethos, 27*, 180–209.

Furukawa, E., Tangney, J., & Higashibara, F. (2012). Cross-cultural continuities and discontinuities in shame, guilt, and pride: A study of children residing in Japan, Korea and the USA. *Self and Identity, 11*, 90–113.

Gao, G. (2001). Intimacy, passion, and commitment in Chinese and US American romantic relationships. *International Journal of Intercultural Relations, 25*, 329–342.

Gao, Y. (2018). *Lu Xun's view of language, his writing, and its relation to modern Chinese litera-ture. The birth of twentieth-century Chinese literature* (G. Li, Trans., pp. 157–180). New York: Palgrave Macmillan.

Getsinger, S. H. (1978). Psychotherapy and the fourth dimension. *Psychotherapy: Theory, Research and Practice, 15*, 216–225.

Goodwin, R., & Lee, I. (1994). Taboo topics among Chinese and English friends. *Journal of Cross-Cultural Psychology, 25*, 325–328.

Gray, S. J. (1988). Towards a theory of cultural influence on the development of accounting sys-tems internationally. *Abacus: A Journal of Accounting, Finance and Business Studies, 24*, 1–15.

Greenberg, M. A., & Stone, A. A. (1992). Emotional disclosure about traumas and its relation to health: Effects of previous disclosure and trauma severity. *Journal of Personality and Social Psychology, 63*, 75–84.

Gudykunst, W. B., & Matsumoto, Y. (1996). Cross-cultural variability of communication in per-sonal relationships. In W. B. Gudykunst, S. Ting-Toomey, & T. Nishida (Eds.), *Communication in personal relationships across cultures* (pp. 19–56). Thousand Oaks: SAGE.

Hagen, L. (2002). Taoism and psychology. In R. P. Olson (Ed.), *Religious theories of personality and psychotherapy: East meets West* (pp. 141–210). New York: Haworth Press.

Hall, S. (1980). Cultural studies: Two paradigms. *Media, Culture and Society, 2*, 57–72.

Hao, W., & Young, D. (2000). Drinking pattern and problems in China. *Journal of Substance Use, 5*, 71–78.

Hao, W., Young, D., Xiao, S., Li, L., & Zhang, Y. (1999). Alcohol consumption and alcohol-related problems: Chinese experience from six area samples, 1994. *Addiction, 94*, 1467–1476.

Hao, W., Su, Z., Liu, B., Zhang, K., Yang, H., Chen, S., Biao, M., & Cui, C. (2004). Drinking and drinking patterns and health status in the general population of five areas of China. *Alcohol and Alcoholism, 39*, 43–52.

Heath, P. J., Vogel, D. L., & Al-Darmaki, F. R. (2016). Help-seeking attitudes of United Arab Emirates students: Examining loss of face, stigma, and self-disclosure. *The Counseling Psychologist, 44*, 331–352.

Heine, S. J. (2001). Self as cultural product: An examination of East Asian and North American selves. *Journal of Personality, 69*, 881–906.

Heine, S. J., Lehman, D. R., Markus, H. R., & Kitayama, S. (1999). Is there a universal need for positive self-regard? *Psychological Review, 106*, 766–794.

Henderson, C., Robinson, E., Evans-Lacko, S., & Thornicroft, G. (2017). Relationships between anti-stigma programme awareness, disclosure comfort and intended help-seeking regarding a mental health problem. *British Journal of Psychiatry, 211*, 316–322.

Higgins, L. T., Zheng, M., Liu, Y., & Sun, C. H. (2002). Attitudes to marriage and sexual behav-iors: A survey of gender and culture differences in China and United Kingdom. *Sex Roles, 46*, 75–89.

Ho, D. Y. F. (1985). Cultural values and professional issues in clinical psychology: Implications from the Hong Kong experience. *American Psychologist, 40*, 1212–1218.

Ho, D. Y. F. (1987). Fatherhood in Chinese culture. In M. E. Lamb (Ed.), *The father's role: Cross-cultural perspectives* (pp. 227–245). Hillsdale: Erlbaum.

Ho, D. Y. F., Fu, W., & Ng, S. M. (2004). Guilt, shame and embarrassment: Revelations of face and self. *Culture and Psychology, 10*, 64–84.

Hofmann, W., Kotabe, H. P., Vohs, K. D., & Baumeister, R. F. (2015). Desire and desire regula-tion. In W. Hofmann & L. F. Nordgren (Eds.), *The psychology of desire (Chap. 3)* (pp. 61–81). New York: Guilford.

Hofstede, G. (1980). *Culture's consequences: International differences in worked related values.* Beverly Hills: Sage.

Hofstede, G. (1984). Cultural dimensions in management and planning. *Asia Pacific Journal of Management, 1*, 81–99.

Hofstede, G. (1991). *Cultures and organizations: Software of the mind* (p. 5). Cambridge: McGraw-Hill.

Hofstede, G. (2001). *Culture's consequences: Comparing values, behaviors, institutions and organizations across nations*. Thousand Oaks: Sage.

Hofstede, G., & Bond, M. H. (1988). The Confucius connection: From cultural roots to economic growth. *Organizational Dynamics, 16*, 5–21.

Holman, E. A., & Silver, R. C. (1998). Getting "stuck" in the past: Temporal orientation and coping with trauma. *Journal of Personality and Social Psychology, 74*, 1146–1163.

Hong, J. J., & Woody, S. R. (2007). Cultural mediators of self-reported social anxiety. *Behaviour Research and Therapy, 45*, 1779–1789.

Huang, Y., Kotov, R., de Girolamo, G., Preti, A., Angermeyer, M., Benjet, C., Demyttenaere, K., de Graaf, R., Gureje, O., Karam, A. N., Lee, S., Lépine, J. P., Matschinger, H., Posada-Villa, J., Suliman, S., Vilagut, G., & Kessler, R. C. (2009). DSM-IV personality disorders in the WHO World Mental Health Surveys. *British Journal of Psychiatry, 195*, 46–53.

Hwang, K.-K. (1999). Filial piety and loyalty: The types of social identification in Confucianism. *Asian Journal of Social Psychology, 2*, 129–149.

Jin, X., & Qi, F. (2009, December 5). *Thoughts on "Questions by Qian Xuesen"*. Guangmingwang. Retrieved October 12, 2018, from http://epaper.gmw.cn/gmrb/html/2009-12/05/nw.D110000gmrb_20091205_1-01.htm?div=-1

Kam, C. C. S., & Bond, M. H. (2008). Role of emotions and behavioural responses in mediating the impact of face loss on relationship deterioration: Are Chinese more face-sensitive than Americans? *Asian Journal of Social Psychology, 11*, 175–184.

Kendall, P. C., & Ingram, R. E. (1989). Cognitive-behavioural perspectives: Theory and research on depression and anxiety. In P. C. Kendall & D. Watson (Eds.), *Anxiety and depression: Distinctive and overlapping features (xviii)* (pp. 27–53). San Diego: Academic Press.

Kirkland, R. (2008). Transcendence and immortality. In F. Pregadio (Ed.), *The Encyclopedia of Taoism* (Vol. I, pp. 91–93). Oxon: Routledge.

Kluckhohn, F. R. (1962). Universal categories of culture. In S. Tax (Ed.), *Anthropology today* (pp. 304–320). Chicago: University of Chicago Press.

Kluckhohn, F. R., & Strodbeck, F. L. (1961). *Variations in value orientation*. Evanston: Row, Paterson and Co.

Kruglanski, A. W., & Webster, D. M. (1996). Motivated closing of the mind: "Seizing" and "freezing". *Psychological Review, 103*, 263–283.

Lam, T. K. (2002). Making sense of SERVQUAL's dimensions to the Chinese customers in Macau. *Journal of Market-Focused Management, 5*, 43–58.

Lang, O. (1946). *Chinese family and society*. New Haven: Yale University Press.

Lau, J. T., Kim, J. H., & Tsui, H. Y. (2008). Prevalence and sociocultural predictors of sexual dysfunction among Chinese men who have sex with men in Hong Kong. *Journal of Sexual Medicine, 5*, 2766–2779.

Laurent, S. M., & Simons, A. D. (2009). Sexual dysfunction in depression and anxiety: Conceptualizing sexual dysfunction as part of an internalizing dimension. *Clinical Psychology Review, 29*, 573–585.

Lebra, T. S. (1976). *Japanese patterns of behavior*. Honolulu: University of Hawaii Press.

Leng, L., & Salzman, M. (2016). The renaissance of confucianism in contemporary China from the perspective of terror management theory. *Sociology and Anthropology, 4*, 52–58.

Lin, Y. T. (1935). *My country and my people* (p. 178). New York: John Day.

Lin, M. H. (1939). Confucius on interpersonal relations. *Psychiatry, 2*, 475–481.

Lindsay-Hartz, J., de Rivera, J., & Mascolo, M. (1995). Differentiating guilt and shame and their effects on motivation. In J. Tangney & K. Fischer (Eds.), *Self-conscious emotions: The psychology of shame, guilt, embarrassment, and pride* (pp. 274–300). New York: Guilford.

Liu, J. (2016). *Zhuangzi and modern Chinese literature*. New York: Oxford University Press.

Lowe, A. C.-T., & Corkindale, D. R. (1998). Differences in "cultural values" and their effects on responses to marketing stimuli: A cross-cultural study between Australians and Chinese from the People's Republic of China. *European Journal of Marketing, 32*, 843–867.

Markus, H. R., & Kitayama, S. (1991). Culture and the self: Implications for cognition, emotion, and motivation. *Psychological Review, 98*, 224–253.

Maslow, A. H. (1943). A theory of human motivation. *Psychological Review, 50*, 370–396.

Maslow, A. H. (1954). *Motivation and personality*. New York: Harper and Row.

Maslow, A. H. (1970a). *Motivation and personality*. New York: Harper and Row.

Maslow, A. H. (1970b). *Religions, values, and peak experiences*. New York: Penguin. (Original work published 1964).

Maslow, A. H. (1971). *The farther feaches of human nature*. Oxford: Viking.

McLeod, S. A. (2007). *Maslow's hierarchy of needs*. Retrieved October 12, 2018, from http://www.simplypsychology.org/maslow.html

Meston, C. M., Trapnell, P. D., & Gorzalka, B. B. (1996). Ethnic and gender differences in sexuality: Variations in sexual behavior between Asian and non-Asian university students. *Archives of Sexual Behavior, 25*, 33–72.

Posey, C., Lowry, P. B., Roberts, T. L., & Ellis, S. (2010). The culture-influenced online community self-disclosure model: The case of working professionals in France and the UK who use online communities. *European Journal of Information Systems, 19*, 181–195.

Pye, L. W. (1972). *China: An introduction* (2nd ed.). Boston: Little Brown.

Rice, C. (1993). *Consumer behavior: Behavioral aspects of marketing*. Oxford: Butterworth Heinemann.

Rosen, D. H., & Crouse, E. M. (2000). The Tao of wisdom: Integration of Taoism and the psychologies of Jung, Erikson, and Maslow. In P. Young-Eisendrath & M. Miller (Eds.), *The psychology of mature spirituality: Integrity, wisdom, transcendence (Chap. 9)* (pp. 95–103). London: Routledge.

Rosenberg, M., Schooler, C., & Schoenbach, C. (1989). Self-esteem and adolescent problems: Modeling. *American Sociological Review, 54*, 1004–1018.

Ryder, A. G., Yang, J., & Heine, S. J. (2002). Somatization vs. psychologization of emotional distress: A paradigmatic example for cultural psychopathology. In *Online readings in psychology and culture* (10th ed.). Bellingham: The Berkeley Electronic Press.

Ryder, A. G., Yang, J., Zhu, X., Yao, S., Yi, J., Heine, S. J., & Bagby, R. M. (2008). The cultural shaping of depression: Somatic symptoms in China, psychological symptoms in North America. *Journal of Abnormal Psychology, 117*, 300–313.

Scarborough, J. (1998). Comparing Chinese and Western cultural roots: Why "East is East and…". *Business Horizons, 41*, 15–24.

Schwarzer, R. (1993). *Measurement of perceived self-efficacy. Psychometric scales for cross-cultural research*. Berlin: Freie Universitat Berlin.

Schwarzer, R., Bäßler, J., Kwiatek, P., Schröder, K., & Zhang, J. X. (1997). The assessment of optimistic self-beliefs: Comparison of the German, Spanish, and Chinese versions of the general self-efficacy scale. *Applied Psychology, 46*, 69–88.

Scott, G., Ciarrochi, J., & Deane, F. P. (2004). Disadvantages of being an individualist in an individualistic culture: Idiocentrism, emotional competence, stress, and mental health. *Australian Psychologist, 39*, 143–154.

Shi, X., Wang, J., & Zou, H. (2017). Family functioning and Internet addiction among Chinese adolescents: The mediating roles of self-esteem and loneliness. *Computers in Human Behavior, 76*, 201–210.

Sirgy, M. J. (1986). A quality-of-life theory derived from Maslow's developmental perspective. *American Journal of Economics and Sociology, 45*, 329–342.

Smith, M. W. (1952). Different cultural concepts of past, present, and future: A study of ego extension. *Psychiatry, 15*, 395–400.

Soenens, B., & Vansteenkiste, M. (2010). A theoretical upgrade of the concept of parental psychological control: Proposing new insights on the basis of self-determination theory. *Developmental Review, 30*, 74–99.

Spears, N., Lin, X., & Mowen, J. C. (2000). Time orientation in the United States, China, and Mexico: Measurement and insights for promotional strategy. *Journal of International Consumer Marketing, 13*, 57–75.

Sprecher, S., & Hendrick, S. S. (2004). Self-disclosure in intimate relationships: Associations with individual and relationship characteristics over time. *Journal of Social and Clinical Psychology, 23*, 857–877.

Sternberg, R. J. (1986). A triangular theory of love. *Psychological Bulletin, 93*, 119–138.

Sternberg, R. J. (1998). *Cupid's arrow: The course of love through time*. London: Cambridge University Press.

Stipek, D. (1998). Differences between Americans and Chinese in the circumstances evoking pride, shame, and guilt. *Journal of Cross-Cultural Psychology, 29*, 616–629.

Stokes, J. P. (1987). The relation of loneliness and self-disclosure. In V. J. Derlega & J. H. Berg (Eds.), *Self-disclosure* (pp. 175–202). New York: Plenum Press.

Suen, L. C. (1983). *The underlying structure of Chinese civilization* [Zhong-guo-wen-hua-di-shen-ceng-jie-gou]. Hong Kong: Yi Shan Publication (in Chinese).

Taylor, S. E., & Brown, J. (1988). Illusion and well-being: Some social psychological contributions to a theory of mental health. *Psychological Bulletin, 103*, 193–210.

Terpstra, V., & David, K. (1985). *The cultural environment of international business*. Cincinnati: Southwestern Publishing.

Tiggemann, M. (2005). Body dissatisfaction and adolescent self-esteem: Prospective findings. *Body Image, 2*, 129–135.

Tomkins, S. S. (1970). Affects as primary motivational system. In M. Arnold (Ed.), *Feelings and emotions* (pp. 101–110). New York: Academic.

Triandis, H. C. (1989). The self and social behavior in differing cultural contexts. *Psychological Review, 96*, 506–520.

Triandis, H. C. (1993). Collectivism and individualism as cultural syndromes. *Cross-Cultural Research, 27*, 155–180.

Triandis, H. C. (2000). Culture and conflict. *International Journal of Psychology, 35*, 145–152.

Triandis, H. C. (2001). Individualism-collectivism and personality. *Journal of Personality, 69*, 907–924.

Triandis, H. C., & Suh, E. M. (2002). Cultural influences on personality. *Annual Review of Psychology, 53*, 133–160.

Triandis, H. C., Bontempo, R., Villareal, M. J., Asai, M., & Lucca, N. (1988). Individualism and collectivism: Cross-cultural perspectives on self-ingroup relationships. *Journal of Personality and Social Psychology, 54*, 323–338.

Tsai, J. L., Ying, Y. W., & Lee, P. A. (2001). Cultural predictors of self-esteem: A study of Chinese American female and male young adults. *Cultural Diversity and Ethnic Minority Psychology, 7*, 284–297.

Tseng, W. S., & Hsu, J. (1970). Chinese culture, personality formation and mental illness. *International Journal of Social Psychiatry, 16*, 5–14.

Tybout, A. M., & Artz, N. (1994). Consumer psychology. *Annual Review of Psychology, 45*, 131–169.

Vogel, D. L., & Wester, S. R. (2003). To seek help or not to seek help: The risks of self-disclosure. *Journal of Counseling Psychology, 50*, 351–361.

Wang, Q. (2016). How not to have nostalgia for the future: A reading of Lu Xun's "Hometown". *Frontiers of Literary Studies in China, 10*, 461–473.

Webster, D. M., & Kruglanski, A. W. (1994). Individual differences in need for cognitive closure. *Journal of Personality and Social Psychology, 67*, 1049–1062.

Wegner, D. M. (1994). Ironic processes of mental control. *Psychological Review, 101*, 34–52.

Wei, M., Russell, D. W., & Zakalik, R. A. (2005). Adult attachment, social self-efficacy, self-disclosure, loneliness, and subsequent depression for Freshman college students: A longitudinal study. *Journal of Counseling Psychology, 52*, 602–614.

Weiner, B. (1992). *Human motivation: Metaphors, theories and research*. Beverly Hills: Sage.

Wicker, F. W., Brown, G., Wiehe, J. A., Hagen, A. S., & Reed, J. L. (1993). On reconsidering Maslow: An examination of the deprivation/domination proposition. *Journal of Research in Personality, 27,* 118–133.

Williams, R. M., Jr. (1970). *American society: A sociological interpretation* (3rd ed.). New York: Knopf.

World Health Organization. (2017). *International classification of diseases* (11th beta Ed.). Retrieved October 12, 2018, from http://www.who.int/classifications/icd/revision/en

Wyrick, R. A., & Wyrick, L. C. (1977). Time experience during depression. *Archives of General Psychiatry, 34,* 1441–1443.

Xiang, Z., Tan, S., Kang, Q., Zhang, B., & Zhu, L. (2017). Longitudinal effects of examination stress on psychological well-being and a possible mediating role of self-esteem in Chinese high school students. *Journal of Happiness Studies.* https://doi.org/10.1007/s10902-017-9948-9.

Yau, O. H. M. (1988). Chinese cultural values: Their dimensions and marketing implications. *European Journal of Marketing, 22,* 44–57.

Yeh, R. S. (1988). On Hofstede's treatment of Chinese and Japanese values. *Asia Pacific Journal of Management, 6,* 149–160.

Yik, M. S. M., Bond, M., & Paulhus, D. (1998). Do Chinese self-enhance or self-efface? It's a matter of domain. *Personality and Social Psychology Bulletin, 24,* 399–406.

Yip, K. S. (2004). Taoism and its impact on mental health of the Chinese communities. *International Journal of Social Psychiatry, 50,* 25–42.

Yu, N. (2012). The metaphorical orientation of time in Chinese. *Journal of Pragmatics, 44,* 1335–1354.

Zhang, J., Conwell, Y., Zhou, L., & Jiang, C. (2004). Culture, risk factors and suicide in rural China: A psychological autopsy case control study. *Acta Psychiatrica Scandinavica, 110,* 430–437.

Zhang, G., Zhao, Y., & Lei, J. (2012). Between a rock and a hard place: Higher education reform and innovation in China. *On the Horizon, 20,* 263–273.

Zhao, L., Yu, X., Zhang, L., & Ren, Z. (2017). Stability of implicit self-esteem among internetaddicted college students in China. *Social Behavior and Personality, 45,* 339–352.

Societal Culture from Late Imperial to Contemporary China: As Indirectly Reflected in A Dream of Red Mansions

Guorong Ma, Mufan Wang, and Wei Wang

1 DRM as a Vector of Chinese Culture

As stated in the previous chapter, culture refers to both the means and values that arise among distinctive social groups and classes, on the basis of their given historical conditions and relationship, through which they handle and respond to the conditions of existence (Hall 1980). Specifically, it is a set of behavioral norms, meanings, and values or reference points utilized by members of a particular society to construct their unique view of the world, and ascertain their identity (Chowdhury 2012). The societal culture refers to a group's distinctive beliefs and normative practices about what is true, valued, and efficient (Sanchez-Burks and Lee 2007). To study societal cultures, literature texts handed down across centuries may provide a rich source of material. Among these literature texts, novels are among the most valuable media for these purposes.

With regard to the study of Chinese culture, especially traditional Chinese culture, A Dream of Red Mansions (DRM) is usually attached with the greatest importance. The fiction is also known as *Hong Lou Meng* (红楼梦), Story of the Stone (石头记), or Dream of the Red Chamber, is one of China's Four Great Classical Novels. The first 80 chapters of the novel (in some versions, Chapters 79 and 80 were not clearly separated but rather compiled together as Chapter 79) are traditionally thought to be finished by Mr. Cao Xueqin (曹雪芹) in the seventeenth to eighteenth century during the Qing Dynasty, whereas the latter 40 episodes were alleged to be the contribution of Mr. Gao E (高鹗) (Chan et al. 2001). Recently, with the discovery of a "new" 28-version of the latter chapters (Anonymous 2014, in

G. Ma · W. Wang (✉)
Department of Clinical Psychology and Psychiatry/School of Public Health,
Zhejiang University College of Medicine, Hangzhou, China
e-mail: drwangwei@zju.edu.cn

M. Wang
Faculty of Psychology, Universidad Complutense de Madrid, Madrid, Spain

© Springer Nature Singapore Pte Ltd. 2019
W. Wang (ed.), *Chinese Perspectives on Cultural Psychiatry*,
https://doi.org/10.1007/978-981-13-3537-2_2

Chinese), some claim that Mr. Cao Xueqin might just be a pen-name which refers to a group of authors, and the leading-author of the writing group is Mr. Wu Weiye (吴伟业, aka Wu Meicun吴梅村). Therefore, the group of authors of DRM is noted as DRM-author here and after.

There are more than 400 named characters described in DRM from virtually every class and profession, e.g., maids-in-waiting, stewards, gardeners, cooks, nuns, actors, officials, members of the imperial family, gamblers and thieves (Gao 2009). The novel offers a precise and detailed observation of life and social structures in the seventeenth to eighteenth century Chinese society and life. Reflective of the society and Chinese culture, themes of the novel include medicine, cuisine, tea custom, festivities, proverbs, opera, music, painting, classic literature, mythology, Confucianism, Buddhism, Daoism, filial piety, funeral rites, etc. Moreover, it is well-known for its grand and beautiful use of poetry and verse.

DRM is long considered a masterpiece of Chinese literature, and is generally acknowledged to be the pinnacle of Chinese fiction. In the 1920s, scholars and devoted readers developed the study of DRM into both a scholarly field and a popular avocation, which encourages researches on the themes, the characters, the versions, and the reciprocal influences mutually with other classical works (e.g., Zhou 1989; Hu 1993; Levy 1999b). Using the criteria of mass and academic appeal, it has been widely acknowledged as one of the world's masterpieces, and comparable to the works of Shakespeare or Goethe (Lin 1935; Levy 1999b). Meanwhile, the influence of the novel's themes and style are evident in many modern Chinese prose works. Many of the cultural features reflected in the novel are still observable in contemporary China or Chinese communities all around the world (Stone 2005). So far, the novel has been translated into many languages including English, and one reliable English version was by an English couple, Mr. Hsien-yi Yang (Chinese English) and Mrs. Gladys Yang (native English) (Yang and Yang 1978). This translation is sometimes referred in the present book in regard to the terms or narrative paragraphs describing psychological world or psychiatric disorders.

Meanwhile, scholars have looked beyond the novel's literary merits alone and have considered it as a highly realistic document of the life of the Chinese nobility, a thinly disguised biographical account of historical, social, and economic events, and a fountain of information on social customs and family structure. For instance, based on its precise and detailed observation of the life and social structures typical of Chinese aristocracy, DRM is used for studying the politics (Zhao 2011), economics (Chan et al. 2001), cultures (Levy 1999a; Liao 2007), religions (Yu 1989; Zhou 2001), social customs (Cooper and Zhang 1993), and psychological disorders (Levy 1994), family structure, even literary taste and *objet d'art* (Spence 1966) of the epoch when it was written. There are also some studies focusing on the psychological world or the psychiatric problems described in the novel, such as those investigating the internal control (Li and Li 1995), bisexuality (Edwards 1990; Yee 1995), homosexuality (Lau and Ng 1989), and the attention deficit/hyperactivity disorder (Levy 1994; Huang and Gillett 2014).

2 Plots and Characters in DRM

Regarding plots, DRM is a far cry from its peers, i.e., The Water Margin (水浒传), The Romance of the Three Kingdoms (三国演义), and The Journey to the West (西游记). These are full of politics, martial encounters, and adventure. The Water Margins describes 108 characters that were persecuted mostly by governmental officials and later behaved in sociopathic ways in the Song (宋) dynasty, thus these people might be characterized by the traits of antisocial personality disorder. The Romance of the Three Kingdoms describes the civil wars at the end of Han (汉) dynasty, and the wisdom used in war-affaires; unfortunately, the wisdom was not used for construction but for destruction of society. The Journey to the West describes a Buddhist pilgrimage by a monk teacher and four prentices for the Buddhist scriptures, and they met countless bogeymen along the journey; the teacher, the prentices, and bogymen might signify the numerous living creatures, who hold the same beliefs of either carnal or spiritual desires as the men in the current society. DRM on the other hand, starts with a frame story (likely because of the high political pressure back then) (Shi 2005). In the story, a sentient Stone, who was abandoned by the god(dess) Nüwa (女娲, might be a homonymic name for Noah in the Old Testament) when he mended the heavens hundreds of thousands years ago, begs a Daoist priest and a Buddhist monk to bring him with them to experience the world. The Stone and his companion, a flower, are then given a chance to learn from the human existence, hence enter the mortal realm.

DRM has two main threads, namely, the tragic love affair of the young and rebellious Mr. Jia Baoyu (贾宝玉) and Miss Lin Daiyu (林黛玉), and the rise and fall of the traditional and decadent families of Jia (贾), Shi (史), Wang (王), and Xue (薛) in those years. The novel especially provides a detailed, episodic record of life in the two branches of the wealthy, aristocratic Jia clan: the Ningguo (宁国府) and Rongguo Houses (荣国府), who reside in two large, adjacent family compounds in Jinling, the capital city. Their statuses came from the achievements of two glorious ancestors, who were made Dukes and given imperial titles, and as the novel begins the two Houses are among the most illustrious families in Jinling city. However, as time goes on, the succeeding generations of males had become increasingly inadequate, and their fortunes were definitely in decline. The central character of the novel is the carefree adolescent male heir of the family, Jia Baoyu, who was born with a magical piece of "jade" in his mouth and spoilt by the doting grandmother Jia (贾母, Lady Dowager), the family matriarch. When staring at a jade in the mouth of Jia Baoyu, Chinese people can easily think of the Chinese character Guo (国, nation or country). This would confer Jia Baoyu the symbol of an authority, i.e., a seal which sucks red ink before executing its role. The red-ink-sucking of a seal is actioned by Jia Baoyu, via his sucking the lip-rouges of young ladies living in the Grand View Garden. However, Jia Baoyu lives in fear of his father, a strict Confucian, and prefers writing poetry and female company to studying the classics. In this life, he has a special bond with his sickly cousin Lin Daiyu, who shares his love of music and poetry. At last, Lin Daiyun hung herself to death, signifying the end of the last emperor of the *Ming* (明) Dynasty, Mr. Zhu Youjian (朱由检). Jia Baoyu gets the chance to marry another one of his cousins, Miss Xue Baochai (薛宝钗), whose grace and intelligence exemplify an ideal woman, but with whom he lacks an emotional connection. From surface, the romantic rivalry and friendship among the three characters against the backdrop of the family's declining fortunes form the main story in the novel. However, the novel wants to show that all efforts, wisdom and intelligence were wasted in the dynasty interchanges, therefore the DRM-author signs "Pages full of fantastic talk, penned with bitter tears; all men call the author mad, none his message hears" (DRM-Chapter 1). The DRM-author was a master of describing characters, and nearly every character is presented in a vivid way, and with his/her own special personality trait. Because of the special nature of the Chinese language, which abounds in homonyms, many names in DRM are polysemous through the association of homonyms or near-homonyms, utilized in a great variety of ways to illuminate various aspects of the novel. Take the family name Jia (贾) for example, it connotes the meaning "false" or "fake", so that Jia Jing (贾敬), which literally means "respect", connotes the meaning "fake respect" (pretend to be respectful), and Jia Zheng (贾政), which literally means "politics" or "administration", connotes "fake righteousness" (pretend to be righteous) (Yang 1996). Moreover, as naming in accord with personality is one of the most fundamental literary devices, it comes as no surprise that many characters' names in the DRM were created in accordance with this principle. This practice not only enhances their personalities, but also foretells their fate and their denouement. Readers may get a deeper understanding of the characters simply by looking at their names (Wo 2008). Table 1 provides a brief introduction to these major characters.

DRM is a domestic novel, with its dramas set almost entirely in the household sphere. Much of the "action" involves the characters holding banquets, giving each other precious presents, putting on plays, composing poetry, sharing clothing, and so on. The DRM-author has a remarkable ability leading the reader into caring about many mundane domestic matters. In first parts of the novel, the outside world mostly intrudes in comic "low life" episodes: a schoolboy riot in the family-clan school (DRM-Chapter 10), a retaliation by Mrs. Wang Xifeng (王熙凤) against unwanted advances from a would-be lover (DRM-Chapter 12), a visit by country bumpkin Granny Liu (刘姥姥, DRM-Chapters 6 and 39), and a blow-back when an actor Mr. Xue Pan (薛蟠) takes a fancy for turns out to be a martial-arts expert (DRM-Chapter 47). There are also visits to temples or the imperial court, trade ventures, and exercises of patronage, but were indirectly narrated. Intertwined with the stories is an ever-present background of tension and conflict over status, involving both the family and the male-female servants. Aunt Zhao (赵姨娘) schemes to raise the status of her own children by using black magic of *Dao* to bring down Wang Xifeng and Jia Baoyu (DRM-Chapter 25). There was also a faction among the domestic staff attempts to unseat the cook (DRM-Chapter 61). Events become darker as the story progresses, involving unhappy marriages and problems with the family finances – the Jia family relies on rents from their land, but are living beyond their means.

Table 1 Brief introductions on the major characters in A Dream of Red Mansions

Character name	Brief introduction of the character
Jia Baoyu (贾宝玉, Mr.)	The main protagonist is about 12 or 13 years old when introduced in the novel. The adolescent son of Mr. Jia Zheng (贾政) and his wife, Lady Wang (王夫人), and born with a piece of luminescent jade in his mouth. Jia Baoyu is the heir apparent to the Rongguo House (荣国府). He was frowned on by his strict Confucian father and does not appreciate the Four Books of classic Chinese education, but rather reads Zhuangzi (庄子) and Story of the Western Wing (西厢记) on the sly. Jia Baoyu is highly intelligent, but dislikes the fawning bureaucrats who frequently appear in his father's house. His romance with Miss Lin Daiyu (林黛玉) forms one of the novel's main plot lines. As a sensitive and compassionate young man, he has a special relationship with many of the women in the house. As the text explains that Jia Baoyu signifies for the authority machine (a seal, which sucks red ink before executing his role; thus, he loves to suck the red lip-rouge of many young girls in the house).
Lin Daiyu (林黛玉, Miss)	The reincarnation of a flower from the frame story. The purpose of her mortal birth is to repay Jia Baoyu with tears for watering her in her previous incarnation. In this life, she is the younger-first cousin and the primary lover of Jia Baoyu. She is the daughter of Mr. Lin Ruhai (林如海), a scholar-official in Yangzhou (or Suchou according some old scriptures) city, and Lady Jia Min (贾敏), Jia Baoyu's paternal aunt. She is sickly, suffering from a respiratory disease, but beautiful in a way that is unconventional. Being fragile emotionally, prone to fits of jealousy, Lin Daiyu is however, an extremely accomplished poet and musician. The novel designates her one of the Twelve Beauties of Jinling, the capital city, and describes her as a lonely, proud and ultimately tragic figure. She hung herself to death at the end, which signifies the death of the last emperor of Ming (明) Dynasty, Mr. Zhu Youjian (朱由检).
Xue Baochai (薛宝钗, Miss)	Jia Baoyu's other first cousin. The only daughter of Aunt Xue (薛姨妈), who is a sister to Jia Baoyu's mother, Xue Baochai is a foil to Lin Daiyu. Lin Daiyu is unconventional and hypersensitive, but Xue Baochai is sensible and tactful. The novel describes her as beautiful and intelligent, but also reserved and were following the rules of decorum. Xue Baochai has a round face, fair skin, large eyes, and she is even more voluptuous figure in contrast to Lin Daiyu's willowy daintiness. She carries a golden locket with her. The golden locket and Jia Baoyu's jade contain inscriptions that appear to complement one another perfectly. Although reluctant to show the extent of her knowledge, she seems to be quite learned and experienced.
Jia Yuanchun (贾元春, Miss)	Jia Baoyu's elder sister by about a decade. Originally one of the ladies-in-waiting in the imperial palace, she later becomes an Imperial Consort, having impressed the Emperor with her virtue and learning. Her illustrious position as a favorite of the Emperor marks the height of the Jia family's powers.
Jia Tanchun (贾探春, miss)	Jia Baoyu's younger half-sister by Concubine Zhao (赵姨娘). Extremely outspoken, she is almost as capable as Wang Xifeng (王熙凤). Wang Xifeng herself compliments her privately, but laments that she was "born in the wrong womb", since concubine children are not respected as much as those by first wives at that time. Jia Tanchun is also a very talented poet, but she later marries into a military family on the South Sea far away from her hometown.

(continued)

Table 1 (continued)

Character name	Brief introduction of the character
Shi Xiangyun (史湘云, Miss)	Jia Baoyu's younger second cousin and Lady Dowager (贾母)'s grandniece. She is also orphaned in infancy similar to Lin Daiyu, and grows up under her wealthy maternal uncle and aunt who treat her unkindly. In spite of this, Shi Xiangyun is openhearted and cheerful, just opposite to Lin Daiyu. A comparatively androgynous beauty, she looks good in men's clothes, and loves to drink. She is also well educated and as talented a poet as Lin Daiyu and Xue Baochai are.
Miaoyu (妙玉, Miss)	A young nun of Buddhist cloisters in the Rongguo House. She was from Suzhou city, and was compelled by her illness to become a nun. She was extremely beautiful and learned, while also extremely aloof, haughty and unsociable, and prominently she is obsessive and compulsive, in cleanliness and orderliness. Her fate is defiled and downhilled after her abduction by bandits.
Jia Yingchun (贾迎春, Miss)	Second female family member of the generation of the Jia household after Jia Yuanchun, Jia Yingchun is the daughter of Mr. Jia She (贾赦), Jia Baoyu's uncle, and a concubine. As a kind-hearted, weak-willed person, Jia Yingchun is said to have a "wooden" character and seems rather apathetic toward all worldly affairs. Although she is very pretty and well-read, she does not compare in intelligence and wit to any of her cousins. To pay back her father's debt, Jia Yingchun was married to an official of the imperial court. Eventually, she becomes a victim of domestic abuse and constant violence at the hands of her cruel, abusive husband, Mr. Sun Shaozu (孙绍祖).
Jia Xichun (贾惜春, Miss)	Jia Baoyu's younger cousin from the Ningguo House (宁国府), but is brought up in the Rongguo House beside Lady Dowager. She is a gifted painter, and also a devout Buddhist.
Wang Xifeng (王熙凤, Mrs.)	Jia Baoyu's elder cousin-in-law, wife to Mr. Jia Lian (贾琏), Jia Baoyu's paternal first cousin), niece to Lady Wang, therefore Wang Xifeng is hence related to Jia Baoyu both by blood and marriage. She is an extremely handsome woman, being capable, clever, humorous, conversable and, at times, vicious and cruel. Being a favorite of Lady Dowager and a confidential assistant to Lady Wang, Wang Xifeng keeps both Lady Wang and Lady Dowager entertained with her constant jokes and amusing chatter, playing the role of the perfect filial daughter-in-law, and rules the entire household with an iron fist. That is, Wang Xifang can be kind-hearted toward the poor and helpless, and also cruel enough to kill on the other.
Jia Qiaojie (贾巧姐, Miss)	Wang Xifeng and Jia Lian's only daughter. After the fall of the house of Jia household, she was saved by Granny Liu (刘姥姥) from being sold into concubinage by her maternal uncle. She marries Ban'er, grandson of Granny Liu, and goes on to lead a happy, uneventful life in the countryside.
Li Wan (李纨, Mrs.)	Jia Baoyu's elder sister-in-law, widow of Jia Baoyu's deceased elder brother, Mr. Jia Zhu (贾珠). Her primary task is to bring up her son, Mr. Jia Lan (贾兰) and look after her female cousins. She is a young widow in her late twenties, and as a mild-mannered woman with no wants or desires, she is the perfect Confucian ideal of a proper mourning widow. She spends her youth upholding the strict standards of behavior.
Qin Keqing (秦可卿, Mrs.)	Daughter-in-law to Mr. Jia Zhen (贾珍). Qin Keqing is apparently a very beautiful and flirtatious woman. She carried on an affair with her father-in-law and brother-in-law and dies before the second quarter of the novel. Her bedroom is bedecked with priceless artifacts belonging to extremely sensual women, both historical and mythological.

(continued)

Table 1 (continued)

Character name	Brief introduction of the character
Lady Dowager (贾母)	The daughter of Marquis Shi (史) of the capital city, Jinling. She is the grandmother to both Jia Baoyu and Lin Daiyu, the highest living authority executing the Rongguo House and the oldest and most respected of the entire clan, yet she is also a doting person. She has two sons, Jia She and Jia Zheng, and a daughter, Jia Min, Lin Daiyu's mother. She helps Lin Daiyu and Jia Baoyu bond as childhood playmates and, later, provides the kindred spirits.
Jia She (贾赦, Mr.)	The elder son of Lady Dowager. He is the father of Mr. Jia Lian (贾琏) and Miss Jia Yingchun. A treacherous and greedy man, and a womanizer, he is jealous of his younger brother whom his mother favors. Later, he is stripped of his title and banished by the government.
Jia Zheng (贾政, Mr.)	Jia Baoyu's father, the younger son of Lady Dowager. He is a disciplinarian and Confucian scholar. He tries to be an upright and decent person, but is out of touch with reality and is a hands-off person at home and in court. Being afraid his one surviving heir will turn bad, he imposes strict rules on Jia Baoyu, and uses occasional corporal punishment. He has a wife, Lady Wang, and two concubines: Zhao and Zhou (周姨娘).
Jia Lian (贾琏, Mr.)	Wang Xifeng's husband and Jia Baoyu's paternal elder cousin, a notorious woman killer whose numerous affairs cause much trouble with his jealous wife Wang Xifeng. His pregnant concubine (Second Sister You, 尤二姐) eventually dies by his wife's engineering. He and his wife often fight over the power of being in charge of most hiring and monetary allocation decisions of Jia family.
Lady Wang (王夫人)	Jia Baoyu's mother. She is the primary being wife of Jia Zheng, a Buddhist, and the daughter of one of the four most prominent families of Jinling. Because of her purported ill-health, she hands over the household management to her niece, Wang Xifeng, as soon as the latter marries into the Jia household, although she retains overall control over Wang Xifeng's affairs so that the latter always has to report to her. Although Lady Wang appears to be kind and doting, she can in fact be cruel and ruthless when her authority is challenged. She pays much attention to Jia Baoyu's maids to make sure that Jia Baoyu does not develop romantic relationships with them. She expelled Qinwen (晴雯, Miss) from Jia household because her suspected affair with Jia Baoyu.
Aunt Xue (薛姨妈)	Jia Baoyu's maternal aunt, sister to Lady Wang and mother to Xue Pan (薛蟠) and Xue Baochai (薛宝钗). She is kindly and affable for the most part, but spoils her son and later finds it hard to control this unruly son.
Xue Pan (薛蟠, Mr.)	Xue Baochai's older brother. He is a dissolute, idle rake who was a local bully in Jinling City, known for his amorous exploits with both men and women, and not particularly well educated. He once killed a man over a servant-girl, but had the manslaughter case hushed up with money.
Granny Liu (刘姥姥)	A country rustic and distant relation to the Wang family, who provides a comic contrast to the ladies of the Rongguo House during two visits. She eventually rescues Jia Qiaojie from her maternal uncle, who wanted to sell her into concubinage.

(continued)

Table 1 (continued)

Character name	Brief introduction of the character
Ping'er (平儿, Mrs.)	Wang Xifeng's chief maid and personal confidante and also concubine to Wang Xifeng's husband, Jia Lian. She follows Wang Xifeng as part of her dowry when Wang Xifeng marries into the Jia household. She assists Wang Xifeng capably, handles her troubles with grace, and appears to have the respect of most of the household servants. She is also one of the very few people who can get close to Wang Xifeng, and wields considerable power in the house as Wang Xifeng's most trusted assistant, but uses her power sparingly and justly. She is very faithful to her mistress, but more soft-hearted and sweet-tempered.
Xiangling (香菱, Mrs.)	The maid of Xue's household (薛家), born Zhen Yinglian (甄英莲, a homophone with "deserving pity"), the kidnapped and lost daughter to Mr. Zhen Shiyin (甄士隐), the country gentleman. Later, her name is changed to Qiuling (秋菱) by Xue Pan (薛蟠)'s spoiled wife, Xia Jingui (夏金桂), who is jealous of her and tries to poison her.
Hua Xiren (花袭人, Miss)	Jia Baoyu's principal maid and his unofficial concubine. She has been Lady Dowager's maid before she was given to Jia Baoyu. She is considerate and forever worries about Jia Baoyu. She is the partner of Jia Baoyu's first adolescent sexual encounter in the real world in DRM-Chapter 5.
Qingwen (晴雯, Miss)	Jia Baoyu's personal maid. She is brash, haughty and the most beautiful maid in the household. Of all of Jia Baoyu's maids, she is the only one who dares to argue with him when reprimanded, but is also extremely devoted to him. Lady Wang later suspected her of having an affair with Jia Baoyu and publicly dismisses her on that account. Qingwen dies of an illness shortly after being expelled from the Jia household.
Yuanyang (鸳鸯, Miss)	Lady Dowager's chief maid.
Mingyan (茗烟, Mr.)	Jia Baoyu's page boy. He knows his master Jia Baoyu like the back of his hand.
Zijuan (紫鹃, Miss)	Lin Daiyu's faithful maid, ceded by Lady Dowager to her granddaughter.
Xueyan (雪雁, Miss)	Lin Daiyu's other maid. She came with Lin Daiyu from Yangzhou (or Suchou) city, and comes across as a young, sweet girl.
Concubine Zhao (赵姨娘)	A concubine of Jia Zheng. She is the mother of Jia Tanchun and Jia Huan (贾环), Jia Baoyu's half-siblings. Concubine Zhao longs to be the mother of the head of the household, which she does not achieve, thus asks Priestess Ma (马道婆) to murder Jia Baoyu and Wang Xifeng with black magic.
Qin Zhong (秦钟, Mr.)	Qin Keqing's younger brother. However, he is the natural son of Mr. Qin Ye (秦业), while Qin Keqing is an adopted daughter. He becomes Jia Baoyu's best friend, and homosexual lover. Qin Zhong and the novice Zhineng (智能) also fall in love with tragic consequences. Qin Zhong dies soon after from a combination of a severe beating administered by his father, sexual exhaustion, and psychological grief and remorse.
Jia Lan (贾兰, Mr.)	Son of Jia Baoyu's deceased older brother Jia Zhu and his virtuous wife Li Wan. Jia Lan is an appealing child throughout the book and at the end succeeds in the imperial examinations to the credit of the family.

(continued)

Table 1 (continued)

Character name	Brief introduction of the character
Jia Zhen (贾珍, Mr.)	Head of the Ningguo House, the elder branch of the Jia family. He has a wife, Lady You (尤氏), a younger sister, Jia Xichun, and many concubines. He is the unofficial head of the clan, since his father has retired. He is extremely greedy and has an adulterous affair with his daughter-in-law, Qin Keqing.
Lady You (尤氏)	Wife of Mr. Jia Zhen. She is the sole mistress of the Ningguo House.
Jia Rong (贾蓉, Mr.)	Son of Mr. Jia Zhen, and the husband of Qin Keqing. He behaves extreme-similarly to his father, and is the Cavalier of the Imperial Guards.
Second Sister You (尤二姐)	Younger sister of Lady You. Jia Lian takes her in secret as his concubine. She was a kept woman before she was married, but after her wedding she becomes a faithful and doting wife to Jia Lian. Because of Wang Xifeng's intrigue, she finally commits suicide by swallowing a large piece of gold.
Lady Xing (邢夫人)	Jia She's wife. She is Jia Lian's stepmother, and she rejects in heart to obey Wang Xifeng's administration of the house.
Jia Huan (贾环, Mr.)	Son of Concubine Zhao. He and his mother are both despised by the family. He shows his vile nature by spilling candle wax, intending to blind his half-brother, Jia Baoyu.
Sheyue (麝月, Miss)	Jia Baoyu's main maid after Hua Xiren and Qingwen. She is beautiful and caring, and a perfect complement to Hua Xiren.
Qiutong (秋桐, Mrs.)	Mr. Jia Lian's other concubine. Originally being a maid of Mr. Jia She, she is given to Mr. Jia Lian as a concubine, and is a very proud and arrogant woman.

From another perspective of view, DRM is remarkable for its "girly" character-istics, which are naturally in accordance with Western feminism and feminist liter-ary (Rao 2005). The portrayal of women was quite a radical departure from earlier literature, such as the other three of the Four Great Classical Novels, where women were primarily subsidiaries to men and treated more likely as a symbol. Women were simplified to be either good-looking but wicked, such as Mrs. Pan Jinlian (潘金莲) in The Water Margin, or omnipotent such as Guanyin (观音) in The Journey to the West. Contrarily, the DRM-author dedicated stories specifically and individually for each female character, such as the scene of burying flowers is specifically for Lin Daiyu (DRM-Chapter 30), chasing butterfly for Xue Baochai (DRM-Chapter 27), tearing up the folding fan for Miss Qinwen (晴雯, DRM-Chapter 31). In these stories, the girls were demonstrated to be well educated. The education for women was increasingly valued in DRM. This can be reflected in the scene in DRM-chapter 3. On her arrival at the Jia household, Lin Daiyu was asked for many times "How old are you, cousin?", "Have you been to schools?" Although the purpose of the education for women is on one hand to prepare them better for raising children, on the other hand to ameliorate the attractiveness of these women and better their chance to marry someone from families of bigger power, because marriage of children was a common way for building up stable relations with other families of power. These purposes are definitely unfair to the women involved according to many social roles they can take. They were not empowered to choose whether to pursuit the power and wealth they were educated for, but rather forced to bear the responsibility for the rise and fall of the family, the glory of the descendants. Nevertheless, all these vivid descriptions in the novel make the readers feel fond of these women even today. Whether this makes the DRM-author some kind of "proto-feminist" is debatable, but the DRM-author was certainly a philogynist ("Danny" 2011), and this "overly" delicate writing of women may also signify that all the intelligent men under royal control in the feudal system are weak as women. That is the reason that Jia Baoyu (standing for authority) are striving to protect the young girls (standing for intelligent men) living in the Grand View Garden. With this knowledge about DRM and the group of authors in mind, we are ready to look into the core components of the culture reflected in the novel.

3 Core Components of Chinese Culture Reflected in DRM

The work of DRM as a whole is robustly realist, and exhibits quite some skepticism about both Confucian values and religions at the heart of Chinese society.

3.1 Confucianism

Confucianism cherishes the ideal of having a society in principles and this school of thought is connected to materialize the ideal in the real world. Despite its acknowledgment of the unattainability of such a goal, it still insists that one should foster the ideal and dedicate oneself to realizing it in the spirit of "doing the impossible" (Tang 2015). With particular emphasis on the importance of the family and social harmony, rather than on an otherworldly source of spiritual values, the core of Confucian is humanistic (Juergensmeyer 2005). In fact, for some scholars, Confucianism is nothing more than a teaching doctrine regarding how to behave oneself, that is to say one should set a demand upon oneself and hold oneself responsible to the world and the nation (Tang 2015). In Confucianism, the family is considered as the basis and the prototype for all social relationships (King and Bond 1985; Lee 1991), and is the foundation of moral society (some discussions over the Chinese beliefs on family is also presented in Chapter "Chinese Family Contributions to Psychological Disorders"). Every member of a family should have a proper relationship with the others and a fixed social role, defined by age, gender and birth order. In sum, the basic tenets of Confucian beliefs to guide family and society are: lord guides retainer, father guides son, and husband guides wife, i.e. the *San Gang* (三纲, the Three Cardinal Guides or the Three Fundamental Bonds). In addition, a young man owed the elders respect, but could also expect protection; therefore, everyone was part of this system. Confucianism also has strict requirements regarding ancestor worship. Ancestors are still family and certainly counted as elders; therefore, they have to be treated with immense respect. The reciprocal obligations in between family members and the base virtue of respect for parents and ancestors are descried as the filial piety. An individual obeyed filial piety and respected their elders, obeyed their parents, assisted the elderly, protected children and treated siblings fairly, therefore the society was harmonious and peaceful (Muscato n.d.). At the beginning of DRM, the novel stated the history of Jia clan, and with the development of the story, it also put lots of stress on the declaration of the relationship between characters, which all shows how much the family structure is valued. In addition, the novel dedicated a large sum of contents on the harmonious relationship and joy in Jia's family, such as the loving mothers and respectful and dutiful descendants, and how Lady Dowager and Lady Wang care for Jia Baoyu and his sisters.

The praise for *Rén* is also fully established in DRM. The worldly concern of Confucianism is the belief that humans are fundamentally good, and teachable, improvable, and perfectible through personal and communal endeavor, especially self-cultivation and self-creation (Tay 2010). *Rén*, as one of the Five Constant Virtues, is the essence of the human being which manifests as compassion (Tay 2010), such as love between friends, forgiveness, sympathy for the weak, helping the poor, doing boldly what is righteous, gratefulness for others' help and so on. Some of the major plots and characters in DRM portray these traits well. Jia Baoyu as the central character of the novel is a concentrated expression of the values and aesthetic ideal of the DRM-author. The trait *Rén* can be seen in Jia Baoyu through his respect for the elderly, consideration for his sisters, respect and tolerance for the maids, sympathy for the poor relative Granny Liu. The plots of Granny Liu coming to Jia household are also important for the story (at least in DRM-Chapters 6 and 39). Granny Liu is a far relative for Lady Wang. She comes to Jia household for three times in DRM. For the first two times, she came for help to get rid of her family's poverty, and the Jia family did offer her a lot of help, partly because Granny Liu managed to please the people from Jia, especially Lady Dowager, but also for the kindness and generosity of the Jia family to the poor. With the help of Jia family, Granny Liu's financial situation gets a lot better, and she was grateful for the help. Her third visit to the Jia happened when she heard the Jia family was confiscated. She did her utmost to return the favor and help, even with the expense of her fields. It was because of the help of Granny Liu, Miss Jia Qiaojie (贾巧姐), the only daughter of Wang Xifeng, was rescued from being sold into concubinage by her maternal uncle. What is reflected in Granny Liu's efforts to help the Jia family is the rule of *Xin* (信) in the Five Constant Virtues, which is also highly praised in Confucianism.

Nevertheless, the DRM-author criticized Confucianism for its promotion of elitism and meritocracy. The Confucianism reinforces unequal, or hierarchical, structure of the society through another one of the Five Constant Virtues, *Li* (Nuyen 2001). While Confucianism acknowledges that all people are born equal, the process of development is such that not all can become *Junzi* (君子, superior man, which means ideal men that are second only to *Shen Ren* 圣人, sage, which means ideal man whose lives are interwoven with the heaven), and only some of the *Junzi* can become a sage. To Confucius, it is the *Junzi* who sustained the functions of government and social stratification through their ethical values (Littlejohn 2010).

Indeed, Confucianism is not committed to equality, but rather seeks to justify social inequality (Nuyen 2001). It uses the Three Cardinal Guides to establish the authority of the King over his ministers and indirectly the authority of the ruling class over the people. Likewise, in the family, the man, as father and husband, is given the position of authority. The Three Cardinal Guides speaks of the inequality in the family, but in practice, the family hierarchy extends to relationships other than to the father and husband: younger siblings are to defer to the older ones and girls to boys, the eldest son takes over the role of the head of the household in the absence of the father and husband (Nuyen 2001). In DRM-Chapter 18, when Jia Yuanchun (贾元春), daughter of Jia Zheng, also the granddaughter of Lady Dowager, returned home to see her family after becoming an Imperial Consort, the family members, including her parents and grandmother, had to bow before her as she has been given a status of the Emperor. The DRM-author also uncovered and criticized the hypocrisy of the hierarchy and social structure with his lash on the inequality between masters and servants. Qinwen, a brash, beautiful, yet devoted maid of Jia Baoyu, died from a serious disease after she was publicly dismissed by Lady Wang for her suspected affair with Jia Baoyu (DRM-Chapters 77 and 78). The DRM revealed the cruelty of hierarchy with the death of Qinwen, but also expressed admiration for the girl for her pure soul and courage of fighting, by implicating that she becomes a goddess of lotus after her death (DRM-Chapter 78), which by the by is an expression of Buddhist thoughts that we will discuss later.

The Confucian culture still holds a great role in the lives of Chinese people today. The aforementioned stress on *Rén* and *Li*, and other virtues of Confucianism still thrives in China and the Chinese communities throughout the world today. For instance, China largely operates as a male-centered society, in which the family name is passed down through the male line. Family plays a fundamental role within Chinese culture and family relationships are still of paramount importance for the Chinese. Moreover, enormous emphasis is placed upon the family and social hierarchy. Following the teachings of the Three Cardinal Guides, the Chinese men continue to occupy a dominant position in the family in terms of decision-making (Lu et al. 2000). A traditional concept of Chinese family involves several generations and immediate families all living under one roof, being a self-sufficient and self-help institution for its members, providing child care and the care for of the elderly, such as the Jia family in DRM. Although it is no longer the case for the modern Chinese society, where most families are nuclear ones with husband and wife living with their children and sometimes their parents, and the Chinese family no longer performs the function of providing mutual help with child care and care for elderly outside their immediate relations, the Chinese continue to emphasize the values of family and to maintain close family links. There is a strong bond between parents, children and other family members. For this reason, children often remain close to the original family in adulthood; those who are required to work away from the home area tend to make regular visits to family a priority, especially during the Chinese new-year or other important festival celebrations.

On the other hand, the hierarchical structure of the society is embodied in the details considered as signs of politeness and respect during social activities. For instance, it is a commonly social practice to introduce the junior to the senior, or the familiar to the unfamiliar. When addressing an elder or person with high status, it is considered highly inappropriate and rude to address the person by given name, while an appropriate way is to address them according to their designation, for example, Mr. Wang, General Zhang, and Doctor Song, etc., are all considered appropriate. As an extension of these beliefs, the Chinese tend to be comfortable with judgments made by those who are wise and compassionate. This leads to personal rather than professional performance appraisal and reward systems, and hence, in the business world, Chinese firms have sought to create a strong culture that guides and encourages actions in the absence of formal policies or procedures. As a result, the intentions of Chinese business leaders commonly remain loosely formulated and subject to opportunistic change (Martinsons and Hempel 1998).

Another example of Confucian culture in modern China is the concepts of *Mianzi* (面子, face) and *Guanxi* (关系, relationship) evolved from Confucian philosophy, and the resultant (or causal) collectivistic worldview of the Chinese. They are still the cornerstones of Chinese social life. The *Mianzi* of a person is an expression for his perceivable dignity and linked to his social status. In China, to give face to someone else can increase your own status and others will think of you as a benevolent and generous person. On the contrary, to take face is considered immature and regarded as sign of a lack of self-control. Another carryover from societal cultural values in Confucianism is the respect for hierarchical authority and equilibrium (harmony) with the system (Avison and Malaurent 2007). As a result, in working environment, a Chinese employee may act less forwardly than their Western counterparts when new opportunities for a raise open up (Iler 2009), just because they believe this may cause harm to their relationship with others. In China, relationships are often considered as more important than laws as those provide a social form of personal safety and influence. If one wants to get to know another one, it is common in China to be introduced by someone else first, one who knows that person already. It works like a transfer of trust. Similarly, when disagreement arises, often a third person is asked to mediate. In general, it can be said that the Chinese emphasize the interpersonal harmony and keeping face as well as maintaining good relations to other people as basic guidelines. These principles lead to Collectivism (Hofstede 1980, 1984), and the latter conversely reinforces the conduct principles. It is common in Asian schools that students wear uniforms to show conformity to the group. While in the classroom, they must stay quiet and follow teachers' instructions. Students acting differently from the rest are viewed as disruptive to the group norm. Collectivistic principles can also be seen in family activities. In families, it is important to follow family traditions, meet family expectations, and strive for family goals (Lai and Tsai 2014).

All these principles to some extent may function positively as they help establish rules and diminish conflicts. However, it should not be neglected that they may also become obstacles to development and to the higher working efficiency. Some functioning styles resulted from the culture, such as informal planning and process modeling, interdependent social and organizational relationships, etc., may ultimately limit the innovation efforts (Woo 2007). There is also some evidence showing that lying is a more acceptable behavior in Collectivist than that in Individualist cultures, if it saves face or helps the in-group member (Triandis 2001). In fact, there are even some traditional ways of lying that are understood as "correct behavior" (Triandis and Suh 2002). Moreover, the conventional thinking of implicitness and indirectness being indicative of thoughtful and humble, and public display of extreme positions and strong emotions being a sign of immaturity and weak-mindedness (Hwang 2009; Ji et al. 2010), may add cost to efficient communications. Besides the influences from Confucianism, those from the Daoist and Buddhist religions also play a strong role in the lives of DRM characters as well as the Chinese people up to the present.

3.2 Daoism and Buddhism

Daoism is an indigenous Chinese religion which is often associated with the *Dao De Jing* (道德经, the Book of the Way and the Book of Virtue), a philosophical and political text purportedly written by Laozi (老子, a pen name for Mr. Li'er 李耳) sometime in the sixth or fifth centuries B.C. (Tang 2015). It is especially important because it is one of the two trends which governed the ideology of the Chinese people for two thousand years. For Chinese culture, philosophy, art and psychology, the greatest influences have been from Confucianism and Daoism. Daoism focuses on the need to live in harmony with the *Dao*. However, one might ask what *Dao* is. Laozi explained that the *Dao* is the source of heaven and earth and in between, and it is elusive and vague, deep and obscure, soundless and formless, thus cannot be seen or touched. It is similar but not equal to what is emphasized in the New Testament, i.e., the truth, or *logos* in Greek. The *Dao* is a source of the universe or the origin of life, which cannot be described by language. According to Laozi, "The *Dao* produced the One. The One produced the Two. The Two produced the Three, and the Three produced the ten thousand things". In other words, the One is the original material force, which produces the Two, i.e., *Yin* (阴) and *Yang* (阳), and "the Three are their blending with the original force which produces ten thousand things" (Tang 2015). Unlike Confucianism, Daoism does not focus on social orders or ritualistic behaviors, but it shares some qualities with Buddhism.

Buddhism was first imported from India to China in the second year B.C. After its introduction into China, Buddhism first attached itself to Daoist necromancy (Tang 2015). Buddhism posits that when the person dies, his/her spirit does not perish but would subsequently take on a new form. This was something totally new that the Chinese people never heard of. Before Buddhism, Chinese people concentrated on human welfare and did not discuss metaphysical questions of the universe and after life. As Confucius said, "You are not yet able to serve people, how could you be able to serve ghosts and spirits?" (*Lun Yu* 论语, Analects). But death and after-life are important issues in human's life, so Chinese people, particularly the ordinary people naturally wish to know what happens after death, which to some extent pushed them to accept the new thoughts of Buddhism (Guang 2013). Buddhism also brought in the thought that for all one's deeds in life, whether good or evil, there will be retribution. One may be reborn as human, gods, ghosts or even animals including insects depending on his or her own karma (which means intentional actions) (Guang 2013). For that reason, one must value the performance of good actions.

When DRM was written, Confucianism, Daoism, and Buddhism had been integrated into the lives of Chinese people for more than 1700 years (Reynolds and Liao 2014), and they were reflected in the major plots and the lives of the major characters created in DRM. Laozi said "Halls filled with gold and jade can never be secured". It is therefore stressed by the Daoism that men should not lay too much stress on money. The DRM also insists the belief in many details of the novel, for instance, in the song "All Good Things Must End" in DRM-Chapter 1, the Daoist chanted "All men long to be immortals, yet to riches and rank each aspires; the great ones of old, where are they now? Their graves are a mass of briars. All men long to be immortals, yet silver and gold they prize; and grub for money all their lives, till death seals up their eyes…" Therefore, one must forget about riches and rank, silver and gold, if he/she wants to be immortal. This is also reflected in Jia Baoyu's hatred of associating with officials and learning something about the world and administration (DRM-Chapter 32). Daoism also emphasizes doing only what is needed in a given situation and nothing more. Daoists rarely initiate action and typically wait to react to the actions of others. In *Dao De Jing*, the sage (in Daoism, the world also means a person who follows the lead of the *Dao*, and he should be the wonderful example of the *Dao*) said: "I take no action, and the people of themselves are transformed. I love tranquility and the people of themselves become correct. I engage in no activity, and the people of themselves become prosperous. I have no desire, and the people of themselves become simple." These thoughts are reflected in DRM, for example, the character of Miss Jia Yingchun. When her nannie, an old woman who started to take care of her since she was very young, was caught for stealing her jewelry, instead of showing some sympathy or maybe anger, she was emotionless and did nothing but turned herself into reading a book (DRM-Chapter 73). Miss Xue Baochai is, on the other hand, an example of characters influenced by Buddhist thoughts. The house of Xue Baochai is surrounded by bamboo that grows straight up toward the sky, and does not have colorful or fragrant flowers to attract people. Most importantly, the inside of a bamboo stalk is empty. All these characteristics match the essence of Buddhist teaching that purity, the "emptiness" or absence of desire and fear lead one to the reality and incorruptibility.

China today is officially an atheist state, religion however still plays a significant role for many Chinese people. It is reported that the Han Chinese that are adherents to Daoist or Confucian Philosophies, accounting for approximately 26% of the country's population. The followers of the Buddhist religion accounting for 6% of the population. The Islam faith has a mere 2% following among the Han Chinese. Only 2% are adherents of Christianity, but it is now becoming a popular alternative in the country (Wee 2018). Nevertheless, a common perception of the Chinese religion is that it is a complex combination of the three teachings of Confucianism, Daoism, and Buddhism (Clart 2007). Contemporary influences of Daoism and Buddhism are presented not only in the religious practices and architectures, but also the language and the routines people take in thinking. As a well-known Chinese linguist said, the Buddhist terminology contributed to Chinese vocabulary tremendously and some of these terms have already embedded in the blood of Chinese language that people do not even know that they are originally from Buddhist literature (Wang 1990, pp. 678–686). For instance, today the Chinese use *Shi Jie* (世界) to mean the "world", but ancient Chinese people used *Tian Xia* (天下) to refer to the same thing. The *Shi Jie* is originally from Buddhist literature, where the *Shi* (世) denotes time and the *Jie* (界) denotes space. Other examples are the terms, such as *Xiang Ru Fei Fei* (想入非非) and *Xin Xin Xiang Yin* (心心相印). The influence of Buddhism further extended to the way Chinese people think. It is noted that the Chinese portrays some intellectual and spiritual traditions that emphasize a relatively cyclical type of reasoning. For example, studies show that relative to Westerners, Easterners understand that change is more natural and inevitable; Easterners feel more comfortable if their surrounding environment changes. In one study, given the task of forecasting growth rates of the world economy and other events, Chinese and American participants were asked whether the current trend would continue or whether it would reverse. The Chinese were found significantly more likely to predict a reversal of the current trend than were Americans, who predicted on average no change in the current trend (Ji et al. 2001). When asked to choose which of several linear and non-linear trends would best predict their happiness over the course of their lifetimes, the Chinese tended to choose non-linear patterns (suggesting that they expected change at several points in time), whereas Americans tended to choose linear patterns (Ji et al. 2001). The difference is to a large extent explained by the impact of Buddhist religion on the Chinese. The Buddhist religion emphasizes that the constant change is inherent in the mental, physical, and social world. However, it should not be neglected that change being important and inevitable is also the key theme in the folk religion of Daoism. From this perspective, the world is inherently unstable and constantly in flux (Tang 2015).

4 Conclusion

Culture is inherently a multilevel construct that exists not only in the minds of individuals, but also in the socially constructed material world. When we talk about Chinese culture, we are largely talking about beliefs and practices that are rooted in the ancient philosophies and religions of China, including primarily Confucianism, Daoism, and Buddhism. Many values in Chinese culture are based upon Confucianism, which stresses duty, sincerity, loyalty, filial piety and honor. In general, the Chinese are a collective society with a need for group affiliation, whether to their family, school, work group, or country. In order to maintain a sense of harmony, they tend to act with decorum at all times and will not do anything to cause someone else a public embarrassment. The novel DRM reveals a huge amount about everyday (aristocratic but also commoner) life in late imperial China (*Ming* 明 and *Qing* 清 dynasties), it tells not only about food and drink, ceremonies, family structures, the gradations of status, illness and medicine, astrology, religion, the legal system, and so on, but also how people interact with each other. Its value as studying material goes beyond literary merits alone. It is considered as a highly realistic document of the life of the Chinese nobility in the seventeenth to eighteenth century, a thinly disguised biographical account of historical, social, and economic events, and a fountain of information on social customs and family structure. To sum up, the DRM is full of evidence of the deeply-rooted traditional beliefs and practices, which offers a magnificent database for the study of Chinese societal culture. In the following two Chapters, basing on DRM, personality structure and personality disorder will be discussed.

References

Anonymous. (2014). *A Dream of Red Mansions in the year of Guiyou [Guiyou ben Shitouji]* (J. J. Jin & X. H. He, Eds.). Beijing: Jiuzhou Publishing House (in Chinese).

Avison, D., & Malaurent, J. (2007). Impact of cultural differences: A case study of ERP introduction in China. *International Journal of Information Management, 27*, 368–374.

Chan, K. H., Lew, A. Y., & Tong, M. Y. J. W. (2001). Accounting and management controls in the classical Chinese novel: A Dream of the Red Mansions. *International Journal of Accounting, 36*, 311–327.

Chowdhury, A. N. (2012). Culture, psychiatry and cultural competence. In L. LAbate (Ed.), *Mental illnesses – Understanding, prediction and control* (pp. 69–104). Rijeka: InTech Open.

Clart, P. (2007). The concept of "folk religion" in the study of Chinese religions: Retrospect and prospects. In Z. Wesolowski (Ed.), *The fourth Fu Jen University International Sinological Symposium: Research on Religions in China: Status quo and Perspectives; Symposium Papers* (pp. 166–203). Taipei: Furen University Press.

Cooper, E., & Zhang, M. (1993). Patterns of cousin marriage in rural Zhejiang and in Dream of the Red Chamber. *Journal of Asian Studies, 52*, 90–106.

Danny Yee's Book Reviews. (2011, November). Retrieved Oct 12, 2018, from http://dannyreviews.com/h/Story_Stone.html

Edwards, L. (1990). Gender imperatives in Honglou meng: Baoyu's bisexuality. *Chinese Literature: Essays, Articles, Reviews, 12*, 69–81.

Gao, Y. (2009). On cultural differences in the two English versions of A Dream of Red Mansions. *Asian Social Science, 5*, 112–117.

Guang, X. (2013). Buddhist impact on Chinese culture. *Asian Philosophy, 23*, 305–322.

Hall, S. (1980). Cultural studies: Two paradigms. *Media, Culture and Society, 2*, 57–72.

Hofstede, G. (1980). *Culture's consequences: International differences in worked related values.* Beverly Hills: Sage.

Hofstede, G. (1984). Cultural dimensions in management and planning. *Asia Pacific Journal of Management, 1*, 81–99.

Hu, W. P. (1993). *A Dream of the Red Mansions abroad.* Beijing: Zhonghua Book Company, in Chinese.

Huang, F., & Gillett, G. (2014). Bao-yu: A mental disorder or a cultural icon. *Journal of Bioethical Inquiry, 11*, 183–189.

Hwang, K.-K. (2009). The development of indigenous counseling in contemporary Confucian communities. *Counseling Psychologist, 37*, 930–943.

Iler, H. (2009). Understanding Chinese culture leads to business success. *Canadian HR Reporter, 22*, 18. Retrieved October 12, 2018, from https://search.proquest.com/docview/220782906?accountid=15198

Ji, L., Nisbett, R. E., & Su, Y. (2001). Culture, change, and prediction. *Psychological Science, 12*, 450–456.

Ji, L.-J., Lee, A., & Guo, T. (2010). The thinking styles of Chinese. In M. H. Bond (Ed.), *Oxford handbook of Chinese psychology* (pp. 155–167). New York: Oxford University Press.

Juergensmeyer, M. (2005). *Religion in global civil society*. New York: Oxford University Press.

King, A. Y., & Bond, M. H. (1985). The Confucian paradigm of man: A sociological view. In W.-S. Tseng & D. Y. H. Wu (Eds.), *Chinese culture and mental health (Chap. 3)* (pp. 29–45). Orlando: Elsevier.

Lai, N. H., & Tsai, H. H. (2014). Practicing psychodrama in Chinese culture. *Arts in Psychotherapy, 41*, 386–390.

Lau, M. P., & Ng, M. L. (1989). Homosexuality in Chinese culture. *Culture, Medicine and Psychiatry, 13*, 465–488.

Lee, S. H. (1991). *Virtues and rights: Reconstruction of Confucianism as a rational communitarianism.* Doctoral dissertation, University of Hawaii.

Levy, D. J. (1994). "Why Bao-yu can't concentrate": Attention deficit disorder in the Story of the Stone. *Literature and Medicine, 13*, 255–273.

Levy, D. J. (1999a). Venerable ancestors: Strategies of ageing in the Chinese novel The Story of the Stone. *Lancet, 354*, 13–16.

Levy, D. J. (1999b). *Ideal and actual in The Story of the Stone*. New York: Columbia University Press.

Li, R. S., & Li, S. H. (1995). An exploratory investigation of internal control concepts in Red Chamber Dream. *Journal of Auding Theory and Practice (China), 8*, 14–17 (in Chinese).

Liao, H. S. (2007). A Chinese Sinthome: Chan, modern subject and politico-semioticizing Dream of the Red Chamber. *American Journal of Semiotics, 23*, 147–171.

Lin, Y. T. (1935). *My country and my people* (p. 178). New York: John Day.

Littlejohn, R. L. (2010). *Confucianism: An introduction*. London: I. B. Tauris.

Lu, Z. Z., Maume, D. J., & Bellas, M. L. (2000). Chinese husbands' participation in household labor. *Journal of Comparative Family Studies, 31*, 191–215.

Martinsons, M. G., & Hempel, P. S. (1998). Chinese business process re-engineering. *International Journal of Information Management, 18*, 393–407.

Muscato, C. (n.d.). *Confucius' ideas on family and society*. Retrieved October 12, 2018, from https://study.com/academy/lesson/confucius-ideas-on-family-society.html#partialRegFormModal

Nuyen, A. T. (2001). Confucianism and the idea of equality. *Asian Philosophy, 11*, 61–71.

Rao, D. (2005). Dream of the Red Chamber and feminist literary criticism. *Journal of Wenzhou Normal College (China), 26*, 34–38 in Chinese.

Reynolds, B. L., & Liao, C. (2014). Translating religion in the Dream of the Red Chamber. *3L: Language, Linguistics, Literature, the Southest Asian Journal of the English Studies, 20*, 101–116.

Sanchez-Burks, J., & Lee, F. (2007). Cultural psychology of workways. In S. Kitayama & D. Cohen (Eds.), *Handbook of cultural psychology* (pp. 346–369). New York: Guilford.

Shi, Y. H. (2005). Beginnings and departures: The Dream of the Red Chamber. *New Zealand Journal of Asian Studies, 7*, 112–133.

Spence, J. D. (1966). *Ts'ao Yin and the K'ang-hsi Emperor: Bondservant and master*. New Haven: Yale University Press.

Stone, A. A. (2005). The Story of the Stone (The Dream of the Red Chamber, Vol. 1: The Golden Days). *American Journal of Psychiatry, 162*, 2412–2413.

Tang, Y. (2015). *Confucianism, Buddhism, Daoism, Christianity and Chinese culture*. Heidelberg: Springer.

Tay, W. L. (2010). Kang Youwei, the Martin Luther of Confucianism and his vision of Confucian modernity and nation. *Secularization, Religion and the State, 17*, 97–109.

Triandis, H. C. (2001). Individualism-collectivism and personality. *Journal of Personality, 69*, 907–924.

Triandis, H. C., & Suh, E. M. (2002). Cultural influences on personality. *Annual Review of Psychology, 53*, 133–160.

Wang, L. (1990). *Anthology of Wang Li – The history of Chinese vocabulary* [Wang Li Wenji – Hanyu cihuishi]. Jinan: Shandong Education Press (in Chinese).

Wee, R. Y. (2018, June 28). Retrieved October 12, 2018, from https://www.worldatlas.com/articles/religious-demographics-of-china.html

Wo, K. H. K. (2008). What gets lost in translation: Language and culture in "Hongloumeng". *LCOM Papers, 1*, 53–63.

Woo, H. S. (2007). Critical success factors for implementing ERP: The case of a Chinese electronics manufacturer. *Journal of Manufacturing Technology Management, 18*, 431–442.

Yang, M. (1996). Naming in Honglou meng. *Chinese Literature: Essays, Articles, Reviews (CLEAR), 18*, 69–100.

Yang, H., & Yang, G. (Trans.). (1978). *A Dream of the Red Mansions*. Beijing: Foreign Languages Press.

Yee, A. C. (1995). Self, sexuality, and writing in Honglou Meng. *Harvard Journal of Asiatic Studies, 55*, 373–407.

Yu, A. C. (1989). The quest of Brother Amor: Buddhist intimations in the Story of the Stone. *Harvard Journal of Asiatic Studies, 49*, 55–92.

Zhao, X. (2011). Court trials and miscarriage of justice in Dream of the Red Chamber. *Law and Literature, 23*, 129–156, 170–171.

Zhou, Z. M. (1989). *Hung Lou Meng – The enchanted world of art*. Taipei: Quan Ya Publishing.

Zhou, Z. (2001). Chaos and the gourd in "the Dream of the Red Chamber". *T'oung Pao Second Series, 87*, 251–288.

Personality Traits Characterized by the Adjectives in A Dream of Red Mansions

Guorong Ma, Junpeng Zhu, Wanzhen Chen, and Wei Wang

1 Introduction

As stated in Chapter "Societal Culture from Late Imperial to Contemporary China: As Indirectly Reflected in A Dream of Red Mansions", a novel, being an extended work that deals with character, action, thought, and so forth, in the form of a story, can offer a rich source for cultural studies. Therefore, not only art and literature specialists but also social scientists, psychologists, and psychiatrists have an interest in the novel, viewing it as a cultural vector. A Dream of Red Mansions (DRM) is valued as a compendium of the Chinese culture and even regarded as a historical document (Yu 1997), and so far have been used for studying many specialties in the society (see Chapter "Societal Culture from Late Imperial to Contemporary China: As Indirectly Reflected in A Dream of Red Mansions"). Ever since its emergence, the novel has been such a success that some even claim that one must read DRM if one wants to understand modern-day China (Stone 2005). It is therefore suggested that the descriptions in the novel were wildly held and concerned in both ancient and contemporary China. Indeed, the terms used in it to depict the distinct and vivid characters and the realistic life scenes are rich in number. Text in

G. Ma · W. Wang (✉)
Department of Clinical Psychology and Psychiatry/School of Public Health,
Zhejiang University College of Medicine, Hangzhou, China
e-mail: drwangwei@zju.edu.cn

J. Zhu
Department of Psychiatry, Zhejiang Provincial People's Hospital, Hangzhou, China

Department of Psychiatry, People's Hospital of Hangzhou Medical College, Hangzhou, China

W. Chen
Department of Social Work, East China University of Science and Technology,
Shanghai, China

© Springer Nature Singapore Pte Ltd. 2019
W. Wang (ed.), *Chinese Perspectives on Cultural Psychiatry*,
https://doi.org/10.1007/978-981-13-3537-2_3

the novel contains a rich source of adjectives, verbs, and motion-event descriptions throughout (Wu 2008).

Therefore, we will continue our journey exploring the relationship between Chinese culture and psychological phenomena by looking into the personality structure embedded in the personality-descriptive adjectives in DRM. Personality consists of stable traits that are observable across ages, genders, and cultures. Generally, traits represent enduring and consistent between-person differences in predispositions for cognitions, emotions, and behaviors (Wilson and Dishman 2015). All living human languages include numerous terms referring to attributes of personality and other human propensities (Dixon 1982).

The psycho-lexical approach means that personality traits are documented in the lexicon, practically in a tangible representation of that lexicon such as a dictionary. Moreover, a kernel characteristic of the approach is that the more a psychological trait is referred to, the more important that characteristic apparently is. Personality psychologists have noted that some terms used in novels are trait-specific (Passakos and de Raad 2009). Lexical approaches have been used in studies of personality structure for a long time (Galton 1884; Digman 1990; Goldberg 1993; de Raad et al. 2014). But conceptions of personality and character may differ across time and culture. Therefore, one of the main goals of the psycho-lexical approach in the study of personality during the last few decades has been the construction of a cross-culturally useful medium for communicating on personality, a generally accepted vocabulary of personality traits. The goal can be achieved following different routes. The most obvious route has been by tracking down trait words from the dictionary, books, letters, audiotapes, or films, listing them, and structuring them (Passakos and de Raad 2009).

Because many of the words describing attributes within any language are synonyms or antonyms with one another, and when applied to describe target persons, these terms are statistically correlated, these attribute terms can be condensed to a much smaller number of basic dimensions (Saucier and Goldberg 2001). Previous study using factor analyses of self- and peer-ratings on the personality-descriptive terms (e.g., adjectives, nouns, and verbs) have revealed various personality structures involving different number of factors. For instance, Saucier et al. (2014) conducted factor analyses of personality lexicons of nine languages of diverse provenance (i.e., Chinese, Korean, Filipino, Turkish, Greek, Polish, Hungarian, Maasai, and Senoufo), and compared their common structure to that of several prominent models in psychology. Their findings showed that a parsimonious bivariate model was substantially convergent across different cultures. The two dimensions (i.e., Social Self-Regulation and Dynamism) provide a common-denominator model involving the two most crucial axes of personality variation, ubiquitous across cultures. However, before Saucier et al. (2014), using similar methodology, de Raad et al. (2010) had found evidence of a structure consisting of three components to stand out as the core of the taxonomies included in the study. The components were named dynamism, affiliation, and order. Using English adjectives, some scholars have demonstrated a five-factor personality structure (Goldberg 1990), including Extraversion, Agreeableness, Conscientiousness, Emotional Stability, and

Intellect/Imagination. The most commonly used five-factor structure is the Big-Five model, namely: (1) Extraversion, Surgency, or Sociability, (2) Neuroticism, Affect, or Emotional Stability, (3) Agreeableness, Altruism, Love, or Compliance, (4) Conscientiousness, Orderliness, Industriousness, Energetic, or Active, and (5) Intellect, Openness to experience, Culture, or Capacity (Costa and Widiger 1994; Saucier and Goldberg 2001). The Big-Five has won relatively great popularity across different cultures. For example, the NEO-PI-R has proven to be structurally reproducible throughout other languages or cultures worldwide (Costa et al. 2001; Yamagata et al. 2006). In spite of its high replicability globally, there has been other evidence showing the model may not always be suitable in other cultures, such as difficulty in constructing in illiterate and indigenous society (Gurven et al. 2013). Hence, other may argue that although the Big-Five has inarguably good universality, more culture uniqueness of trait structure still worth finding out (Church 2016).

Psycho-lexical studies conducted in contemporary Chinese society have yielded convergent findings. Yang and Bond (1990) examined the relation between indigenous and imported constructs of the personality perception, derived a five-factor structure from both the emic Chinese descriptors and the imported American descriptors. The five factors extracted from the Chinese terms were respectively: Social Orientation-Self centeredness, Competence-Impotence, Expressiveness-Conservation, Self control-Impulsiveness, and Optimism-Neuroticism. In Chapter "Personality Traits in Contemporary China: A Lexical Approach", we will test a large adjective pool of personality-related adjectives on the university students in Northern, Southern, Western and Eastern China, and also disclosed five factors, namely: Intelligent, Emotional, Conscientious, Unsocial, and Agreeable. However, Zhou et al. (2009) used 413 terms with the highest frequency and administered them to two independent large samples in China for self-ratings and peer ratings to explore the emic Chinese personality structure. The results indicated that a seven-factor structure was the most informative structure relatively salient across subsamples of self-ratings and peer ratings, across original and ipsatized data, and across differences in variable selections. These factors were namely: Extraversion, Conscientiousness/Diligence, Unselfishness, Negative Valence, Emotional Volatility, Intellect/Positive Valence, and Dependency/Fragility. One reason for the discrepancy might be the different term pools used in these studies. These pools may cover different aspects of the Chinese culture and these aforementioned findings were primarily derived using terms selected from dictionary.

On the other hand, literary works can be helpful in achieving a full understanding of personality traits and their facets, and many literature texts that are handed down across time could provide rich, trait-relevant information of different eras (Compadre et al. 1985; Passakos and de Raad 2009). Scholars have studied ancient Chinese documents to learn about personality descriptors in ancient China. For instance, Yang (2005) examined the ancient Chinese personality terms in *Shi Ji* (史记, the Historical Records, a monumental history of ancient China and the world finished around 94 B.C. by the Han dynasty official Mr. Sima Qian (司马迁) after having been started by his father, Sima Tan (司马谈). The work covers the world as it was then known to the Chinese and a 2500-year period from the age of the legendary

Yellow Emperor to the reign of Emperor Hanwu (汉武帝) in the author's own time; "Records" (n.d.). He identified a four-factor structure, namely: *Rén* (仁, meaning benevolence, mercifulness or graciousness), *Zhi* (智, intelligence or wisdom), *Yong* (勇, courage), and *Yin* (隐, being a hermit). These factors are similar to some contemporary personality descriptions to some extent (e.g., *Rén* likely represents Agreeableness, *Zhi* represents Intellect, *Yong* represents Emotional stability, and *Yin* represents Introversion). However, *Shi Ji* is primarily biography of ancient heroes or personages (Kern 2015), rather than of ordinary people. One might wonder what the personality structures of general people look like in ancient times. Whether there is a clear picture of personality structure if we use words chosen from a novel, such as DRM, instead of historical literature study material?

Therefore, we designed the present study to elucidate the possible implicit structures of personality by examining the trait-descriptive adjectives in the novel. Inspired by contemporary efforts in understanding the ancient personality descriptions (reviewed by Millon 2012), we invited a group of well-educated matriculating university students to evaluate some personality-related adjectives used in the novel.

2 Methods

Seven contributors of the book including four coauthors of this chapter (all native Chinese speakers; 4 women and 3 men; 2 PhD holders, 4 PhD and 1 MSc candidates in clinical psychology) served as judges to decide which adjectives to be included in the study. They independently examined the 80-chapter version of DRM in search for any adjective that is person-descriptive. The latter chapters found in other versions of the novel were neglected for their distinctions from the preceding 80 chapters in writing style. In principle, the judges used questions such as, "What kind of person is he/she? He/she is [adjective]" and "What do you think of this person? He/she is [adjective]", to help determine whether an adjective referred to states or traits. The resulting 557 adjectives were compiled and approved by three authors of this article. Adjectives were removed from the list if less than two judges voted that they were personality descriptive. Finally, 493 adjectives were retained to the word pool. Because DRM was written about 300 years ago, it contains certain adjectives that are difficult for contemporary people to comprehend. For these adjectives each, a short explanation was attached immediately after.

Seven hundred and thirty-two Chinese university students (474 women, mean age 20.42 years with 1.46 SD, range = 17–39 years; 258 men, 20.71 ± 1.48 SD, range = 18–32 years) majoring in Arts, Education, Foreign Languages, Mechanics, and Medicine, were invited to participate in the present study. Participants judged each of the 493 adjectives on a 5-point rating scale: (1) very unlike me, (2) moderately unlike me, (3) somewhat like and unlike me, (4) moderately like me, (5) very like me. All participants were found to be free of and had no history of somatic or psychiatric disorders.

Due to the influence of individual differences in the overall elevation of responses, a bipolar-scattered construct may easily (or misleadingly) emerge. Therefore, ipsatization, as a partialling procedure to avoid the erroneous interpretation (ten Berge 1999) and used in several personality studies (e.g., Saucier and Goldberg 1996; Boies et al. 2001; Ashton et al. 2004), has been used in the present study. The method also fits into our present study where some adjectives are of negative valence.

Afterward, the data were submitted to the principal component analysis, and factor loadings were rotated orthogonally using the varimax normalized method. Once factor solutions were obtained, top adjectives with highest loadings on each target factor and without significant cross-loadings on other factors were selected for further analyses. Based on the top adjectives for each factor (scale), the internal reliability (Cronbach's alpha coefficient) of each scale was calculated. Mean scale scores in women and men were also calculated, and their differences were submitted to a two-way ANOVA plus a post-hoc analysis by Duncan's multiple new range test. Pearson's correlation was used to search for possible relations among these scale scores.

3 Results

The principal component analysis of the answers to the 493 items disclosed 20 factors whose eigenvalues were greater than 3.0. The first seven factors accounted for 8.9%, 4.5%, 2.9%, 2.2%, 1.9%, 1.4%, and 1.3% of the variance respectively (Fig. 1).

The five-factor structure was clearer (term examples are shown in Table 1). The first factor was defined most strongly by terms such as officious and spiteful,

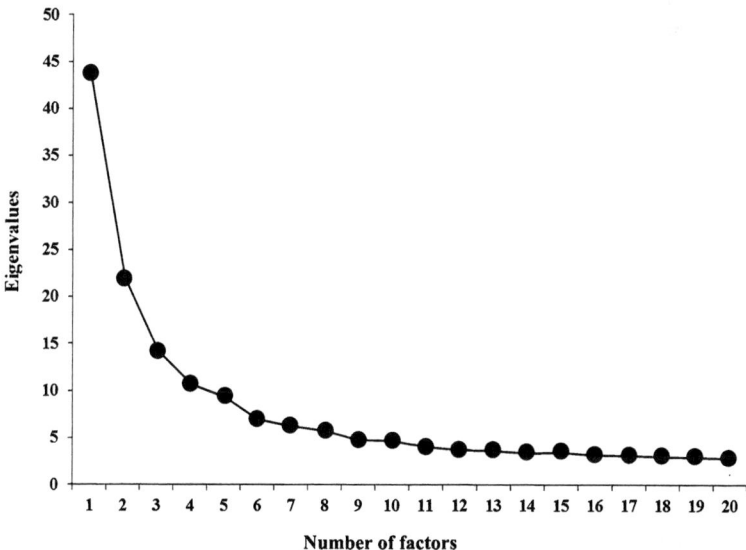

Fig. 1 Scree plot of eigenvalues obtained from factor analysis of 493 Chinese terms. (After Zhu et al. 2015)

Table 1 Loadings of the top 20 adjectives (Chinese plus English translation) on each factor in 732 participants

Chinese (DRM-Chapter appeared)	English translation	Factor 1 Wicked	2 Intelligent	3 Sociable	4 Conscientious	5 Frank
多蛊多妒 (56)	Officious and spiteful	0.62				
奸淫凶恶 (1)	Adulterous and fierce	0.60				
淫奔无耻 (66)	Shameless and wantonly	0.60				
黑心 (25, 37, 62)	Black-hearted	0.60				
歹毒 (74)	Sinister and vicious	0.60				
无耻老辣 (65)	Brazen and shrew	0.59				
狂三诈四 (39)	High-handed and cheating	0.59				
歪心邪意 (20)	Wicked and sly	0.56				
骄奢淫荡 (5)	Arrogant, extravagant and lascivious	0.55				
丧伦败行 (69)	Incestuous and relationship-upsetting	0.54				
为非作歹 (57)	Outrage-perpetrating	0.54				
暴虐 (2)	Brutal	0.53				
脏心烂肺 (63)	Dirty-minded	0.53				
赚骗无节 (58)	Always profiting and cheating	0.52				
狐媚魇道 (44)	Vamp-acting	0.52				
放荡弛纵 (19)	Reckless and headstrong	0.51				
邪谬 (2)	Absurd	0.50				
心里歹毒 (65)	Crafty and vicious	0.50				
见利忘义 (56)	Friendship-forgetting for profit	0.50				
利欲熏心 (56)	Mercenary	0.48				
足智多谋 (68)	Clever and resourceful		0.56			
聪明 (2, 5, 6, 9, 10, 12, 19, 29, 35, 39, 43, 44, 52, 54, 57, 66, 67, 71, 76, 77, 78)	Smart		0.55			
聪敏 (2, 21, 48, 49, 54, 56, 57, 74, 78)	Sensible and clever		0.55			

(continued)

Table 1 (continued)

Chinese (DRM-Chapter appeared)	English translation	Factor 1 Wicked	2 Intelligent	3 Sociable	4 Conscientious	5 Frank
伶牙俐齿 (73)	Glib		0.53			
敏捷 (50)	Quick-witted		0.53			
聪俊灵秀 (2)	Purely intelligent		0.53			
伶俐 (6, 19, 24, 27, 33, 39, 42, 43, 44, 48, 52, 54, 57, 58, 67, 74, 77, 78)	Sharp-witted		0.51			
智慧 (19, 29)	Intelligent		0.51			
有智谋 (46)	Strategically resourceful		0.51			
精明 (5)	Talented		0.50			
嘴巧 (54)	Smooth-spoken		0.50			
拘板庸涩 (78)	Stereotyped and pedantic		−0.51			
沉默 (3)	Demure		−0.51			
蠢笨 (24)	Stupid and clumsy		−0.51			
钝愚 (22)	Dull and stupid		−0.54			
无能无为 (21, 24, 36, 58, 65)	Incapable and useless		−0.55			
愚 (1)	Stupid		−0.56			
笨嘴笨腮 (54)	Inarticulate		−0.58			
心拙口笨 (30)	Inept and tongue-tied		−0.59			
呆头呆脑 (48)	Stupid-looking		−0.59			
和蔼可亲 (75)	Amiable			0.50		
慈爱 (13)	Kind			0.48		
宽柔 (33)	Lenient and gentle			0.46		
至善至贤 (77)	Being a paragon of virtue			0.46		
贤惠 (47, 49, 68, 69)	Virtuous and kind			0.43		
贤淑 (1)	Virtuous and educated			0.43		
温存和气 (35)	Gentle and amiable			0.42		
随和 (7, 22)	Easy-going			0.41		
和顺 (5, 55, 65, 78)	Obedient			0.40		
体贴 (9, 17, 18, 29, 32, 34, 51, 52, 57, 58, 78)	Considerate			0.40		
乖巧 (21)	Clever and cute			0.40		
慈软 (16)	Generous and soft			0.39		

(continued)

Table 1 (continued)

Chinese (DRM-Chapter appeared)	English translation	Factor 1 Wicked	2 Intelligent	3 Sociable	4 Conscientious	5 Frank
宽洪大量 (68, 69, 71)	Magnanimous and broad-minded			0.38		
心性高强 (10)	Highly strung			−0.40		
怪僻 (41)	Eccentric			−0.41		
傲慢 (4)	Insolent			−0.43		
左性 (47, 57)	Wayward			−0.43		
轻狂 (8, 31, 37, 54, 55, 57, 59, 74, 75)	Extremely frivolous			−0.43		
心高 (46, 72)	Highly ambitious			−0.45		
高傲 (58)	Haughty			−0.49		
斯斯文文 (7, 19)	Refined and elegant				0.50	
安静 (3, 16, 54, 77)	Quiet				0.48	
谨慎 (33, 55, 56, 59, 61)	Careful				0.48	
细心 (10, 34, 47, 48, 54, 74, 78)	Cautious				0.47	
文雅 (2)	Elegant				0.45	
稳重 (22, 57)	Steady				0.44	
细致 (38, 43, 45, 57)	Painstaking				0.43	
知书达礼 (54, 57)	Civilized and well-bred				0.43	
恭肃严整 (3)	Respectful and solemn				0.42	
娴雅 (4)	Naturally refined				0.41	
谨肃 (66)	Prudent				0.40	
精细 (55, 66)	Meticulous				0.40	
疯疯癫癫 (1, 3, 66, 67, 74)	Crazy and lunatic				−0.40	
口没遮拦 (49)	Talking too freely				−0.40	
顽劣 (2, 3)	Stubborn and roguish				−0.42	
不防头 (7, 22, 34,)	Careless				−0.44	
草莽 (3)	Uncultivated and refractory				−0.44	
憨皮 (30)	Naughty				−0.45	
淘气 (2, 7, 9, 11, 19, 23, 24, 26, 30, 31, 35, 40, 42, 45, 48, 54, 56, 58, 59, 60, 61, 62, 78, 80)	Mischievous				−0.46	

(continued)

Table 1 (continued)

Chinese (DRM-Chapter appeared)	English translation	Factor 1 Wicked	2 Intelligent	3 Sociable	4 Conscientious	5 Frank
冒撞 (5, 12, 19, 34, 36, 60, 75)	Tactless				−0.52	
大胆 (32, 34, 52, 55, 63, 68, 69)	Bold					0.50
响快 (6, 46)	Straightforward					0.49
刚强 (63)	Stern					0.48
有胆量 (24, 64, 72)	Plucky					0.47
刚烈 (66)	Upright and unyielding					0.46
简捷爽利 (73)	Quick and efficient					0.44
刚硬 (16, 36, 79)	Firm					0.44
直率 (16)	Frank					0.41
痛快 (10, 38, 54)	Straightforward and simple					0.41
天不怕地不怕 (34, 45)	Absolutely fearless					0.36
蝎蝎螫螫 (51, 52, 67)	Fussy					−0.38
习猜忌 (27)	Oversensitive					−0.39
畏头畏尾 (75)	Widely fearful					−0.39
畏事 (75)	Timid					−0.39
惧贵怯官 (14)	Awed by nobles and officials					−0.43
胆小 (9, 39, 72, 74, 77)	Cowardly					−0.43
怯懦 (19)	Timid and weak					−0.45
积粘 (46)	Sticky					−0.45
没胆量 (74)	Weak					−0.50
婆婆妈妈 (11, 77)	Old-womanish					−0.50

After Zhu et al. (2015)
Note: a word might appear more than once in a DRM-Chapter; adjectives with a cross-loading (absolute value) higher than 0.30 were omitted

adulterous and fierce, shameless and wantonly, black-hearted, and sinister and vicious versus propriety-abiding (factor loading, −0.36), devout (−0.34), and prudent (−0.34). The last three terms with less heavy loadings on the opposite pole were not shown in Table 1. The factor was named as Wicked after terms with high loadings. When scrutinizing individual answers, we identified a low-mean-response pattern. Most participants (about 77.12%) chose 1 ("very unlike me"), whereas far fewer chose 2 (about 13.83%, "moderately unlike me"), 3 (about 3.43%, "somewhat like and unlike me"), 4 (about 1.47%, "moderately like me"), or 5 (about 0.32%, "very like me").

The second factor in the five-factor solution was defined by terms such as clever and resourceful, smart, intelligent, sharp-witted, and so forth. This factor was then named Intelligent. The third factor included terms such as amiable, kind, lenient and gentle, easy-going, obedient and considerate, virtuous and educated, haughty, highly ambitious, insolent, eccentric, extremely frivolous, wayward, and highly strung on the other pole. It was then named Amiable. The fourth factor clearly represented Conscientious, was highly connected with prudent, painstaking, careful, cautious, meticulous, steady, and elegant versus tactless, careless, crazy and lunatic, mischievous, naughty, and stubborn and roguish. Some terms, such as civilized and well-bred, refined and elegant, and uncultivated and refractory, implied that this factor was education-related. The fifth factor, named Frank, was loaded with stern, firm, frank, bold, plucky, straightforward, quick and efficient, and absolutely fearless versus old-womanish, cowardly, timid and weak, sticky, fussy, and oversensitive. Adjectives loaded on this factor (Frank) were also loaded on the intellect-related factor in the two- or three-factor solution. With the top 10 items of each factor for calculating factor scores, the correlations between the four factors in the four-factor solution and the five factors in the five-factor solution were between 0.09 (Factor 3 in the four-factor solution and Factor 5 [Frank] in the five-factor solution) and 0.97 (the Factor 2 in the four-factor solution and Factor 1 [Wicked] in the five-factor solution).

As seen in the scree plot of the eigenvalues, there was a clear level-off after the fifth factor (see Fig. 1). Because the five-factor solution was much clearer and understandable than either the six or the seven factor solutions, we selected the five-factor model for further analyses. Table 1 illustrates the top 20 adjectives with highest loadings (absolute values) on the target factor (scale) and cross-loadings (absolute values) below 0.30 on other non-target factors.

The internal reliability of each scale was calculated with the top 20 adjectives. They are respectively 0.93 for Wicked, 0.90 for Intelligent, 0.84 for Sociable, 0.86 for Conscientious, and 0.86 for Frank. Two-way ANOVA detected a significant gender effect, $F(1, 730) = 4.15$, $MSE = 182.8$, $p < 0.05$, on the five scale scores. Men scored higher on Wicked ($p < 0.01$, 95% confidence interval (CI) = [2.20, 4.90]) and Conscientious ($p < 0.05$, 95% CI = [0.50, 3.70]), and lower on Amiable ($p < 0.01$, 95% CI = [−5.16, −2.24]) than women did (Fig. 2). Moreover, in all participants (n = 732), some scales were significantly intercorrelated. For example, Wicked was negatively correlated with Amiable ($r = −0.45$), whereas Intelligent was positively correlated with Frank ($r = 0.53$; Table 2).

4 Discussion

We selected 493 personality-descriptive adjectives from DRM, a novel written about 300 years ago, and identified different factor-solution models. The one- and two-factor solutions were similar to the ones reported earlier by de Raad et al. (2010) and Zhou et al. (2009), and the three- and four-factor solutions raised factors

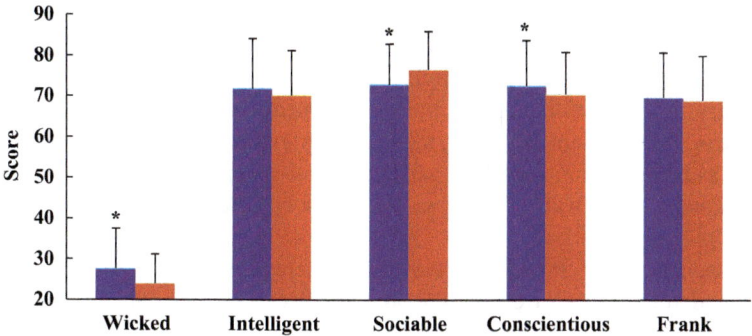

Fig. 2 Personality scale scores in men (violet bars, n = 258) and women (red bars, n = 474). * p < 0.05 vs. women. (After Zhu et al. 2015)

Table 2 Intercorrelations between the five factors based on the top 20 adjectives for each factor (n = 732)

	Intelligent	Sociable	Conscientious	Frank
Wicked	−0.29	−0.45	−0.32	−0.29
Intelligent		0.32	0.23	0.53
Sociable			0.39	0.25
Conscientious				0.06

After Zhu et al. (2015)
Note, all factors were significantly correlated with each other except Frank and Conscientious (p < 0.05)

similar to the ones reported by Saucier (2009) and Zhou et al. (2009). In the six-factor solution, the factors Wicked, Intelligent, and Conscientious were similar to those reported in previous studies (Saucier 2009; Zhou et al. 2009). The sixth factor was comparable with the dependency/fragility trait as reported by Zhou et al. (2009), and the other two factors in the solution reflected the agreeableness trait. However, our six-factor solution did not fit well into the six-factor model proposed by Saucier (2009). Our seven-factor solution also did not fit well into the previously reported seven-factor model, although the results of our seven-factor solution were comparable with those of Saucier (2003).

The five-factor solution presents a relatively clearer picture of personality structure. The first factor, Wicked, may be an artificial structure due to social unacceptability related response bias. However, it corresponds to the negative pole of Agreeableness (Peabody and de Raad 2002; Saucier and Goldberg 1996) and of *Rén*, as noted in *Shi Ji* (Yang 2005). It also resembles the Negative Valence, (Dis) Honesty (Ashton et al. 2000; Saucier 2009; Zhou et al. 2009), or Integrity Values (Szirmák and de Raad 1994). Highly evaluative terms, such as wicked and black-hearted, manifest patterns discernible in the emotional expression, thinking, or behavior (Saucier 2009; Zhou et al. 2009; Ashton et al. 2014). The negative attributes are important because they provide the threshold between acceptable and unacceptable, and between socially tolerable and intolerable behavior (Saucier 2003). As East Asians are believed to show more avoidant motivations (Heine and Buchtel 2009), the factor Wicked might reflect people's concern for their own safety. It was also in line with the reasoning, that Wicked was negatively correlated with Amiable in our study. Interestingly, men scored significantly higher on Wicked than women, as is the case in one of our studies of anti-social personality traits in China (see Chapter "Adjectival Descriptors for Antisocial Personality Trait in Chinese Culture").

The second factor, Intelligent, which represents the quality of being talented, clever, and reflective, corresponds to the Intellect (Saucier and Goldberg 1996; Zhou et al. 2009), Intelligent (see Chapter "Personality Traits in Contemporary China: A Lexical Approach"), and *Zhi* (Yang 2005) reported previously. Intelligence is a trait dimension that affects almost every aspect of an individual's life (Costa and McCrae 1994; deYoung et al. 2012). This factor also reflects wisdom, an attribute that is highly valued and might be the foundation of all other virtues (Thompson 2007). Interestingly, terms relating to communication skills also loaded on this factor. Sharing feelings with each other through language is one of the primary functions of the Chinese community; it helps to maintain existing personal relationships, reinforce role and status differences, and above all preserve harmony within the group (Gao 1998). Indeed, Intelligent is a highly treasured trait among Chinese people (Zhou et al. 2009).

The third factor, Amiable, corresponded to Agreeableness (Saucier and Goldberg 1996; Ashton et al. 2014) and Agreeable (see Chapter "Personality Traits in Contemporary China: A Lexical Approach") in previous models. McCrae and Costa (1989) showed that the interpersonal circumplex was defined by the two dimensions of Extraversion and Agreeableness. Avoidance in friendships was also characterized by these two personality traits (Marušić et al. 2011). Self, in a collectivistic culture (Earley 1989; Kwan 2009; Tjosvold et al. 2010), is not an independent entity and complete by itself, it is relational and defined by the surrounding personal encounters (Gao 1998). It is thus understandable that the Amiable trait is connected with agreeable and extravert tendencies in our study. Consistent with that, women scored higher than men on Agreeableness (Costa et al. 2001; Cuddy et al. 2015) and Extraversion (Feingold 1994). In the present study, women scored higher than men did on Amiable.

The fourth factor, Conscientious, representing careful, steady, and solemn attributes, corresponds to Conscientiousness in the Big-Five (Saucier and Goldberg 1996; Zhou et al. 2009) and Conscientious in the Chinese Adjective Descriptors of Personality (see our work to be described in Chapter "Personality Traits in Contemporary China: A Lexical Approach"). Terms such as refined and elegant, and civilized and well-bred were also loaded on this factor. This outcome is in line with the practicing of *Rěn*, which refers to self-restraint and self-discipline on a personal level (Chen and Chung 1994). The related disciplines also help to explain the correlation between Amiable and Conscientious found in the present study. Moreover, as breadwinners in a male-dominated society (Chia et al. 1994; Marshall 2008; Hyde 2014), Chinese men had to take more social and familial responsibilities, which required them to be more conscientious. The last factor, Frank, representing bold, stern, and fearless characteristics, corresponds generally to the Yong as noted in *Shi Ji* (Yang 2005) and the Emotional stability trait as previously illustrated (Zhou et al. 2009). The trait is closely related to courage, which guarantees the practicing *Rěn* together with wisdom (Chen 2010). These connections might also explain the correlation between Frank and Intelligent found in the present study.

Nevertheless, as this is was only a preliminary study, one should bear in mind some limitations of our design. First, the adjective pool was taken only from DRM, a novel written in the seventeenth to eighteenth century, rather than from a genuine lexical-design. Therefore, it remains unknown how much the writing style of the DRM-author had influenced the personality descriptions. In addition, although the novel contains a large number of characters and character descriptions that took place in everyday life, the adjectives used might not be exhaustive of that era. Second, we did not include terms from other novels as controls, nor other independent measures. Studies on other literary works of the same era might serve as a wonderful comparison in future study. Third, we did not use a personality questionnaire. Therefore, whether these personality traits identified in the present study are cross-cultural remains to be seen. Furthermore, the factor Wicked, which displayed a low-mean-response property, might also suffer from this third response style limitation, despite having a satisfactory internal reliability (0.93).

Overall, the results of the present study show that this design was effective. The personality factors identified with words used in DRM were comparable to those reported in the literature. This implies that an excellent novel such as DRM can help us better understand the structure of personality and personality disorders that exist in society. Future study should elucidate the importance of this trait in modern life and people's mentality. Similarly, attention should be paid to the Intelligent trait, one that might play a significant role in modern psychiatry. For instance, the concept of wisdom of ancient India has helped in the development of psychotherapies in modern Indian society (Jeste and Vahia 2008). The Amiable trait in our finds covers both Agreeableness and Extraversion among the Big-Five, and focuses on interpersonal relationships. The Frank trait in our study is also a mixture of Extraversion and Emotional Stability. Based on these results, personality psychologists might pay more attention to the role of a different worldview and emphasize personal relationships in Chinese personality traits. In the next chapter, narrations about personality disorders in DRM will be discussed.

References

Ashton, M. C., Lee, K., & Son, C. (2000). Honesty as the sixth factor of personality: Correlations with Machiavellianism, primary psychopathy, and social adroitness. *European Journal of Personality, 14,* 359–368.

Ashton, M. C., Lee, K., Perugini, M., Szarota, P., de Vries, R. E., di Blas, L., & de Raad, B. (2004). A six-factor structure of personality-descriptive adjectives: Solutions from psycholexical studies in seven languages. *Journal of Personality and Social Psychology, 86,* 356–366.

Ashton, M. C., Lee, K., & de Vries, R. E. (2014). The HEXACO honesty-humility, agreeableness, and emotionality factors: A review of research and theory. *Personality and Social Psychology Review, 18*, 139–152.

Boies, K., Lee, K., Ashton, M. C., Pascal, S., & Nicol, A. A. M. (2001). The structure of the French personality lexicon. *European Journal of Personality, 15*, 277–295.

Chen, L. (2010). Courage in the analects: A genealogical survey of the Confucian virtue of courage. *Frontiers of Philosophy in China, 5*, 1–30.

Chen, G. M., & Chung, J. (1994). The impact of Confucianism on organizational communication. *Communication Quarterly, 42*, 93–105.

Chia, R. C., Moore, J. L., Lam, K. N., Chuang, C. J., & Cheng, B. S. (1994). Cultural differences in gender role attitudes between Chinese and American students. *Sex Roles, 31*, 23–30.

Church, A. T. (2016). Personality traits across cultures. *Current Opinion in Psychology, 8*, 22–30.

Compadre, C. M., Pezzuto, J. M., Kinghorn, A. D., & Kamath, S. K. (1985). Hernandulcin: An intensely sweet compound discovered by review of ancient literature. *Science, 227*, 417–419.

Costa, P. T., Jr., & McCrae, R. R. (1994). *NEO Personality Inventory-Revised (NEO-PI-R) manual*. Odessa: Psychological Assessment Resources.

Costa, P. T., Jr., & Widiger, T. A. (1994). *Personality disorder and the five-factor model of personality*. Washington: American Psychological Association.

Costa, P. T., Jr., Terracciano, A., & McCrae, R. R. (2001). Gender differences in personality traits across cultures: Robust and surprising findings. *Journal of Personality and Social Psychology, 81*, 322–331.

Cuddy, A. J., Wolf, E. B., Glick, P., Crotty, S., Chong, J., & Norton, M. I. (2015). Men as cultural ideals: Cultural values moderate gender stereotype content. *Journal of Personality and Social Psychology, 109*, 622–635.

de Raad, B., Barelds, D. P. H., Levert, E., Ostendorf, F., Mlačić, B., di Blas, L., Hřebíčková, M., Szirmák, Z., Szarota, P., Perugini, M., Church, A. T., & Katigbak, M. S. (2010). Only three factors of personality description are fully replicable across languages: A comparison of 14 trait taxonomies. *Journal of Personality and Social Psychology, 98*, 160–173.

de Raad, B., Barelds, D. P., Timmerman, M. E., de Roover, K., Mlačić, B., & Church, A. T. (2014). Towards a pan-cultural personality structure: Input from 11 psycholexical studies. *European Journal of Personality, 28*, 497–510.

deYoung, C. G., Grazioplene, R. G., & Peterson, J. B. (2012). From madness to genius: The Openness/Intellect trait domain as a paradoxical simplex. *Journal of Research in Personality, 46*, 63–78.

Digman, J. M. (1990). Personality structure: Emergence of the five-factor model. *Annual Reviews of Psychology, 41*, 417–440.

Dixon, R. M. W. (1982). *Where have all the adjectives gone? And other essays in semantics and syntax*. New York: Mouton.

Earley, P. C. (1989). Social loafing and collectivism: A comparison of the United States and the People's Republic of China. *Administrative Science Quarterly, 34*, 565–581.

Feingold, A. (1994). Gender differences in personality: A metaanalysis. *Psychological Bulletin, 116*, 429–456.

Galton, F. (1884). Measurement of character. *Fortnightly Review, 36*, 179–185.

Gao, G. (1998). "Don't take my word for it" – Understanding Chinese speaking practices. *International Journal of Intercultural Relations, 22*, 163–186.

Goldberg, L. R. (1990). An alternative "description of personality": The Big-Five factor structure. *Journal of Personality and Social Psychology, 59*, 1216–1229.

Goldberg, L. R. (1993). The structure of phenotypic personality traits. *American Journal of Psychology, 48*, 26–34.

Gurven, M., von Rueden, C., Massenkoff, M., Kaplan, H., & Vie, M. L. (2013). How universal is the big five? Testing the five-factor model of personality variation among forager-farmers in the Bolivian Amazon. *Journal of Personality and Social Psychology, 104*, 354–370.

Heine, S. J., & Buchtel, E. E. (2009). Personality: The universal and the culturally specific. *Annual Reviews of Psychology, 60*, 369–394.

Hyde, J. S. (2014). Gender similarities and differences. *Annual Review of Psychology, 65*, 373–398.

Jeste, D. V., & Vahia, I. V. (2008). Comparison of the conceptualization of wisdom in ancient Indian literature with modern views: Focus on the Bhagavad Gita. *Psychiatry, 71*, 197–209.

Kern, M. (2015). The "Masters" in the Shiji. *T'oung Pao, 101*, 335–362.

Kwan, K. L. K. (2009). Collectivistic conflict of Chinese in counseling: Conceptualization and therapeutic directions. *Counseling Psychologist, 37*, 967–986.

Marshall, T. C. (2008). Cultural differences in intimacy: The influence of gender-role ideology and individualism-collectivism. *Journal of Social and Personal Relationships, 25*, 143–168.

Marušić, I., Kamenov, Ž., & Jelić, M. (2011). Personality and attachment to friends. *Drustvena Istrazivanja, 20*, 1119–1137.

McCrae, R. R., & Costa, P. T., Jr. (1989). The structure of interpersonal traits: Wiggins's circumplex and the five-factor model. *Journal of Personality and Social Psychology, 56*, 586–595.

Millon, T. (2012). On the history and future study of personality and its disorders. *Annual Reviews of Clinical Psychology, 8*, 1–19.

Passakos, C. G., & de Raad, B. (2009). Ancient personality: Trait attributions to characters in Homer's Iliad. *Ancient Narrative, 7*, 75–95.

Peabody, D., & de Raad, B. (2002). The substantive nature of psycholexical personality factors: A comparison across languages. *Journal of Personality and Social Psychology, 83*, 983–997.

Records of the Grand Historian. (n.d.). Retrieved October 12, 2018, from https://en.wikipedia.org/wiki/Records_of_the_Grand_Historian

Saucier, G. (2003). An alternative multi-language structure for personality attributes. *European Journal of Personality, 17*, 179–205.

Saucier, G. (2009). Recurrent personality dimensions in inclusive lexical studies: Indications for a Big Six structure. *Journal of Personality, 77*, 1577–1614.

Saucier, G., & Goldberg, L. R. (1996). Evidence for the Big Five in analyses of familiar English personality adjectives. *European Journal of Personality, 10*, 61–77.

Saucier, G., & Goldberg, L. R. (2001). Lexical studies of indigenous personality factors: Premises, products, and prospects. *Journal of Personality, 69*, 847–879.

Saucier, G., Thalmayer, A. G., Payne, D. L., Carlson, R., Sanogo, L., Ole-Kotikash, L., Church, A. T., Katigbak, M. S., Somer, O., Szarota, P., Szirmak, Z., & Zhou, X. (2014). A basic bivariate structure of personality attributes evident across nine languages. *Journal of Personality, 82*, 1–14.

Stone, A. A. (2005). The Story of the Stone (The Dream of the Red Chamber, Vol. 1: The Golden Days). *American Journal of Psychiatry, 162*, 2412–2413.

Szirmák, Z., & de Raad, B. (1994). Taxonomy and structure of Hungarian personality traits. *European Journal of Personality, 8*, 95–117.

ten Berge, J. M. F. (1999). A legitimate case of component analysis of ipsative measures, and partialling the mean as an alternative to ipsatization. *Multivariate Behavioral Research, 34*, 89–102.

Thompson, K. O. (2007). The archery of "wisdom" in the stream of life: "Wisdom" in the four books with Zhu Xi's reflections. *Philosophy East and West, 57*, 330–344.

Tjosvold, D., Wu, P., & Chen, Y. F. (2010). The effects of collectivistic and individualistic values on conflict and decision making: An experiment in China. *Journal of Applied Social Psychology, 40*, 2904–2926.

Wilson, K. E., & Dishman, R. K. (2015). Personality and physical activity: A systematic review and meta-analysis. *Personality and Individual Differences, 72*, 230–242.

Wu, J. (2008). Translating cultures: A linguistic reading of a dream of red mansions. *Meta: Translators' Journal, 53*, 507–527.

Yamagata, S., Suzuki, A., Ando, J., Ono, Y., Kijima, N., Yoshimura, K., Ostendorf, F., Angleitner, A., Riemann, R., Spinath, F. M., Livesley, W. J., & Jang, K. L. (2006). Is the genetic structure of human personality universal? A cross-cultural twin study from North America, Europe, and Asia. *Journal of Personality and Social Psychology, 90*, 987–998.

Yang, B. (2005). A factor analysis of the ancient Chinese personality structure. *Psychological Science (China), 28*, 668–672. (in Chinese)

Yang, K. S., & Bond, M. H. (1990). Exploring implicit personality theories with indigenous or imported constructs: The Chinese case. *Journal of Personality and Social Psychology, 58*, 1087–1095.

Yu, A. C. (1997). *Rereading the stone: Desire and the making of fiction in "Dream of the Red Chamber"*. Princeton: Princeton University Press.

Zhou, X., Saucier, G., Gao, D., & Liu, J. (2009). The factor structure of Chinese personality terms. *Journal of Personality, 77*, 363–400.

Zhu, J., Chen, W., Fan, H., Zhang, B., Liao, K., Li, X., Xu, Y., & Wang, W. (2015). Personality traits characterized by adjectives in a famous Chinese novel of the 18th century: A Dream of Red Mansions. *SAGE Open*. https://doi.org/10.1177/2158244015592011.

Narrations of Personality Disorders in A Dream of Red Mansions

Hongying Fan, Wanzhen Chen, and Wei Wang

1 Introduction

Since cultural phenomena are somewhat reflected in literary work, the novel – A Dream of Red Mansions (DRM), might also be regarded as an appropriate material source when drawing the outline of personality disorders in the background of Chinese culture, or in succession of traditional Chinese culture. The culture encompasses diverse and sometimes competing schools of thought, including Confucianism, Daoism, Buddhism, etc., and a host of other regional cultures. The Confucianism is undisputedly the most influential thought, which forms the foundation of the Chinese cultural tradition and still provides the basis for the norms of Chinese interpersonal behavior (Pye 1972). In Confucianism, rules are spelled out for the social behavior of each individual, governing the entire range of human interactions in society. The elementary teaching of Confucius is distilled in *Wu Chang*: *Rén, Yi, Li, Zhi*, and *Xin* (see Chapter "Hierarchical Needs and Psychological Disorders in China"). Confucius further defined five basic human relations and their principles, *Wu Lun: Zhong, Xiao, Rén* (忍), *Ti*, and *Xin* (see Chapter "Hierarchical Needs and Psychological Disorders in China"). Thus, relationships were structured to deliver optimal benefits for both parties. For each relation, certain behavior principles must be followed to ensure a harmonious society.

Nevertheless, the obsession with maintaining harmony in society and family systems ultimately brings about the excessive power distance and rigid rules, at the

H. Fan · W. Wang (✉)
Department of Clinical Psychology and Psychiatry/School of Public Health, Zhejiang University College of Medicine, Hangzhou, China
e-mail: drwangwei@zju.edu.cn

W. Chen
Department of Social Work, East China University of Science and Technology, Shanghai, China
e-mail: cwzdyzj@ecust.edu.cn

© Springer Nature Singapore Pte Ltd. 2019
W. Wang (ed.), *Chinese Perspectives on Cultural Psychiatry*,
https://doi.org/10.1007/978-981-13-3537-2_4

price of flexibility and professionalism (Chan et al. 2001). On the other hand, the obsession also displays a characteristic of Chinese culture through ancient and modern times, which is the Collectivism in contrast with the Individualism. In collectivistic culture, where socialization goals are to preserve group harmony and cooperation, people place high emphasis on conformity, submissiveness, and group orientation (Triandis 1995). However, in individualistic culture, high value is placed on the individual self, such that children are reared to a goal of the essence for their promotion of independence, freedom, and autonomy (Trommsdorff and Essau 1999). Thus, scholars considered that more overtly social norms existed in collectivistic culture for the sake of preserving social harmony (Essau et al. 2011). Based on this assumption, the association between social anxiety and cultural norms have been investigated and compared in the context of collectivistic and individual societies. For instance, Heinrichs et al. (2006) have found that collectivistic countries permitted more social reticence and withdrawn behaviors, and exhibited greater levels of social anxiety and more fear of blushing, than individualistic countries. Similarly, Schreier et al. (2010) have replicated the result described above in Asian and individualistic countries, which corroborate the assumption empirically. Moreover, another study has shown the prevalence of common anxiety disorders in a collectivistic society, Japan, where people commonly have a strong fear of offending others or disrupting interpersonal harmony than those in an individual society (Asnaani et al. 2010).

Among these five basic human relations, (a) three are family relations, which clearly show the importance of family in Chinese society and account for its paternalism; (b) the first two relations, filial piety and loyalty, are generally deemed the most important; (c) when they are applied to management, the first and last relations stand out, leading to the birth of a paternalistic management style in China (Hsiao et al. 1990); (d) Confucius always used only the male versions of language to define family relations. This paternal character is clearly expressed in the Chinese system of property inheritance (Fan 2000). The close interpersonal relationships supported by Confucianism results in Chinese collectivistic culture, which tends to embrace interdependence, family security, social hierarchies, co-operation, and lower levels of competition and is opposite to individualistic culture which emphasizes independence, freedom, high levels of competition and pleasure (Triandis 1989, 1993, 2001). Moreover, a collective orientation also implies a tendency to submit to one's individual fate-fatalism (Chan 1967), whereas the individualistic orientation, in the quest for freedom, implies a desire to seek control over one's fate. Allik and McCrae (2004) have stated that Individualism is dominant in both European and American cultures, which Western people are outgoing, open to new experience, and antagonistic; the Asian (including Chinese) and African people are introverted, traditional, and compliant. Furnham and Cheng (1999) also have shown that Chinese and Japanese people are less extraverted than British people are.

Further, in collectivist societies, paternalism acts as a vital role of the risk factor to mental health especially of family members as well. Paternalism and legal moralism reigns supreme in family and its extension, institutions, because collectivist societies would like to sacrifice individual interests for common good and social harmony (Bhugra 2004, 2005). As for male dominance, it could be related to psychological and behavioral problems. Males are spotted quicker to establish hierarchies of dominance by pushing others around, to become the leader, so that they tend to have lower empathizing skills (Strayer 1980). In a comprehensive review, Levinson (1989) concluded that when men hold the economic and decision-making power of the family, wife-beating is more common. It has also been admitted that rape and sexual assault are connected with male dominance (Sorenson and Siegel 1992). A possible interpretation is that males have more maladjusted portion than females, such as attention-deficit/hyperactivity disorder, both provocative and impulsive forms of solitary aggressive, oppositional defiant, and avoidant disorders (McDermott 1996). There are many studies holding the standpoint that domestic violence, as a presentative of the gender issue, could be regarded as an exemple of patriarchy and male dominance over women (Dobash and Dobash 1979; Johnson 1995; Walker 2000). Therefore, we might wonder, whether the special traditional Chinese culture, including paternalism, male dominance and Collectivism, had a great influence on the ancient personality characteristics and especially lead to some kinds of personality disorders from an ancient epoch on.

On the other hand, parental bonding styles are closely related to personality in many cultures. Poor parental bonding, such as lack of maternal care and low paternal overprotection, was associated with a psychopathic personality (Gao et al. 2010; Xu et al. 2016). Two externalizing problems – aggressive and delinquent – were characterized by low maternal care, paternal over-protection, and low maternal overprotection (Hiramura et al. 2010). In China, patients with personality disorder scored lower on parental Care but higher on parental Freedom Control and Autonomy Denial (Yu et al. 2007; Zheng et al. 2011).

Scholars have some attempts on finding a historical and stable Chinese personality structure by examining the ancient Chinese language terms relating to personality. For example, Yang (2005) has focused on a history book named *Shi Ji*, and found four factors: *Rén, Zhi, Yong,* and *Yin* (see Chapter "Personality Traits Characterized by the Adjectives in A Dream of Red Mansions"). Moreover, by analyzing nearly five hundred personality-descriptive adjectives, in Chapter "Personality Traits Characterized by the Adjectives in A Dream of Red Mansions", a structure of five factors was identified, namely Wicked, Intelligent, Sociable, Conscientious and Frank from the novel DRM. In contemporary, it is even more productive that the personality structures are described by the taxonomical pool. For instance, Chinese adjectival descriptors were applied to describe a five-factor normal personality trait structure, Intelligent, Emotional, Conscientious, Unsocial and Agreeable (see Chapter "Personality Traits in Contemporary China: A Lexical Approach"). The personality structures described in ancient and contemporary eras share some similarities, which confirm that history is often indicative of the future. The question therefore arises whether the ancient Chinese culture and the family environment have left some hints on the development of personality structures of that epoch. However, there have been few studies on the disordered personality traits of ancient Chinese. Therefore, we focused on exploring the personality disorders in traditional Chinese culture. As history is often indicative of the future, the findings might help to track historical culture composition in personality disorders of modern society and seek the special personality disorders in Chinese which might differ from other cultures. Answering this question might help trace the cognitive and behavioral imprints in the development of personality, and offer some profound clues for management of the contemporary personality disorders.

Therefore, our strategy is to look for a reliable vector of ancient scenarios to characterize personality disorders in Chinese culture. Being valued as a compendium of Chinese culture (Levy 1999), and even taken as historical documents (Yu 1997), DRM was specially chosen for this study again. Seen from the literature, there are also some studies focusing on the psychological world or the psychiatric problems described in DRM (see Chapter "Societal Culture from Late Imperial to Contemporary China: As Indirectly Reflected in A Dream of Red Mansions"). In the novel for instance, a few playboys in an affluent household, such as Jia Baoyu and Xue Pan, philander with their convoy of pages, school boys, visiting actors, as well as with various women (Lau and Ng 1989).

Up to the present, there is no study about the disordered personality traits in DRM or in ancient Chinese culture. With rich social and family environment sources, and detailed character descriptions (including speech, behaviors, and psychological scopes), DRM might provide some information about personality disorders and their related culture/family factors in the seventeenth to eighteenth century. However, narrations of a character might not be enough to form a personality disorder diagnosis, such as to meet all the necessary criteria proposed in the Diagnostic and Statistical Manual of Mental Disorders, Fifth Edition (DSM-5; American Psychiatric Association 2013), they might offer some hints of disorder personality traits, such as those dimensionally classified in the DSM-5 Section III (personality disorders or trait-specified). While a fitting to DSM-5 Section III criteria avoids the excessive heterogeneity within diagnoses, excessive diagnostic comorbidity, inadequate coverage, arbitrary boundaries with normal psychological functioning, and an inadequate scientific foundation (Livesley 2001; Trull and Durrett 2005; Widiger and Trull 2007; Clark 2007). Thereupon, we have hypothesized that the personality-related, information-bearing terms/ phrases and sentences/paragraphs in DRM are used as peer-reports; and based on these narrations, (1) some main characters in the novel are diagnosed into personality disorders or trait-specified in the DSM-5 Section III, and (2) there are connections between the cultural, societal, or family factors and the putative personality disorders.

2 Methods

Similar to the approaches used in Chapter "Personality Traits Characterized by the Adjectives in A Dream of Red Mansions", in the current study, we chose the 80-chapter version of DRM, and the latter DRM-chapters of other versions were ignored for their different style of writing from the preceding 80 DRM-chapters. The original first 80 DRM-Chapters in Chinese were carefully compared with their translations in English (Yang and Yang 1978; Beijing: Foreign Languages Press). The character names translated into English by Yang and Yang (1978) were updated in the contemporary Chinese Pinyin (see the introduction of DRM and the characteristics in the novel in Chapter "Societal Culture from Late Imperial to Contemporary China: As Indirectly Reflected in A Dream of Red Mansions"). Because of the detailed and large variety of character descriptions (including speech, behaviors, psychological scope) as take place in everyday life, especially for the main characters, it invites analysis of their possible personality disorders. Eight contributors of this book (judges) including the three co-authors of this chapter were involved in selecting and voting on the personality-descriptive terms (adjectives)/ phrases, and sentences/paragraphs in DRM, and in further comparing them with the personality disorder criteria described in the DSM-5 Section III (American Psychiatric Association 2013).

2.1   The Judges

All judges were majoring in Clinical Psychology or Psychiatry, functioned to select and vote on the descriptions of personality trait (adjectives/phrases, and sentences/paragraphs), and to compare and vote on the descriptions for their DSM-5 criteria-fitting. Two judges were PhD, and two MSc holders, three were PhD and one MSc candidates. In addition, two judges were junior psychiatrists, and one senior psychiatrist.

2.2   The Personality-Related Descriptions

For a personality description of a given DRM character, the judges used interrogative sentences to help identify and determine whether the description referred to impairment in personality functioning or pathological personality traits. Each judge independently examined the first 80 DRM-Chapters to search for the personality-descriptive adjectives/phrases, and sentences/paragraphs. For instance, for adjectives, the judges used questions such as, "What kind of person is he/she? He/she is [adjective]" and "What do you think of this person? He/she is [adjective]" to help determine whether an adjective referred to states or traits. Altogether 141 adjectives/ phrases and 241 sentences/paragraphs were identified after an exhaustive search by each author.

Each description was afterwards voted on by seven judges independently and labeled as "qualified" if it received more than four "yes" votes. If a description received three "yes" and three "no" votes, the seventh judge (one of the PhD holders) made a preliminary decision, which had to be confirmed by the senior judge later. Finally, 93 adjectives/phrases and 188 sentences/paragraphs survived after voting.

2.3 The Comparisons with DSM-5 Criteria

For each DRM character, his/her personality-related descriptions were carefully compared with the DSM-5 Section III criteria (American Psychiatric Association 2013). In brief, for each personality disorder, we examined criteria for the impairments of personality functioning: Identity, Self-direction, Empathy and Intimacy. We also examined the pathological personality traits (25 facet traits from five higher-order trait domains): *negative affectivity* (emotional lability, anxiousness, separation insecurity, perseveration, submissiveness, hostility, restricted affectivity [lack of], and suspiciousness); *detachment* (restricted affectivity, depressivity, suspiciousness, withdrawal, anhedonia, and intimacy avoidance); *antagonism* (hostility, manipulativeness, deceitfulness, grandiosity, attention seeking, and callousness); *disinhibition* (irresponsibility, impulsivity, rigid perfectionism [lack of], distractibility, and risk taking); and *psychoticism* (unusual beliefs and experiences, eccentricity, and cognitive and perceptual dysregulation). If a specific personality type was not indicated but personality dysfunction was present, we designated a trait-specified for that situation.

Once again, each description for the main DRM characters was voted on by seven judges independently and labeled as "qualified" if it fitted either into an impairment in personality functioning, or a pathological personality trait. If a description received three "yes" and three "no" votes, the seventh judge (one of the PhD holders) made a preliminary decision, which had to be confirmed by the senior judge later. Afterwards, DRM characters matched with the descriptions and the DSM-5 section III criteria appeared, and their gender, age (up to DRM-Chapter 80), name-showing frequency, and numbers of DRM-Chapter bearing important information (with specific plot) are illustrated in Table 1.

3   Results

After the summary on the personality-descriptive adjectives/phrases and sentences/paragraphs of each character in DRM, we found following main characters who might meet criteria for a specific personality disorder or a trait-specified (Table 2). The relevant personality-descriptive narrations of each character for the diagnosis are shown in Appendix Table 1. Table 1 (in Chapter "Societal Culture from Late Imperial to Contemporary China: As Indirectly Reflected in A Dream of Red Mansions") presented detailed descriptions of major characters of the novel. Although Jia Huan (贾环) and Xia Jingui (夏金桂)'s antisocial personality is not yet fully matched due to their young ages (less than 18 years old up to DRM-Chapter 80), we also diagnosed them with a trend of the disorder. They had shown some prodromal signs and symptoms that might foretell a future diagnosis of personality disorders in their putative adulthood.

Table 1 Name-appearing frequency, number of information-bearing DRM-chapters (with specific plot), gender, and age (up to DRM-Chapter 80) of the matched DRM characters

Name	Name-appearing Frequencies	DRM-chapters	Gender	Age (year)
Concubine Zhao (赵姨娘)	101	19	Female	30 ± (?)
Jia Baoyu (贾宝玉)	2625	78	Male	15
Jia Huan (贾环)	103	22	Male	13
Jia Jing (贾敬)	20	7	Male	66
Jia Rui (贾瑞)	73	4	Male	20+ (?)
Jia Xichun (贾惜春)	88	29	Female	13
Jia Yucun (贾雨村)	116	12	Male	40+ (?)
Lin Daiyu (林黛玉)	947	62	Female	14
Miaoyu (妙玉)	48	6	Female	21
Qingwen (晴雯)	302	34	Female	17
Wang Xifeng (王熙凤)	1253	67	Female	25
Xia Jingui (夏金桂)	58	2	Female	17
Xue Baochai (薛宝钗)	689	63	Female	17
Xue Pan (薛蟠)	244	20	Male	23

After Fan et al. (2018)

Table 2 Possible impairments in personality functioning, pathological personality traits, personality disorder or trait specified in each DRM character

Character Name	Impairments in personality functioning	Pathological personality traits	Personality disorder	Trait-specified
Concubine Zhao (赵姨娘)	Self-direction; Empathy; Intimacy	*Antagonism* (manipulativeness, callousness, deceitfulness, hostility); *Disinhibition* (risk taking, impulsivity)	Antisocial	
Jia Baoyu (贾宝玉)	Identity; Self-direction; Intimacy	*Psychoticism* (cognitive and perceptual dysregulation, unusual beliefs and experiences, eccentricity); *Detachment* (withdrawal)	Schizotypal	Distractibility
	Identity; Intimacy	*Negative affectivity* (emotional lability, separation insecurity, depressivity); *Disinhibition* (impulsivity)	Borderline	
Jia Huan (贾环)	Self-direction; Empathy; Intimacy	*Antagonism* (deceitfulness, hostility); *Disinhibition* (irresponsibility)	(Probable) Antisocial	
Jia Jing (贾敬)	Identity; Self-direction	*Psychoticism* (unusual beliefs and experiences, eccentricity); *Detachment* (restricted affectivity, withdrawal).	Schizotypal	

(continued)

Table 2 (continued)

Character Name	Impairments in personality functioning	Pathological personality traits	Personality disorder	Trait-specified
Jia Rui (贾瑞)	Self-direction; Intimacy	*Antagonism* (manipulativeness, callousness, deceitfulness, hostility); *Disinhibition* (risk taking, impulsivity)	Antisocial	
Jia Xichun (贾惜春)	Self-direction; Intimacy			Callousness
Jia Yucun (贾雨村)	Identity; Self-indirection; Intimacy	*Antagonism* (manipulativeness, callousness, deceitfulness, hostility); *Disinhibition* (risk taking, irresponsibility)	Antisocial	
Lin Daiyu (林黛玉)	Identity; Empathy; Intimacy	*Negative Affectivity* (emotional lability, anxiousness, separation insecurity, depressivity); *Disinhibition* (impulsivity); *Antagonism* (hostility)	Borderline	Grandiosity Suspicious
Miaoyu (妙玉)	Empathy; Intimacy	*Antagonism* (grandiosity, attention seeking)	Narcissistic	Withdrawal; Hostility; Grandiosity
	Empathy; Intimacy	*Disinhibition* (rigid perfectionism); *Detachment* (intimacy avoidance, restricted affectivity)	Compulsive-obsessive	
Qingwen (晴雯)	Empathy; Intimacy		(Probable) Antisocial (Probable) Borderline	Hostility; Impulsivity
Wang Xifeng (王熙凤)	Identity; Self-direction; Empathy; Intimacy	*Antagonism* (grandiosity, attention seeking)	Narcissistic	Unusual beliefs and experiences; Suspiciousness
	Self-direction; Empathy	*Antagonism* (manipulativeness, callousness, deceitfulness, hostility); *Disinhibition* (risk taking, irresponsibility)	Antisocial	
Xia Jingui (夏金桂)	Self-direction; Empathy; Intimacy	*Antagonism* (manipulativeness, callousness, deceitfulness, hostility); *Disinhibition* (risk taking, impulsivity)	(Probable) Antisocial	Emotional lability
Xue Baochai (薛宝钗)				*Antagonism*
Xue Pan (薛蟠)	Self-direction; Empathy	*Antagonism* (manipulativeness, callousness, deceitfulness, hostility); *Disinhibition* (risk taking, impulsivity, irresponsibility)	Antisocial	

After Fan et al. (2018)

For antisocial personality disorder, Xue Pan (薛蟠), one cousin of Jia Baoyu, might typically meet the related criteria. Xue Pan comes from a scholarly family of Jinling, who has lost his father while still a child. As the only son and heir of the family, he was thoroughly spoiled by his mother, with the result that he has grown up good for nothing (老大无成, DRM-Chapter 4). He always fails to conform to lawful and ethical behaviors, with an egocentric, callous lack of concern for others, and was accompanied by deceitfulness, manipulativeness, hostility, callousness, irresponsibility, and impulsivity.

On the basis of the limited information with the first 80 DRM-chapters, Xue Baochai (薛宝钗), the younger sister of Xue Pan (and born of the same parents), might not receive an antisocial diagnosis. However, she might potentially meet the criteria of the *antagonism* domain. Growing up with his troublesome brother, she has learned to masquerade as a non-malicious girl and has achieved some of her goals in the dark.

Jia Huan (贾环) was the half-brother of Jia Baoyu, born from Concubine Zhao (赵姨娘) and Jia Zheng. He might receive a diagnosis of the antisocial personality disorder trend. He is payed less attention and lacks family education due to his humble origins as the son of a concubine. Jia Huan was described to have a vulgar and common appearance, contrasting so strongly with Jia Baoyu, who has a striking charm and an air of distinction (神彩飘逸, 秀色夺人, DRM-Chapter 23). He was spineless (没气性的, DRM-Chapter 20), shameless/mean and sneaky (下流, DRM-Chapter 20), having no self-respect (不尊重, DRM-Chapter 20), and often letting others to warp his mind and to teach him the sneaky ways (歪心邪意, DRM-Chapter 20). Jia Huan had specific features of deceitfulness, hostility and irresponsibility, along with impairments in coherent personal goals and close relationships.

Concubine Zhao (赵姨娘), mother of Jia Huan, might also be labeled as antisocial personality disorder. It was not a blessing for the woman who was half master and half servant to bear a boy. As noted above, her son would live under the pressure of Jia Baoyu, who was the son of Jia Zheng's principal wife, and the first heir to Jia household. Concubine Zhao and her son sensed being despised and neglected by masters and servants in Jia household all the time, cultivating the personality features of manipulativeness, callousness, deceitfulness, hostility, risk taking, and impulsivity.

In addition, Jia Yucun (贾雨村), a careerist on the climb, might also meet the criteria of antisocial personality disorder. He is highly learned but so anxious about high official titles with a high salary that he dared not to uphold justice and punish Xue Pan, as mentioned above, a good-for-nothing young man from a wealthy family, who killed a man. Jia Yucun was brewing plots for the sake of money which resulted in disintegration of families, yet he had nothing to repent of.

Jia Rui (贾瑞), with his parents died long before, was the eldest grandson of Jia Dairu (贾代儒). He was a venerable Confucian scholar, running the school of Jia household, raised by the strict discipline of his grandfather. Thus, Jia Rui got too far out of line on the contrary, and he was an unscrupulous, grasping scoundrel who often used his position in the school to fleece the boys (最是个图便宜没行止的人,

DRM-Chapter 9). Furthermore, he tried to fornicate with one of his elder cousins Wang Xifeng (王熙凤), who was the wife of Jialian (贾琏). The antisocial personality features he had were manipulativeness, callousness, deceitfulness, hostility, risk taking, and impulsivity.

For borderline personality disorder, the emotional Lin Daiyu (林黛玉) might meet the criteria. Intelligent and pretty, she received good education because her parents would make up for their loss of a son and help themselves forget their sorrow. The mother of Lin Daiyu was the only and most loved daughter of Lady Dowager; however, she died when Lin Daiyu was young. Later, Lady Dowager sent for Lin Daiyu and brought her up to live in Rongguo House. Lin Daiyu always regarded herself as a guest in the house, so she was insecure and lacking in confidence to others including her lover Jia Baoyu. The borderline personality features she had were an unstable self-image and interpersonal relationships, and maladaptive traits of emotional lability, separation insecurity, depression, hostility, and impulsivity.

For narcissistic personality disorder, Wang Xifeng (王熙凤) might be diagnosed as suffering from the disorder. She was the niece of Lady Wang, also the wife of Jia Lian, son of Jia She (贾赦, uncle of Jia Baoyu). Wang Xifeng had been educated like a boy, and thus was given a schoolroom name – Xifeng. She was described as extremely good-looking and a clever talker, so resourceful and astute that not a man in ten thousand was a match for her (男人万不及一, DRM-Chapter 2). She had a variable and vulnerable self-esteem, and an overt grandiosity, with attempts at regulation through attention and approval seeking. The descriptions about her might comply with the diagnosis of antisocial personality disorder, for instance, she had a maladaptive trait in the domains of *antagonism* and *disinhibition*, contributing to the malignant narcissism. In addition, Wang Xifeng had suspiciousness, and once had unusual beliefs and experiences as a result of the secret harmful action performed by Concubine Zhao and Priestess Ma (马道婆).

The main character of DRM, Jia Baoyu (贾宝玉), was also the most complicated one concerning personality features, who was described as remarkably mischievous yet very clever. He was born into the world with a piece of clear, brilliantly colored jade in his mouth, with inscriptions on the jade. Therefore, Lady Dowager, who was the almost complete authority's owner over the extended household, had doted on him and regarded him as her darling. The whole clan not only indulged Jia Baoyu more than a beautiful son, but also considered him privileged to inherit the wealthy household normally. He was even allowed to live with his beloved sisters and girl cousins in the Grand View Garden. However, his father Jia Zheng was very strict with him because of his heir status. Jia Baoyu was asked to prepare to fulfill his social obligations for the sake of undertaking the affair of the family line and bringing glory to its name. Under the circumstance, he got plainly spoiled and used to seek the all-powerful protection of the indulgent Lady Dowager from his rigid father. These two totally contrary and conflict nursing patterns might give rise to the features of two types of personality disorder, such as the schizotypal and borderline.

Xia Jingui (夏金桂), the wife of Xue Pan, was another specially described female in DRM who seemed to be totally negative. Quite good-looking and educated, she had just turned 17 when making her debut, being comparable to Wang Xifeng in regard to her ability and craftiness. Her father died when she was a child, just like her husband Xue Pan, with no brothers either. Her widowed mother spoiled her since she was the only daughter, doting on her and falling in with all her whims. It was inevitable that the over-indulgence made her like a brigand (盗跖, DRM-Chapter 79). With a self-grandiosity, callousness, and lack of concern for others, she displayed maladaptive traits of *antagonism* and *disinhibition*. Based on the information, we might diagnose Xia Jingui as suffering from trends of antisocial and narcissistic personality disorders.

For the schizotypal personality disorder, Jia Jing (贾敬) might be one sufferer. He was the younger son of Jia Daihua (贾代化), the elder son of the Duke of Ningguo (宁国公), and he had inherited the Duke title. Unfortunately, he was too wrapped up in Daoism to taking any interest in anything but distilling elixirs. Owing to having a son Jia Zhen (贾珍) when he was younger, Jia Jing was relinquished the Duke title so that he could give his entire mind to becoming an immortal. Jia Jing washed his hands of all mundane matters to chase unrealistic goals, accompanied by his unusual beliefs and experiences and avoidant behaviors.

Qingwen (晴雯) was one of the intimate maidservants of Jia Baoyu, who was also pretty and intelligent. Marked by impairments in empathy and intimacy, accompanied by her maladaptive traits of hostility and impulsivity, she had exposed the tendency of antisocial personality disorder.

For the obsessive-compulsive personality, Miaoyu (妙玉) might meet the criteria. She was delicate as a child, coming from a family of scholars and officials in Suzhou city. Though her relatives bought many substitute novices for her, her health was not improved, until she joined the Buddhist order keeping hair practice. The pity is that her parents were dead at her debut, leaving behind her only having two old nurses and one maid to look after her. She had become widely read and well-versed in the sutras, as well being very good-looking. Miaoyu has remarkable rigid perfectionism, in consort with intimacy avoidance, restrictiveness, withdrawal hostility, and grandiosity.

Jia Xichun (贾惜春) was the young daughter of Jia Jing, who was good at drawing. Although descriptions of her were comparatively less, her preference for Buddhism referred her to the impairment of self-direction and intimacy. Meanwhile her callousness was also evident, pointing to a diagnosis of schizoid personality disorder (DSM-5, Section II).

There were also many other females described in DRM we want to focus on, who were all poor (可怜, DRM-Chapter 80), soft and weak (软弱, DRM-Chapter 69), and might be related to the anxiousness and submissiveness (*negative affectivity*). They might have low self-esteem and problems in maintaining intimate relationship, such as Xiangling (香菱, a concubine of Xue Pan), Second Sister You (尤二姐, a concubine of Jia Lian), and Jia Yingchun (贾迎春, one of the sisters of Jia Baoyu). Taking Xiangling for example, she had to follow Xia Jingui's unreasonable orders, and tolerate Xue Pan's beating with no resistance (DRM-Chapter 80). Further, they all had to marry someone they did not like: Xiangling to Xue Pan (DRM-Chapter 3), Second Sister You to Jia Lian (DRM-Chapter 65), and Jia Yingchun to Sun Shaozu (孙绍祖, DRM-Chapter 80). Therefore, they might be diagnosed to meet the criteria of avoidant personality disorder with a submissiveness trait. In contrast, their husbands had revealed themselves high levels of irresponsibility (*disinhibition*), callousness, and manipulation (*antagonism*).

4 Discussion

Throughout summarizing copious and precise descriptions in detail for each DRM character, we could apply to the DSM-5 Section III – defined antisocial, borderline, narcissistic, obsessive-compulsive, and schizotypal personality disorders to Jia Baoyu, Wang Xifeng, Lin Daiyu, Xue Pan, Concubine Zhao, Jia Rui, Miaoyu, and Jia Jing, among which antisocial personality disorder was the most frequently diagnosed one. More impairments the characters presented were in their interpersonal functionings than self-functionings. Maladaptive traits in *antagonism* domain were the most depicted, mainly embodied with Wang Xifeng, Lin Daiyu, Qingwen, Xue Pan, Jia Yucun, Jia Huan, Concubine Zhao, Jia Xichun, Jia Rui, Xia Jingui, and Miaoyu.

The ancient Chinese society placed a great deal of emphasis on the family system, from which all social characteristics were seen to derive (Lin 1935, p. 175). Then the paternalism plays an important role in Chinese daily life. Dominated by elders and men, traditional Chinese families are authoritarian and hierarchical (Lang 1946; Ho 1987). The hierarchy in the family is constantly braced up by legal and moral rules, like filial piety for younger generations. Chinese parents are responsible for governing, i.e., teaching and disciplining, their children (e.g., Hsu 1981), and children are encouraged to pledge obedience and reverence to their parents. Therefore, child achievement is closely linked to the reputation of the family. For instance, it is commonly believed that the failure of a child in social and academic performance might generate disgrace and shame to parents and ancestors (Luo 1996). Thus, it is imperative for parents, especially the father, who always presents less care but extreme strict, having the most responsibility to maintain and enhance the reputation of the family, to give assistance to children in order to achieving to the highest level; at the same time, the mother is submissive to father and has less effects (Ho 1987). On the other side, personality disorder is closely linked to the poor parent-child interactions and problematic parenting practices (Laulik et al. 2013), probably being the case in ancient China remarkably. It is obvious that parental neglect and a lack of family cohesion were associated with the development of schizoid and dependent personality disorders respectively (Lieberz 1989; Head et al. 1991). Thus, the excessive authoritarian even assault, altogether with the doting of Lady Dowager, might accelerate the improvement of *psychoticism* and *negative affectivity* (separation insecurity) in Jia Baoyu. Then again, Jia Rui, controlled and taught with rigor by his grandfather, might also be another sufferer. The antisocial personality is connected to experiences of low parental care and maternal over-protection (Reti et al. 2002), which was exemplified by Xue Pan, Xia Jingui, and Jia Huan. Such personality is correlated with a parental loss in childhood as well (Reich 1986; Patterson et al. 1989), which again exemplified by Xue Pan and Xia Jingui. Unpredictable and intrusive care-giving is associated with borderline personality disorder (Paris et al. 1994; Reich and Zanarini 2001), which might be applicative with the case for Lin Daiyu. Wang Xifeng was educated as a boy from her child-hood, which might contribute to her expanded self-esteem leading to the narcissism (Levy et al. 2007). Besides, the insecure, disorganized and unresolved adult attach-ment patterns (Lyddon and Sherry 2001; Crittenden and Newman 2010) might cause the disorders of Jia Huan and Jia Xichun.

Emphasizing the family and the preservation of social harmony is a negation of Individualism, which leads to Collectivism, as the existence of a relatively higher degree of interdependence among individuals (Hofstede 1980, 1984). In accordance with the hypothesis of Gray (1988), societies those are inclined to hold Collectivism, or have a long power distance, are more prone to prefer statutory or centralized control. In such a situation, self-direction might be easily lost in virtue of the trend towards bullying individuals into submission in their fate-fatalism (Chan 1967). Confucian culture has a high regard for learning and academic achievement, and emphasis on effort to achieve academically, of which the collectivist aspect under-scores relationships, family closeness, and social harmony. As a result, individuals attempt to achieve their personal success and ulterior honor of their family and society (Huang and Leung 2005; Mok 2006). The individual and his/her family have ambiguous boundaries, that the self-achievement is likewise regarded as the family achievement. Thus, it is clearer to see that Jia Baoyu was resistant to or escaped from the obligation, which led to the assaults of Jia Zheng. After that, the assaults in turn contributed to *negative affectivity* and *disinhibition* found in Jia Baoyu.

The preference for Daoism or Buddhism additionally, would lead to unrealistic goal setting, avoidance of social contact, and compulsive behaviors, typically as in cases of Jia Jing and Miaoyu. The Daoism, for instance, advocating self-transcendence, integrated with the Law of Nature, inaction, and infinite frame of reference, taking the place of social attainment, self-development, progressive endeavor, and personal interpretation (Yip 2004). Nevertheless, most descriptions of the DRM characters were on the basis of their daily activities and their commu-nications with each other. The self-dominated activities of Jia Jing and Miaoyu were not comprehensive in DRM. On the other hand, we could find that most descriptions of the characters were based on their daily life, communicating with each other, which might also strongly due to the Chinese collectivistic culture with the exis-tence of a relatively higher degree of interdependence among individuals (Hofstede 1980, 1984). Therefore, more interpersonal impairments would be detected once a personality disorder appears.

As the most-described trait in DRM, *Antagonism* has been found to be the mostly described trait domain in DRM. Forgiveness is a part of Confucian philosophy, whereas Chinese people appear to be less forgiving towards underachievement and misbehaviors than Europeans do, and the Chinese people are likely to disagree with statements that express toughness, maliciousness, and proviolence more strongly (Stankov 2010), which might be affected by the obsession with preserving harmony in society (Chan et al. 2001). As free expression of negative emotions might disrupt relationships, collectivists often tend to control such emotions inward (Triandis 2000), which however, might in turn lead to an excessive suppression and a later pathological-rebound. Moreover, Collectivism is relatively higher and simpler in conformity than Individualism is (Triandis 1993; Bond and Smith 1996), likewise involving more rigid rules. Nevertheless, this might be extremely boring and unbearing for high sensation seekers who are easily distracted by novelty things (Zuckerman et al. 1978). Therefore, *disinhibition* appears more frequently in males, especially the higher sensation seekers (Wang et al. 2000). Moreover, Collectivism laid stress on the experience of living, and particularly cared for getting along with others, i.e., the dependence (Diaz-Guerrero 1979; Triandis and Suh 2002). Thereupon, the trait *detachment* was the correspondingly less described one in DRM.

As mentioned before, due to male dominance (Fan 2000) and collective orientation (Chan 1967) in Chinese culture, most females showed increased trend to submit to their individual fate-fatalism. Although in DRM, some females took center stage and were frequently shown be more capable than their male counterparts, especially Wang Xifeng and Xia Jingui, with their means not so similar, which might have caused avoidant proneness for the poor females. Xiangling attempted to avoid but had bared abuse from her male host – Xue Pan, unfortunately, she was hit and failed in the end. Quite the reverse, most males in the DRM were philandering and irresponsible though they had more autonomy.

Furthermore, there is another focal idea namely the value, which reflects culture with concentration. In China, most cultural values are laudable, yet some could make hidden troubles (Yang 1987; Fan 2000). Governing by leaders rather than by law created the circumstance that individuals in a position of authority, as Xue Pan, Wang Xifeng, Jia Yucun and other characters in DRM, could do anything they wanted but did not pay the fiddler. To maintain interpersonal relations, tolerance of others, harmony with others, and propriety, people are expected to swallow their feelings, while exceed negative emotions could result in more stress and frustration. This might explain the phenomenon (also described in DRM) – people present as a gentleman on the surface but engage in bad things on the back.

There were still some limitations of the current study design that we must bear in mind. First of all, every DRM character was evaluated by the contemporary eight judges, whose overall levels of personality functioning might not be precise. Second, we examined many other characters in DRM, with their information available insufficient. For instance, Hua Xiren (花袭人), a personal maid of Jia Baoyu, had shown herself on the stage frequently, but the detailed narrations about her behavior and psychological world were inadequate. Third, the diagnoses were only on the basis of the novel narrations, and the writing techniques and styles of a literature might not correspond precisely to the real life. Fourth, the complete descriptions about the characters were reported from the first 80 DRM-chapters, thus, our current conclusion might not be generalized. In this respect, more information of the characters might be sought from the remaining 28 DRM-chapters (as recently published – Anonymous 2014). At last, we have only considered personality disorders diagnosed by criteria in DSM-5 Section III, whereas other psychiatric problems such as the bipolar disorder, dissociative identity disorder, or schizophrenia were not recorded.

This study implicated both the similar and the special personality disorders or features that might exist in ancient China. We have studied the ancient Chinese scenarios from the contemporary standpoint, and a variety of thoughts from other cultures has distributed over China, but the majority of Chinese culture and its centered Chinese values have been retained (Yang 1987). The antisocial personality disorder fictionalized in DRM was apparent in the seventeenth to eighteenth century, that the existence of this personality disorder reflected the cross-culture and time consistency of personality disorder. The study also implicates the importance of family in the development of personality traits in Chinese society. On the other hand, owing to the special traditional Chinese culture, self-direction would be difficult in some degree and interpersonal impairments would stand out with the personality disorder. Nowadays, people are influenced by Chinese culture in every aspect of the society with numerous traditional factors. Only when the harmful factors are fully revealed can Chinese culture reject the dross and assimilate the fine essence, thus the reductions of personality disorders or other psychological disorders can be realized. There was a high level of *Antagonism* in the characters and special submissiveness for most females that time. The current study has revealed the drawbacks of Daoism, Buddhism, and hierarchy, male dominance, and Collectivism under the influence of Confucianism in personality disorders, (e.g., Daoism or Buddhism would lead to unrealistic goal setting, and avoidance of social contact), but the structure of Chinese culture and its concrete effect on other psychological disorders are still an unknown terrain. Answering these questions will contribute to disclose the association between Chinese culture (both ancient and contemporary) and psychological disorders. So far, around the novel DRM, we have discussed the specific influence on personality traits and personality disorders by Chinese culture. In next chapter, we would like to pay more attention to personality disorders, concretely emphasizing the relationship between their features and Chinese culture. Further, we could make it available to understand and treat the disorders from the root of the culture, for people in China, Japan, Singapore, South Korea, Thailand, and other countries all over the world, given that Chinese culture has been one of the most influential ones worldwide (Wu and Jia 1992).

References

Allik, J., & McCrae, R. R. (2004). Toward a geography of personality traits: Patterns of profiles across 36 cultures. *Journal of Cross-Cultural Psychology, 35*, 13–28.
American Psychiatric Association. (2013). *Diagnostic and statistical manual of mental disorder* (5th ed.). Washington, DC: American Psychiatric Association.

Anonymous. (2014). *A Dream of Red Mansions in the year of Guiyou [Guiyou ben Shitouji]* (J. J. Jin & X. H. He, Eds.). Beijing: Jiuzhou Publishing House (in Chinese).

Asnaani, A., Richey, J. A., Dimaite, R., Hinton, D. E., & Hofmann, S. G. (2010). A cross-ethnic comparison of lifetime prevalence rates of anxiety disorders. *Journal of Nervous and Mental Disease, 198*, 551–555.

Bhugra, D. (2004). Migration, distress and cultural identity. *British Medical Bulletin, 69*, 129–141.

Bhugra, D. (2005). Cultural identities and cultural congruency: A new model for evaluating mental distress in immigrants. *Acta Psychiatrica Scandinavica, 111*, 84–93.

Bond, R., & Smith, P. B. (1996). Culture and conformity: A meta-analysis of studies using Asch's (1952b, 1956) line judgment task. *Psychological Bulletin, 119*, 111–137.

Chan, W. (1967). The individual in Chinese religions. In C. A. Moore (Ed.), *The Chinese mind: Essentials of Chinese philosophy and culture*. Honolulu: University of Hawaii Press.

Chan, K. H., Lew, A. Y., & Tong, M. Y. J. W. (2001). Accounting and management controls in the classical Chinese novel: A Dream of the Red Mansions. *International Journal of Accounting, 36*, 311–327.

Clark, L. A. (2007). Assessment and diagnosis of personality disorder: Perennial issues and an emerging reconceptualization. *Annual Review of Psychology, 58*, 227–257.

Crittenden, P. M., & Newman, L. (2010). Comparing models of borderline personality disorder: Mothers' experience, self-protective strategies, and dispositional representations. *Clinical Child Psychology and Psychiatry, 15*, 433–452.

Diaz-Guerrero, R. (1979). The development of coping style. *Human Development, 22*, 320–331.

Dobash, R. E., & Dobash, R. P. (1979). *Violence against wives: A case against the patriarchy*. New York: Free Press.

Essau, C. A., Ishikawa, S. I., Sasagawa, S., Sato, H., Okajima, I., Otsui, K., Georgiou, G. A., O'Callaghan, J., & Michie, F. (2011). Anxiety symptoms among adolescents in Japan and England: Their relationship with self-construals and social support. *Depression and Anxiety, 28*, 509–518.

Fan, Y. (2000). A classification of Chinese culture. *Cross Cultural Management, 7*, 3–10.

Fan, H., Chen, W., Shen, C., Qin, Y., Zhu, J., Xu, Y., Gao, Q., & Wang, W. (2018). Narrations of personality disorders in a Chinese famous novel in the eighteenth century – A Dream of Red Mansions. *Journal of Psychiatry: Open Access, 21*, 440.

Furnham, A., & Cheng, H. (1999). Personality as predictor of mental health and happiness in the East and West. *Personality and Individual Differences, 27*, 395–403.

Gao, Y., Raine, A., Chan, F., Venables, P. H., & Mednick, S. A. (2010). Early maternal and paternal bonding, childhood physical abuse and adult psychopathic personality. *Psychological Medicine, 40*, 1007–1016.

Gray, S. J. (1988). Towards a theory of cultural influence on the development of accounting systems internationally. *Abacus: A Journal of Accounting, Finance and Business Studies, 24*, 1–15.

Head, S. B., Baker, J. D., & Williamson, D. A. (1991). Family environment characteristics and dependent personality disorder. *Journal of Personality Disorders, 5*, 256–263.

Heinrichs, N., Rapee, R. M., Alden, L. A., Bögels, S., Hofmann, S. G., Oh, K. J., & Sakano, Y. (2006). Cultural differences in perceived social norms and social anxiety. *Behaviour Research and Therapy, 44*, 1187–1197.

Hiramura, H., Uji, M., Shikai, N., Chen, Z., Matsuoka, N., & Kitamura, T. (2010). Understanding externalizing behavior from children's personality and parenting characteristics. *Psychiatry Research, 175*, 142–147.

Ho, D. Y. F. (1987). Fatherhood in Chinese culture. In M. E. Lamb (Ed.), *The father's role: Cross-cultural perspectives* (pp. 227–245). Hillsdale: Erlbaum.

Hofstede, G. (1980). *Culture's consequences: International differences in worked related values*. Beverly Hills: Sage.

Hofstede, G. (1984). Cultural dimensions in management and planning. *Asia Pacific Journal of Management, 1*, 81–99.

Hsiao, F. S. T., Jen, F. C., & Lee, C. F. (1990). Impacts of culture and communist orthodoxy on Chinese management. In J. Child & M. Lockett (Eds.), *Advances in Chinese industrial studies (Vol. 1 (Part A))* (pp. 301–314). Greenwich: JAI Press.

Hsu, F. L. K. (1981). *Americans and Chinese: Passage to differences* (3rd ed.). Honolulu: University Press of Hawaii.

Huang, R., & Leung, F. K. S. (2005). Deconstructing teacher-centeredness and student centeredness dichotomy: A case study of a Shanghai mathematics lesson. *Mathematics Educator, 15*, 35–41.

Johnson, M. P. (1995). Patriarchal terrorism and common couple violence: Two forms of violence against women. *Journal of Marriage and the Family, 57*, 283–294.

Lang, O. (1946). *Chinese family and society*. New Haven: Yale University Press.

Lau, M. P., & Ng, M. L. (1989). Homosexuality in Chinese culture. *Culture, Medicine and Psychiatry, 13*, 465–488.

Laulik, S., Chou, S., Browne, K. D., & Allam, J. (2013). The link between personality disorder and parenting behaviors: A systematic review. *Aggression and Violent Behavior, 18*, 644–655.

Levinson, D. (1989). *Family violence in cross-cultural perspective*. Newbury Park: Sage.

Levy, D. J. (1999). *Ideal and actual in The Story of the Stone*. New York: Columbia University Press.

Levy, K. N., Reynoso, J. S., Wasserman, R. H., & Clarkin, J. F. (2007). Narcissistic personality disorder. In W. O'Donohoue, K. A. Fowler, & S. O. Lilienfeld (Eds.), *Personality disorders towards the DSM-V* (pp. 233–277). Thousand Oaks: Sage.

Lieberz, K. (1989). Children at risk for schizoid disorders. *Journal of Personality Disorders, 3*, 329–337.

Lin, Y. T. (1935). *My country and my people* (p. 178). New York: John Day.

Livesley, W. J. (2001). Conceptual and taxonomic issues. In W. J. Livesley (Ed.), *Handbook of personality disorders: Theory, research, and treatment* (pp. 3–38). New York: Guilford.

Luo, G. (1996). *Chinese traditional social and moral ideas and rules*. Beijing: The University of Chinese People Press, in Chinese.

Lyddon, W., & Sherry, A. (2001). Developmental personality styles: An attachment theory conceptualization of personality disorders. *Journal of Counseling and Development, 79*, 405–414.

McDermott, P. A. (1996). A nationwide study of developmental and gender prevalence for psychopathology in childhood and adolescence. *Journal of Abnormal Child Psychology, 24*, 53–66.

Mok, I. A. C. (2006). Shedding light on the East Asian learner paradox: Reconstructing student-centredness in a Shanghai classroom. *Asia Pacific Journal of Education, 26*, 131–142.

Paris, J., Zweig-Frank, H., & Guzder, J. (1994). Psychological risk factors for borderline personality duiroder in female patients. *Comprehensive Psychiatry, 35*, 301–305.

Patterson, G. R., DeBaryshe, B. D., & Ramsey, E. (1989). A developmental perspective on antisocial behavior. *American Psychologist, 44*, 329–335.

Pye, L. W. (1972). *China: An introduction* (2nd ed.). Boston: Little Brown.

Reich, J. (1986). The relationship between early life events and DSM-III personality disorders. *Hillside Journal of Clinical Psychiatry, 8*, 164–173.

Reich, D. B., & Zanarini, M. C. (2001). Developmental aspects of borderline personality disorder. *Harvard Review of Psychiatry, 9*, 294–301.

Reti, I. M., Samuels, J. F., Eaton, W. W., Bienvenu Iii, O. J., Costa, P. T., Jr., & Nestadt, G. (2002). Adult antisocial personality traits are associated with experiences of low parental care and maternal overprotection. *Acta Psychiatrica Scandinavica, 106*, 126–133.

Schreier, S., Heinrichs, N., Alden, L., Rapee, R. M., Hofmann, S. G., Chen, J., Oh, K. J., & Bögels, S. (2010). Social anxiety and socialnorms in individualistic and collectivistic countries. *Depression and Anxiety, 27*, 1128–1134.

Sorenson, S. B., & Siegel, J. M. (1992). Gender, ethnicity, and sexual assault: Findings from a Los Angeles study. *Journal of Social Issues, 48*, 93–104.

Stankov, L. (2010). Unforgiving Confucian culture: A breeding ground for high academic achievement, test anxiety and self-doubt? *Learning and Individual Differences, 20*, 555–563.

Strayer, F. F. (1980). Child ethology and the study of preschool social relations. In H. C. Foot, A. J. Chapman, & J. R. Smith (Eds.), *Friendship and social relations in children* (pp. 235–265). Piscataway: Transaction Publishers.

Triandis, H. C. (1989). The self and social behavior in differing cultural contexts. *Psychological Review, 96*, 506–520.

Triandis, H. C. (1993). Collectivism and individualism as cultural syndromes. *Cross-Cultural Research, 27*, 155–180.

Triandis, H. C. (1995). *Individualism and collectivism: New directions in social psychology.* Boulder: Westview Press.

Triandis, H. C. (2000). Culture and conflict. *International Journal of Psychology, 35*, 145–152.

Triandis, H. C. (2001). Individualism-collectivism and personality. *Journal of Personality, 69*, 907–924.

Triandis, H. C., & Suh, E. M. (2002). Cultural influences on personality. *Annual Review of Psychology, 53*, 133–160.

Trommsdorff, G., & Essau, C. A. (1999). Japanese and German adolescents'control orientation: Across-cultural study. In G. Trommsdorff, W. Friedlmeier, & H. J. Kornadt (Eds.), *Japan in transition – A comparative view on social and psychological aspects* (pp. 198–211). Lengerich: Pabst Science Publishers.

Trull, T. J., & Durrett, C. A. (2005). Categorical and dimensional models of personality disorder. *Annual Review of Clinical Psychology, 1*, 355–380.

Walker, L. (2000). *The battered woman syndrome* (2nd ed.). New York: Springer.

Wang, W., Wu, Y. X., Peng, Z. G., Lu, S. W., Yu, L., Wang, G. P., Fu, X. M., & Wang, Y. H. (2000). Test of sensation seeking in a Chinese sample. *Personality and Individual Differences, 28*, 169–179.

Widiger, T. A., & Trull, T. J. (2007). Plate tectonics in the classification of personality disorder: Shifting to a dimensional model. *American Psychologist, 62*, 71–83.

Wu, C., & Jia, S. (1992). Chinese culture and fertility decline. *Chinese Journal of Population Science, 4*, 95–103, in Chinese.

Xu, Y., Lin, L., Yang, L., Zhou, L., Tao, Y., Chen, W., Chai, H., & Wang, W. (2016). Personality disorder and perceived parenting in Chinese students of divorced and intact families. *Family Journal, 24*, 70–76.

Yang, K. (1987). Chinese values and the search for culture-free dimensions of culture. *International Journal of Psychology, 18*, 143–164.

Yang, B. (2005). A factor analysis of the ancient Chinese personality structure. *Psychological Science (China), 28*, 668–672. (in Chinese).

Yang, H., & Yang, G. (Trans.). (1978). *A Dream of the Red Mansions.* Beijing: Foreign Languages Press.

Yip, K. S. (2004). Taoism and its impact on mental health of the Chinese communities. *International Journal of Social Psychiatry, 50*, 25–42.

Yu, A. C. (1997). *Rereading the stone: Desire and the making of fiction in "Dream of the Red Chamber".* Princeton: Princeton University Press.

Yu, R., Wang, Z., Qian, F., Jang, K. L., Livesley, W. J., Paris, J., Shen, M., & Wang, W. (2007). Perceived parenting styles and disordered personality traits in adolescent and adult students and in personality disorder patients. *Social Behavior and Personality, 35*, 587–598.

Zheng, L., Chai, H., Chen, W., Yu, R., He, W., Jiang, Z., Yu, S., Li, H., & Wang, W. (2011). Recognition of facial emotion and perceived parental bonding styles in healthy volunteers and personality disorder patients. *Psychiatry and Clinical Neurosciences, 65*, 648–654.

Zuckerman, M., Eysenck, S. B., & Eysenck, H. J. (1978). Sensation seeking in England and America: Cross-cultural, age, and sex comparisons. *Journal of Consulting and Clinical Psychology, 46*, 139–149.

Cultural Contribution to Personality Disorders in China

Jiawei Wang and Wei Wang

1 Introduction

As mentioned in Chapter "Narrations of Personality Disorders in A Dream of Red Mansions", personality disorders comprise a set of diagnostic categories characterized by inflexible, pervasive and enduring patterns of cognition, affect, behavior and social interaction. These patterns emerge by early adulthood, are evident across a wide range of contexts and deviate from local cultural norms (American Psychiatric Association 2013). Thus, the accurate diagnosis and treatment of personality disorders depend largely on how a society judges a certain behavior. Culture is described as the collection of values, beliefs, behaviors, customs, and attitudes that distinguish a society, which is complex and multi-dimensional (Fan 2000). The cultural diversity is underestimated worldwide, which may lead to misinterpretations when recognizing the problematic patterns of behaviors from the normative one. The Chinese culture, one of the earliest ancient civilizations, profoundly influences the formation and development of personality of the Chinese from generation to generation. The representatives of the Chinese culture, such as the Confucius tradition and Collectivism, also affect the prevalence and presentation of personality disorders deeply. Previous chapters have highlighted the features of personality traits or personality disorders by the personality-descriptive terms (adjective)/phrases, or by narrative text, in the famous novel DRM, which is a compendium of Chinese culture. In this chapter, we will look for the evidence how Confucianism and Collectivism influence on the formation of personality and personality disorders and which characteristics in Confucianism and Collectivism served as the basis of personality disorders in China.

J. Wang · W. Wang (✉)
Department of Clinical Psychology and Psychiatry/School of Public Health, Zhejiang University College of Medicine, Hangzhou, China
e-mail: drwangwei@zju.edu.cn

© Springer Nature Singapore Pte Ltd. 2019
W. Wang (ed.), *Chinese Perspectives on Cultural Psychiatry*,
https://doi.org/10.1007/978-981-13-3537-2_5

2   Characteristics of Chinese Culture

Chinese culture has consistent and specific core values, and it contributes to the constitution of the basic identity of Chinese people. China, mainly consisted of the Han nationality, used to be the centrality and sovereignty based on its agricultural economy for a long history, has a history of 5000 years and same language. The core of Chinese culture is relatively stable for a long time in mainland and overseas Chinese people, underlying their daily life experience and relationships.

The traditional Chinese culture is consisted of diverse schools of thought, like Confucianism, Daoism, Buddhism, etc. Yet, Confucianism, the most influential thought, established the foundation of the Chinese tradition, continually provides the norms of social and interpersonal behaviors (Pye 1972). As noted in Chapter "Hierarchical Needs and Psychological Disorders in China", Five Constant Virtues: humanity, righteousness, propriety, wisdom and faithfulness, is the basic teaching of Confucius. The Confucius also defines *Wu Lun* – the Five Cardinal Relationships as: between ruler and minister, between father and son, between husband and wife, between brothers, and between friends; and defines the principles for each relation.

As a traditional agricultural society, the family tends to be located in certain places and preserves its spatial coherence. As a consequence, family hierarchy is extremely concerning interpersonal relationships in Chinese culture. People think highly of the connections with other persons and social institutions. In Chinese culture, individual's identity is always defined as a member in a group of "sociocentric" selves. While for Westerners, an individual's identity may be defined quite independently of the group. The closely related one with the notion of relational identity is collective identity, wherein an individual's identity, is defined by membership in the reference group to which he/she belongs. In the extreme, the individual is not regarded as a separate being, but as a member of the larger group. For Westerners, an individual's identity may be defined quite independently of the group. For Asians, however, individual identity tends to be interwoven with collective identity. Each member partakes of the attributes of the group. Each shares the pride that group claims, and bears the burden of its collective humiliation. All these seem unique to Chinese society, for instance, Schwartz (1994) found that Hong Kong scored relatively high on conservatism, whereas former West Germany scored high on autonomy when rating the culture-level dimensions of value. In China indeed, Confucian stresses the relationship between self and others, while the conception of freedom is considered as deviant behaviors.

Chinese society is governed by etiquette and sentiment as well as by law. The Confucian system of ethics defines proper behavior among people. The great emphasis on propriety leaves little room for the unbridled expression of emotions and feelings. It is considered shameful to show open affection in public, hence what is seen as social withdrawal or shyness in Western culture may be seen as courtesy or gentleness in Eastern culture (Cai et al. 2011). The extreme rigidity of prescriptions for proper conduct tolerates no deviation from the norm and thus inhibits the development of individuality. In Chinese way of life, emphasis is put on individual's appropriate place and behavior among his fellowmen. Confucianism tends to apprise people who view behavior in terms of whether it meets or fails to meet some external moral or social criteria instead of individual needs, sentiments, or volition. Deviation from prescribed behavior often causes the deviant person to feel ashamed.

3   Normal Personality Trait and Culture

Personality or individual differences, defined psychologically as habitual patterns of behavior, thought, and emotion, is relatively stable over time and situations, differs across individuals (e.g., some people are outgoing whereas others are not). Various personality-related ideas and theories have existed for a long history in China. The terms "human nature", "disposition" and "character" used by Chinese ancient ideologists have more or less include the meaning of personality. Personality trait is in contrast to states, which are more transitory dispositions. Personality researchers have reached a consensus that personality traits can be established as a higher-order structure. Among the best established models, the Big-Five Model is the most prominent one (John and Srivastava 1999; please also see Chapter "Personality Traits Characterized by the Adjectives in A Dream of Red Mansions").

According to the Big-Five Model, personality traits are developed during childhood and reach maturation in adulthood, which are stable within an individual (McCrae and Costa 1999). However, research nowadays have shown that personality traits would keep changing in adulthood even in old age. Several cross-sectional and longitudinal studies concerning personality-trait change in adulthood have demonstrated that these traits differ by age (Roberts and Mroczek 2008; Durbin et al. 2016). Therefore, there are plasticity features of personality traits, the personality change is complex and ongoing, and many factors might affect the change process.

The culture can provide social members with solutions to problems of both external adaptation and internal integration. The value of a culture shapes people's enduring beliefs and attitudes and guides their conducts, which in most situations are the criteria and norms to judge a certain behavior. Definitely, not all people of a culture hold exactly the same values (Hofstede 1984). Different traditions and practices including social, religious, and family values tend to influence the development and formation of individual personality, whether normal or disordered (Ronningstam et al. 2018). From contextual perspective, personality traits are multiply determined, and one important factor is the social contexts, which include social roles and life events (Roberts et al. 2003). Cultural variation may also influence gene-environment interactions and pathology leading to personality disorders.

There are interactions between personality and culture, i.e., culture is an active agent which plays an important role in shaping individual's personalities, and the general personality traits in turn affect his spirits and behaviors, leading to their further change to environment. The influence of culture on personality is well-illustrated through linkages with Individualism or Collectivism. Most developed and industrialized regions, such as the United States, Europe, and Australia are typically regarded as individualistic, and developing regions, such as the Asia and Africa are collectivistic (Oyserman et al. 2002). People in a collectivistic society, who value tradition, sociability and interdependence, might receive social support and feelings of belonging. On the contrary, people in individualistic society, who value competition, hedonism and self-reliance, often foster the pursuit of self-actualization. On the other hand, both Individualism and Collectivism are believed to have some disadvantages when considering the psychological health (Triandis and Gelfand 1998), for instance, the over emphasis on self would lead to social isolation (Triandis 2001). Collectivism and traditional cultures may create conditions resulting in depression and anxiety, especially when an individual does not meet the social obligations. Previous results have shown that Individualism was positively correlated with scales for paranoid, schizoid, narcissistic, borderline and antisocial personality disorders, while collectivism was associated with the low report of symptoms on these scales (Caldwell-Harris and Aycicegi 2006).

4   Current Clinical-Definitions of Personality Disorder

Along these years, there has been a debate on whether personality disorders are discrete clinical conditions or arbitrary distinctions compared to normal personality functioning (Samuel and Widiger 2008). However, many scholars have established a dimensional rather than categorical classification of personality disorders (Trull and Durrett 2005; Livesley and Jang 2005).

The most generally acknowledged diagnostic systems of psychological disorder at present, including the Diagnostic and Statistical Manual of Mental Disorders, Fifth Edition (DSM-5, American Psychiatric Association 2013) and the International Classification of Diseases, 11th beta version (ICD-11; World Health Organization 2017) represent the personality disorders in a categorical way. The definitions may vary somewhat in different systems. But the acknowledged personality disorders have three clusters of characteristics that share common themes or elements as follows. Cluster A includes paranoid, schizoid, and schizotypal personality disorders, and individuals with these disorders often appear odd or eccentric (Esterberg et al. 2010). Cluster B includes antisocial, borderline, histrionic, and narcissistic personality disorders, and individuals with these disorders often appear dramatic, emotional, or erratic (Livesley and Schroeder 1991). Cluster C includes avoidant, dependent, and obsessive-compulsive personality disorders, and individuals with these disorders often appear anxious or fearful (Freeman et al. 2004). It should be noted that this clustering system, although useful in some research and educational situations, has serious limitations and has not been consistently validated.

While most people recognize traits of themselves in many different personality disorders, a person who qualifies for a personality disorder diagnosis will exhibit most traits of the disorder, and these traits cause significant life problems to the individual. Personality disorders classified according to DSM-5 (American Psychiatric Association 2013) can also be regarded as maladaptive variants of the personality traits described with the Big-Five Model. The alternative dimensional models have much in common and together appear to cover the important areas of personality dysfunction. The disordered personality traits listed in the Section III of the DSM-5 (American Psychiatric Association 2013) can be organized hierarchically as follows: negative affectivity, detachment, antagonism, disinhibition, and psychoticism (Wright et al. 2012). Widiger and Simonsen (2005) also provided evidence of four broad bipolar domains and a fifth potential domain as following: extraversion to introversion, antagonism to compliance, constraint to impulsivity, negative affect to emotional stability, and unconventionality to closedness to experience. Similarly, empirical investigations have shown that Emotional Dysregulation of the Dimensional Assessment of Personality Pathology was positively correlated with NEO-PI-R Neuroticism; Inhibitedness negatively with Extraversion; Dissocial Behavior negatively with Agreeableness; and Compulsivity positively with Conscientiousness (Schroeder et al. 1992; Livesley and Jang 2005). Cultural research demonstrated good support for the validity of four dimensions of the Big-Five Model in Asian populations, again with the exception of Openness to experiences (Ryder et al. 2014). However, a group of Chinese scholars have identified further evidence supporting the fifth disordered personality, the Peculiarity Seeking, covering openness to experience, and impulsive sensation seeking (Chai et al. 2012).

5 Personality Disorder and Chinese Culture

The diagnosis of personality disorders occurs within prevailing cultural expectations, which is highly dependent on the concept of the self and values, the way of emotion experience and of how a society views certain behaviors. Multiple conceptional and nosological descriptions of personality disorders are usually controversial among different cultures. When people suffered from personality disorder, the life adversities they experienced were closely associated with social status, and the reactions and responses to their symptoms from surrounding and social contexts might mitigate or amplify their impaired functioning. Therefore, the way how behavioral differences are perceived, interpreted, and managed by individuals of different national cultures need to be well considered when the physician reaches a diagnosis (Fink et al. 2006).

The Cultural Formulation Interview in DSM-5 (American Psychiatric Association 2013) focuses on how aspects of individuals' background, developmental experiences, and current social contexts can affect their perspective on psychiatric condition. When dealing with patients from different ethnic backgrounds, it is important to consider to what extent certain customs and habits, religious conceptions and political convictions originate from the respective culture. In addition, the diagnostic system emphasizes that personality disorders should not be confounded with problems in context with the acculturation process of immigrants (Do 2011). Fortunately, studies comparing community prevalence, types of symptoms, and cohort effects in different countries would help us demonstrate the influence of social and cultural factors.

5.1   Epidemiological Studies in Chinese Culture

There is limited epidemiological data on the prevalence of personality disorders in different cultures. A screening survey across 13 countries by the World Health Organization (Huang et al. 2009) has identified a prevalence estimate of around 6% for personality disorders. While in general, the prevalence of Cluster A disorders was 5.7%, of Cluster B 1.5%, of Cluster C 6.0%, and of any personality disorder 9.1% (Huang et al. 2009). The prevalence sometimes varied with demographic and socioeconomic factors (Huang et al. 2009). Data from the 2001–2002 National Epidemiologic Survey on Alcohol and Related Conditions suggest that approximately 15% of American adults have at least one personality disorder. Up to present, there are no exact data about the prevalence of personality disorders in Chinese. The prevalence of personality disorders in China was lower compared with Western countries (Tang and Huang 1995), and the prevalence of antisocial personality disorder in Taiwan was about 0.2%, and in the United States about 3%, which might be due to a specific cultural tendency where the Taiwanese neglect antisocial behaviors to offer socially desired answers (Hwu et al. 1986; Compton et al. 1991). However, the data might be challenged later since Asian and mixed-race patients were more likely to have a personality disorder diagnosis than Americans were (Wu et al. 2013).

5.2   Personality Disorder Types in Chinese Culture

There is little research on the cultural characteristic of a specific personality disorder. In this subsection, we briefly introduce 10 types of personality disorder in relation to the cultural context of Chinese vs. Western.

5.2.1   Paranoid, Schizoid, and Schizotypal Personality Disorders

Cluster A personality disorders including the paranoid, schizoid, and schizotypal types, are regarded as the schizophrenia spectrum (Asarnow et al. 2001). The major commonality of the cluster is that the affected individuals generally have very weak or nonexistent social attachments and odd/eccentric behavior (Esterberg et al. 2010). Cognitive theorists believe the disorders are a result of an underlying belief that other people are unfriendly, and of a lack in self-awareness in combination.

Paranoid personality disorder is predominantly characterized by suspiciousness, self-reference, pathological jealousy and exquisite sensitivity (Triebwasser et al. 2013). The paranoid beliefs in adulthood is related to traumatic events occurring during childhood (i.e., history of maltreatment, physical, social or psychological abuse), which even are threatening to the inner models of the self to some extent (Carvalho et al. 2016). Regarding the Chinese culture, there has been many conspiracy theorists in history who asserted that the world is filled with dirty tricks; or in another word, life is a war, no matter in the fields of business, officialdom, academic or love affair. For example, the reform of Mr. Wang Anshi (王安石, a premier level official) was one of the famous political reforms in *Song* (宋) dynasty, but it failed in the end. From the perspective of personality, Wang Anshi was described as *"Gang Bi Zi Yong"* (刚愎自用), which means that he was so self-willed and conceited that he never acted upon others' advices and appointed sycophants who hypocritically supported his ideas. His distrust and suspicious to others even include his friends such as Mr. Sima Guang (司马光), might account to the failure of his radically-political reform.

Schizoid personality disorder is characterized by a lack of interest in social relationships, a tendency towards a solitary or sheltered lifestyle, secretiveness, emotional coldness, detachment, and apathy (Triebwasser et al. 2012). As the famous saying suggests, "Hustling for benefit, all come; bustling for benefit, all leave." There exists a common mental state of Chinese: callousness, emotional coldness, merciless attitude towards losers as a result of the traditional pursuit of fame and fortune. For example, Mr. Kong Yiji (孔乙己) was portraited by Mr. Lu Xun (鲁迅) as an alcoholic failed scholar who frequently appeared in a tavern. Though failed to pass the imperial examination, Kong Yiji arrogantly filled his speech with muddled classical tags, refused to perform menial work, and stole to avoid starvation. He was treated with cruelty and contempt by the other customers and suffered with the fickleness of the feudal society.

Schizotypal personality disorder is characterized by social and interpersonal deficits marked by acute discomfort with, and reduced capacity for, close relationships as well as by cognitive or perceptual distortions and eccentricities of behavior (Siever et al. 2013). Schizotypal personality disorder shows a common but different degrees of attentional impairment (Roitman et al. 1997), and it corresponds to the trait of inhibition, defined as intimacy problems, restricted expression, social avoidance and withdrawal (Wang et al. 2004). Other studies have demonstrated that the Chinese from single-parent family, who were related to the less self-esteem and family support, scored significantly higher on the schizotypal scales (Huang et al. 2007; Wang et al. 2017).

5.2.2 Antisocial Personality Disorder

Patients with antisocial personality disorder present a psychopathic pattern of behaviors: a low moral sense, disregard and violation of others' rights, and aggressive acts. Along with a history of crime, legal problems are common in a group of antisocial personality disorder patients (Glenn et al. 2013). The sociocultural contexts influence the presentation and diagnosis of antisocial personality disorder due to various cultural-norms (Lock 2008). An external source of control, such as the law, traditional standards, or religion differs a lot across cultures. Compared to Western countries, the erosion of collective standards in eastern countries might be more implicit so it is different to identify the individual with latent antisocial personality disorder from their previously prosocial behavior (Fabrega 2002).

Most research have demonstrated that the socioeconomic status, family structure, exposure to violence, and parenting behaviors are the risk factors for antisocial behaviors (Paris 1996; Morcillo et al. 2011). As for the traditional Chinese family, antisocial personality disorder is more likely from family which have their own characteristics, e.g., strong and authoritative parents, high expectations to children, and prized family devotion. Rich examples of antisocial personality disorder are described in another popular novel, the Water Margin, one of the Four Great Classical Novels of Chinese literature. It tells a group of 108 outlaws gather at Mount Liang to form a sizable army before they are eventually granted amnesty by the government and sent on campaigns to resist foreign invaders and suppress rebel forces in the *Song* dynasty. Most characters in this novel are unsatisfied with the reality and institution of society and have a history of committing serious crimes. The explosive emotion, impulsive behavior, and hostility to the "unfair" society of these characters have revealed an antisocial tendency in all Chinese feudal dynastics.

5.2.3 Borderline Personality Disorder

Patients with borderline personality disorder are characterized by impairments in emotion regulation, including affective instability especially in the social context, difficulty in anger-control, impulsivity, suicidal tendencies (Lieb et al. 2004). Therefore, these patients encounter problems of interpersonal relationships. Compared to adulthood, the borderline symptoms in adolescence are closely associated with greater anger-hostility, lower self-esteem, poorer quality of life, lower occupational functioning, social impairment and less partner involvement, especially in women (Rüsch et al. 2007).

Unfortunately, the diagnosis of borderline personality disorder has been overlooked by the Chinese psychiatric community for nearly a century. The Chinese psychiatrists claimed that some diagnostic criteria of borderline personality disorder are not appropriate in the Chinese cultural context, which values collectivistic identities and interpersonal relationships, and these criteria are likely to characterize the fear of abandonment. Consequently, borderline personality disorder has not formally been included as a diagnosis in the Chinese Classification of Mental Disorders, Third Revision (CCMD-3, Chinese Society of Psychiatry 2001). Indeed, the impulsivity is one of most important criteria of borderline personality disorder, which can be manifested as a behavioral problem resulting in reckless driving or substance abuse in most western countries, but less described in the scholastic literature in

China. The reason behind it might be that Chinese people used to have less car-ownership and stricter drug-control more than a decade ago.

Given the rapidity of social change in China over the past few years, the techno-logical development, increased urbanization rate, and one-child policy, have been disrupting traditional Chinese family systems and weakening interpersonal relation-ships, which raise the attention to the borderline personality disorder now. Recent epidemiological data show that the prevalence of borderline personality disorder is up to 8.4% in high school students (Wang et al. 2013; Cheng et al. 2010), and around 1~7% in clinical samples (Yang et al. 2000).

The negative interpersonal effects of behavioral problems in borderline personal-ity disorder might be particularly pronounced in a culture that values emotional control. The Chinese tradition of enduring on the other hand might make the behav-ioral problems more disharmony in social condition. A study (Keng et al. 2018) conducted in the Singaporean context, which consists of largely ethnic Chinese, has shown unique factor structures of borderline personality disorder symptomology: the three-factor solution came out from the well-established measure, the McLean Screening Instrument, consisting of affect dysregulation, self-disturbances, and behavioral and interpersonal dysregulation. In western studies, the third factor could be separated into two factors, i.e., the behavioral and interpersonal dysregulations (Selby and Joiner 2008). The difference may suggest that the collectivistic culture shed lights on the interpersonal difficulties, and the related behavioral problems in borderline personality disorder. Within family for example, where everyone live closely and share a kinship, the interpersonal relationship suffers a lot from the behavioral problems of a given member.

Studies conducted in China have demonstrated a strong association between early trauma experiences (e.g., child abuse) and severity of symptoms of borderline personality disorder (Huang et al. 2012; Zhang et al. 2012). Conformity is one of the factors contributing to the associations. The conformity which refers to the extent of an individual to endorse to norms plays a mediation role between childhood trauma and symptoms of borderline personality disorder. Individuals who view the self as a part of a large group rather than an individualized identity, which is the typical char-acteristic in the collectivistic Chinese cultural context, are vulnerable to childhood trauma. These traumatic experiences in turn, create further difficulties and troubles for the individual and the society. On the other hand, following the conformity rule, East Asians frequently suppress their emotions, therefore they are less likely to express their feelings and have lower behavioral reactivity to external emotion stim-uli compared to European Americans (Chentsova-Dutton et al. 2007).

5.2.4 Narcissistic Personality Disorder

Narcissistic personality disorder shows a long-term pattern of abnormal behavior, which is characterized by exaggerated self-importance, an excessive need for admi-ration and affirmation, and a lack of empathy (American Psychiatric Association 2013). Although many individuals have some narcissistic traits, only high levels of narcissism can be manifested as a pathological form, and diagnosed as narcissistic personality disorder. Grandiosity, self-centeredness, as well as attention-seeking are the most used adjectives to describe this disorder.

The higher levels of narcissism are frequently found in individualistic culture, and narcissistic individuals have pronounced independent trait (Foster et al. 2003). As a consequence, the prevalence of narcissistic personality disorder is higher in Western (more individualistic) than in Eastern cultures (Stinson et al. 2008). In the context of American culture, narcissists rated themselves as more dominant, independent and creative, which showed an egoistic and self-concerned phenomena, but less caring, moral and kind, which are precious qualities in Eastern cultures (Campbell et al. 2002).

The narcissism might be replaced by *"Mianzi"* (also see Chapter "Societal Culture from Late Imperial to Contemporary China: As Indirectly Reflected in A Dream of Red Mansions") in Chinese. The over-emphasis on *"Mianzi"* is one of the characteristics of the Chinese people, or one important part of Chinese culture. A typical example is shown in the Chinese drinking culture along history. One popular drinking-culture in Chinese is exchanging toasts at daily gathering to warm up the atmosphere even today. If I buy you a drink, you have to accept it otherwise you will hurt my *"Mianzi"*. This face-saving action is connected tightly with the normal narcissism which is a self-affirmation rather than an evaluation by others. Pathological narcissism in addition, exaggerates the self's worth and feelings so that the self refuses to accept criticism or advice.

5.2.5 Histrionic Personality Disorder

The histrionic personality disorder is characterized by a pattern of excessive attention-seeking, exaggerated expression of emotions, self-dramatization, egocentricity, self-indulgence, lack of consideration for others, and easily hurt feelings (American Psychiatric Association 2013). Psychoanalytic theories state that the authoritarian or distant attitudes of parents have a potential influence on the development of histrionic personality disorder of a child (Bienenfeld 2007). Cultural comparison studies have shown that Chinese parents practiced have more authoritarian style comparing to American parents, which might account for the social values and norms of the stricter family hierarchy in China (Porter et al. 2005).

The histrionic personality disorder patients are characterized with behaviors as "excessive" in reference to a social understanding of normal personality. In the traditionally conservative Chinese society, individuals are expected to behave in a conservative, restraint manner and are more prone to emotions arisen from guilt and shame, especially for women (Chen and Li 2000; Bedford 2004). The phenomena might account for the reason that the diagnosis of the histrionic personality disorder has been rarely assigned to a traditional Chinese person.

5.2.6 Avoidant Personality Disorder

The avoidant personality disorder displays a pattern of social inhibition, feelings of inadequacy, and hypersensitivity to negative evaluation (American Psychiatric Association 2013). Patients with avoidant personality disorder are characterized by a long-standing, pervasive and active withdrawal from social relationships, and they are easily to be hurt by criticism and disapproval. These patients also often feel extremely abashed in front of other people, and they often keep distance from other people.

Such interpersonal behavior patterns are cultural bounded ones, especially those of the low self-esteem and feeling of shame. People in East Asian cultures have more vulnerable self-esteem and report lower self-esteem and psychological well-being compared to Western cultures (Spencer-Rodgers et al. 2004; Heine and Hamamura 2007). The shame feeling in Western culture usually comes from the discrepancy between individual's own ego ideal and behavior, the Asian type of shame on the other hand, comes from the concern about how other people view the individual's behavior (Simonsen 2012). As a member of society group, Easterners fear that once the shortcomings are aware by other people, including strangers, relatives, and close friends, they might be separately treated by that group.

The avoidant trait has been described since ancient Chinese epoch. Under the influence of traditional Confucian thought, scholars are aiming to be an official to realize their aspiration. However, many famous writers and poets were highly critical of their society which leads to a deep contradiction in choosing official career or being a hermit. As a representative, Mr. Tao Yuanming (陶渊明) tried to be an official more than once but failed to adapt himself to politics and social reality. His famous remark, like "Bu Wei Wu Dou Mi Zhe Yao" (不为五斗米折腰, one cannot make curtsies for the salary of five bushels of rice), encourages many people to withdraw from society and to live in solitude. Their life style, from other aspects, reflects the avoidant attitude towards reality. Similarly, Cynicism, being characterized by a general distrust of others' motives, rejects all conventions, religion, manners, housing, dress, or decency, instead, it advocates the pursuit of virtue in accordance with a simple and idealistic way of life.

The collectivistic characteristics of the emotional restraint and interpersonal sensitivity, such as the obedient, conforming, and respectful interpersonal style, and the belief in a submissive harmony with nature at the expense of individuality, help to explain the frequent culture-bound avoidant personality disorder among Asians especially Chinese.

5.2.7 Dependent Personality Disorder

The dependent personality disorder patients have a pattern of submissive and clinging behavior which is related to an excessive need to be taken care of. The disorder is characterized by excessive fear and anxiety, which are related to the inability to function independently, for instance, being related to a strong willingness to subordinate own needs to those of others, and to a lack of self-confidence (American Psychiatric Association 2013).

The desire of dependence mostly falls into the categories of physiological and safety needs according to Maslow's Hierarchy of Needs Theory (see Chapter "Hierarchical Needs and Psychological Disorders in China"). During personality development, the attachment style, self-esteem, and identity, which are related to the desire of dependence, are influenced by parental child-rearing behaviors (Johnson et al. 2011). Previous studies have shown that dependent traits tended to increase in children with overprotective or authoritarian parents (Brook et al. 2003). The risk for a child to develop dependent personality disorder is even higher in this kind of family, since the rearing style would reduce the capability of autonomy and the child would be less powerful and competent when he grows up.

Cultural differences profoundly complicate the diagnosis of dependent personality disorder regarding dependency and autonomy (Bornstein 1998). In East Asian culture, with Confucianism, the dependence or submission is regarded as the proper behavior fitting social roles and obligation. Moreover, the conformity to the in-group norm and harmony are more adaptive to this collectivist cultures. Interestingly, such a conduct is usually discouraged in the West, where people are focusing on self-reliance, autonomy, individuation, and assertive social skills (Tabbat 1976).

In an ancient family of China, each person acted as a member of a big clan, which had a rigid feudal hierarchy regulating every aspect of daily life. Therefore, regarding the parental bonding styles in China, parents are likely to exert control and protection over their children and intend to establish their authority to get the obedience of their kids (Lin and Fu 1990). Parents often encourage their young children to stay close and to be dependent on them (Ho 1986). For example, most Chinese kids sleep in the same bed or in the same room with their parents, and those children who are sensitive, cautious, and behaviorally restrained are praised as "good kids" (Chen et al. 1998).

5.2.8 Obsessive-Compulsive Personality Disorder

Obsessive-compulsive personality disorder is a pattern of preoccupation with orderliness, perfectionism, and control at the expense of flexibility, openness, and efficiency (American Psychiatric Association 2013). In one study (Fineberg et al. 2007), the disorder was described by eight overt features such as the rigidity, miserliness, perfectionism, overattention to detail, excessive devotion to work, inability to discard worn or useless items, hypermorality, and inability to delegate tasks.

The high standards to self, cognitively and affectively, often lead to maladaptive discrepancy. While the orderliness and perfectionism are closely associated with self-evaluations. People from East Asian countries score lower on self-evaluations than do those from Western countries (Schmitt and Allik 2005). It might be due to that the cultural norms of modesty are stronger in East Asians than those in North America and Western Europe (Markus and Kitayama 1991).

The Chinese people admit that the rule of Conformity is the major rule for self-restraint. Consequently, the minority is subordinate to the majority. In conforming to majority, individual must restraint self to seek the common ground and stick to the convention. Similarly, the Confucian puts forth ways of determination, study, self-constraint, self-revision, and retrospection when cultivating personality. Unfortunately, conformity emphasizes on non-individuality, resulting in stereo-typed life style and thinking modes, thus in a compulsive tendency, or even compulsive symptoms.

Once again, in collectivistic China, a person constructs an interdependent self in the social context, including the attitude and evaluation from others (Matsumoto 1999). People are motivated to find a way to fit in with relevant others, to fulfill and create obligation, and in general to become part of various interpersonal relationships. As a consequence, sensitive individuals who are afraid of criticism from others tend to be preoccupied with details to an extreme extent and to behave overcautiously to make sure that they can complete the task flawlessly.

6   Conclusion

Studies regarding the symptomatology of personality disorders in China are few, and these limited research suffer from methodological and conceptual flaws. The first limitation is that the sample sizes are small; the second one is the culture issues embedded in diagnostic criteria which are mainly defined by western views and explanations instead of by eastern ones. Cross-cultural studies on personality traits also indicate that the trait definitions are linked with local norms. Bearing these in mind, clinicians might have broadened their views to the sociocultural context when they assess, describe, diagnose and communicate findings with others about personality traits or disorders. Of course, clinicians are also located in the cultural contexts which are potentially leading them to the diagnostic misunderstandings or the provision of suboptimal treatment.

Nonetheless, research on culture and personality disorder will be successful to the extent to expand possibilities for effective intervention and prevention of these complex and troublesome patterns of maladaptive behavior. Future research might be continuously focused on personality traits (see Chapter "Personality Traits in Contemporary China: A Lexical Approach") or personality disorders in Chinese culture.

References

American Psychiatric Association. (2013). *Diagnostic and statistical manual of mental disorder* (5th ed.). Washington, DC: American Psychiatric Association.

Asarnow, R. F., Nuechterlein, K. H., Fogelson, D., Subotnik, K. L., Payne, D. A., Russell, A. T., Asamen, J., Kuppinger, H., & Kendler, K. S. (2001). Schizophrenia and schizophrenia-spectrum personality disorders in the first-degree relatives of children with schizophrenia: The UCLA family study. *Archives of General Psychiatry, 58*, 581–588.

Bedford, O. (2004). The individual experience of guilt and shame in Chinese culture. *Culture and Psychology, 10*, 29–52.

Bienenfeld, D. (2007). Personality disorders. *Psychiatric Annals, 37*, 84–85.

Bornstein, R. F. (1998). Dependency in the personality disorders: Intensity, insight, expression, and defense. *Journal of Clinical Psychology, 54*, 175–189.

Brook, J. S., Brook, D. W., & Whiteman, M. (2003). Maternal correlates of toddler insecure and dependent behavior. *Journal of Genetic Psychology, 164*, 72–87.

Cai, H., Sedikides, C., Gaertner, L., Wang, C., Carvallo, M., Xu, Y., O'Mara, E. M., & Jackson, L. E. (2011). Tactical self-enhancement in China: Is modesty at the service of self-enhancement in East Asian culture? *Social Psychological and Personality Science, 2*, 59–64.

Caldwell-Harris, C. L., & Aycicegi, A. (2006). When personality and culture clash: The psychological distress of allocentrics in an individualist culture and idiocentrics in a collectivist culture. *Transcultural Psychiatry, 43*, 331–361.

Campbell, W. K., Rudich, E. A., & Sedikides, C. (2002). Narcissism, self-esteem, and the positivity of self-views: Two portraits of self-love. *Personality and Social Psychology Bulletin, 28*, 358–368.

Carvalho, C. B., da Motta, C., Pinto-Gouveia, J., & Peixoto, E. (2016). Influence of family and childhood memories in the development and manifestation of paranoid ideation: Influence of family and childhood memories. *Clinical Psychology and Psychotherapy, 23*, 397–406.

Chai, H., Xu, S., Zhu, J., Chen, W., Xu, Y., He, W., & Wang, W. (2012). Further evidence for the fifth higher trait of personality pathology: A correlation study using normal and disordered personality measures. *Psychiatry Research, 200*, 444–449.

Chen, X., & Li, B. (2000). Depressed mood in Chinese children: Development significance for social and school adjustment. *International Journal of Behavioral Development, 24*, 472–479.

Chen, X., Hastings, P. D., Rubin, K. H., Chen, H., Cen, G., & Stewart, S. L. (1998). Child-rearing attitudes and behavioral inhibition in Chinese and Canadian toddlers: A cross-cultural study. *Developmental Psychology, 34*, 677–686.

Cheng, H., Huang, Y., Liu, B., & Liu, Z. (2010). Familial aggregation of personality disorder: Epidemiological evidence from high school students 18 years and older in Beijing, China. *Comprehensive Psychiatry, 51*, 524–530.

Chentsova-Dutton, Y. E., Chu, J. P., Tsai, J. L., Rottenberg, J., Gross, J. J., & Gotlib, I. H. (2007). Depression and emotional reactivity: Variation among Asian Americans of East Asian descent and European Americans. *Journal of Abnormal Psychology, 116*, 776–785.

Chinese Society of Psychiatry. (2001). *The Chinese classification and diagnostic criteria of mental disorders, version 3 (CCMD-3)*. Jinan: Chinese Society of Psychiatry (in Chinese).

Compton, W. M., Heizer, J. E., Hwu, H., Yeh, E., McEvoy, L., Tipp, J. E., & Spitznagel, E. L. (1991). New methods in cross-cultural psychiatry: Psychiatric illness in Taiwan and the United States. *American Journal of Psychiatry, 148*, 1697–1704.

Do, L. L. T. N. (2011). American Psychiatric Association Diagnostic and Statistical Manual of Mental Disorders (DSM-IV). In S. Goldstein & J. A. Naglieri (Eds.), *Encyclopedia of child behavior and development* (pp. 84–85). Boston: Springer.

Durbin, C. E., Hicks, B. M., Blonigen, D. M., Johnson, W., Iacono, W. G., & McGue, M. (2016). Personality trait change across late childhood to young adulthood: Evidence for nonlinearity and sex differences in change. *European Journal of Personality, 30*, 31–44.

Esterberg, M. L., Goulding, S. M., & Walker, E. F. (2010). Cluster A personality disorders: Schizotypal, schizoid and paranoid personality disorders in childhood and adolescence. *Journal of Psychopathology and Behavioral Assessment, 32*, 515–528.

Fabrega, H. (2002). Evolutionary theory, culture and psychiatric diagnosis. In M. Maj, W. Gaebel, J. J. López-Ibor, & N. Sartorius (Eds.), *Psychiatric diagnosis and classification*. London: Wiley.

Fan, Y. (2000). A classification of Chinese culture. *Cross Cultural Management, 7*, 3–10.

Fineberg, N. A., Sharma, P., Sivakumaran, T., Sahakian, B., & Chamberlain, S. (2007). Does obsessive-compulsive personality disorder belong within the obsessive-compulsive spectrum? *CNS Spectrums, 12*, 467–482.

Fink, G., Neyer, A. K., & Kölling, M. (2006). Understanding cross-cultural management interaction: Research into cultural standards to complement cultural value dimensions and personality traits. *International Studies of Management and Organization, 36*, 38–60.

Foster, J. D., Campbell, W. K., & Twenge, J. M. (2003). Individual differences in narcissism: Inflated self-views across the lifespan and around the world. *Journal of Research in Personality, 37*, 469–486.

Freeman, A., Pretzer, J., Fleming, B., & Simon, K. M. (2004). Avoidant, dependent, and obsessive-compulsive personality disorders. In *Clinical applications of cognitive therapy* (2nd ed., pp. 287–325). Boston: Springer.

Glenn, A. L., Johnson, A. K., & Raine, A. (2013). Antisocial personality disorder: A current review. *Current Psychiatry Reports, 15*, 1–8.

Heine, S. J., & Hamamura, T. (2007). In search of East Asian self-enhancement. *Personality and Social Psychology Review, 11*, 4–27.

Ho, D. Y. F. (1986). Chinese patterns of socialization: A critical review. In M. H. Bond (Ed.), *The psychology of the Chinese people*. New York: Oxford University Press.

Hofstede, G. (1984). The cultural relativity of the quality of life concept. *Academy of Management Review, 9*, 389–398.

Huang, X., Ling, H., Yang, B., & Dou, G. (2007). Screening of personality disorders among Chinese college students by personality diagnostic questionnaire-4+. *Journal of Personality Disorders, 21*, 448–454.

Huang, Y., Kotov, R., de Girolamo, G., Preti, A., Angermeyer, M., Benjet, C., Demyttenaere, K., de Graaf, R., Gureje, O., Karam, A. N., Lee, S., Lépine, J. P., Matschinger, H., Posada-Villa, J., Suliman, S., Vilagut, G., & Kessler, R. C. (2009). DSM-IV personality disorders in the WHO World Mental Health Surveys. *British Journal of Psychiatry, 195*, 46–53.

Huang, J., Yang, Y., Wu, J., Napolitano, L. A., Xi, Y., & Cui, Y. (2012). Childhood abuse in Chinese patients with borderline personality disorder. *Journal of Personality Disorders, 26*, 238–254.

Hwu, H.-G., Yeh, E.-K., & Chang, L.-Y. (1986). Chinese diagnostic interview schedule: I. Agreement with psychiatrist's diagnosis. *Acta Psychiatrica Scandinavica, 73*, 225–233.

John, O. P., & Srivastava, S. (1999). The Big Five trait taxonomy: History, measurement, and theoretical perspectives. In L. A. Pervin & O. P. John (Eds.), *Handbook of personality: Theory and research* (2nd ed., pp. 102–138). New York: Guildford.

Johnson, J. G., Liu, L., & Cohen, P. (2011). *Parenting behaviours associated with the development of adaptive and maladaptive offspring personality traits*. Los Angeles: SAGE.

Keng, S. L., Lee, Y., Drabu, S., Hong, R. Y., Cyi, C., Csh, H., & Rcm, H. (2018). Construct validity of the mclean screening instrument for borderline personality disorder in two singaporean samples. *Journal of Personality Disorders, 32*, 1–20.

Lieb, K., Zanarini, M. C., Schmahl, C., Linehan, M. M., & Bohus, M. (2004). Borderline personality disorder. *Lancet, 364*, 453–461.

Lin, C. C., & Fu, V. R. (1990). A comparison of child-rearing practices among Chinese, immigrant Chinese, and Caucasian-American parents. *Child Development, 61*, 429–433.

Livesley, W. J., & Jang, K. L. (2005). Differentiating normal, abnormal, and disordered personality. *European Journal of Personality, 19*, 257–268.

Livesley, W. J., & Schroeder, M. L. (1991). Dimensions of personality disorder: The DSM-III-R cluster B diagnoses. *Journal of Nervous and Mental Disease, 179*, 320–328.

Lock, M. P. (2008). Treatment of antisocial personality disorder. *British Journal of Psychiatry, 193*, 426–427.

Markus, H. R., & Kitayama, S. (1991). Culture and the self: Implications for cognition, emotion, and motivation. *Psychological Review, 98*, 224–253.

Matsumoto, D. (1999). Culture and self: An empirical assessment of Markus and Kitayama's theory of independent and interdependednt self-construal. *Asian Journal of Social Psychology, 2*, 289–310.

McCrae, R. R., & Costa, P. T., Jr. (1999). A five-factor theory of personality. In L. A. Pervin & O. P. John (Eds.), *Handbook of personality: Theory and research* (2nd ed., pp. 139–153). New York: Guildford.

Morcillo, C., Duarte, C. S., Shen, S., Blanco, C., Canino, G., & Bird, H. R. (2011). Parental familism and antisocial behaviors: Development, gender and potential mechanisms. *Journal of the American Academy of Child and Adolescent Psychiatry, 50*, 471–479.

Oyserman, D., Kemmelmeier, M., & Coon, H. M. (2002). Cultural psychology, a new look: Reply to bond (2002), fiske (2002), kitayama (2002), and miller (2002). *Psychological Bulletin, 128*, 110–117.

Paris, J. (1996). Antisocial personality disorder: A biopsychosocial model. *Canadian Journal of Psychiatry, 41*, 75–80.

Porter, C. L., Hart, C. H., Yang, C., Robinson, C. C., Olsen, S. F., Zeng, Q., Olsen, J. A., & Jin, S. (2005). A comparative study of child temperament and parenting in Beijing, China and the western United States. *International Journal of Behavioral Development, 29*, 541–551.

Pye, L. W. (1972). Culture and political science: Problems in the evaluation of the concept of political culture. *Social Science Quarterly, 53*, 285–296.

Roberts, B. W., & Mroczek, D. (2008). Personality trait change in adulthood. *Current Directions in Psychological Science, 17*, 31–35.

Roberts, B. W., Robins, R. W., Trzesniewski, K. H., & Caspi, A. (2003). *Personality trait development in adulthood* (Handbook of the life course). Boston: Springer.

Roitman, S. E., Cornblatt, B. A., Bergman, A., Obuchowski, M., Mitropoulou, V., Keefe, R. S. E., Silverman, J. M., & Siever, L. J. (1997). Attentional functioning in schizotypal personality disorder. *American Journal of Psychiatry, 154*, 655–660.

Ronningstam, E. F., Keng, S. L., Ridolfi, M. E., Arbabi, M., & Grenyer, B. F. (2018). Cultural aspects in symptomatology, assessment, and treatment of personality disorders. *Current Psychiatry Reports, 20*, 22.

Rüsch, N., Lieb, K., Göttler, I., Hermann, C., Schramm, E., Richter, H., Jacob, G. A., Corrigan, P. W., & Bohus, M. (2007). Shame and implicit self-concept in women with borderline personality disorder. *American Journal of Psychiatry, 164*, 500–508.

Ryder, A. G., Sun, J., Dere, J., & Fung, K. (2014). Personality disorders in Asians: Summary, and a call for cultural research. *Asian Journal of Psychiatry, 7*, 86–88.

Samuel, D. B., & Widiger, T. A. (2008). A meta-analytic review of the relationships between the five-factor model and DSM-IV-TR personality disorders: A facet level analysis. *Clinical Psychology Review, 28*, 1326–1342.

Schmitt, D. P., & Allik, J. (2005). Simultaneous administration of the rosenberg self-esteem scale in 53 nations: Exploring the universal and culture-specific features of global self-esteem. *Journal of Personality and Social Psychology, 89*, 623–642.

Schroeder, M. L., Wormworth, J. A., & Livesley, W. J. (1992). Dimensions of personality disorder and their relationships to the Big Five dimensions of personality. *Psychological Assessment, 4*, 47–53.

Schwartz, S. H. (1994). Are there universal aspects in the structure and contents of human values? *Journal of Social Issues, 50*, 19–45.

Selby, E. A., & Joiner, T. E. (2008). Ethnic variations in the structure of borderline personality disorder symptomatology. *Journal of Psychiatric Research, 43*, 115–123.

Siever, L. J., Bernstein, D. P., & Silverman, J. M. (2013). Schizotypal personality disorder. *Journal of Personality Disorders, 27*, 652–679.

Simonsen, E. (2012). Culture and diagnosis: Considering avoidant personality disorder: A commentary on the case by toshimasa maruta et al. *Personality and Mental Health, 6*, 271–272.

Spencer-Rodgers, J., Peng, K., Wang, L., & Hou, Y. (2004). Dialectical self-esteem and east-west differences in psychological well-being. *Personality and Social Psychology Bulletin, 30*, 1416–1432.

Stinson, F. S., Dawson, D. A., Goldstein, R. B., Chou, S. P., Huang, B., Smith, S. M., Ruan, W. J., Pulay, A. J., Saha, T. D., Pickering, R. P., & Grant, B. F. (2008). Prevalence, correlates, disability, and comorbidity of DSM-IV narcissistic personality disorder: Results from the wave 2 national epidemiologic survey on alcohol and related conditions. *Journal of Clinical Psychiatry, 69*, 1033–1045.

Tabbat, B. K. (1976). The anatomy of dependence by Takeo Doi, MD. A discussion. *Bulletin of the Menninger Clinic, 40*, 660–664.

Tang, S. W., & Huang, Y. (1995). Diagnosing personality disorders in China. *International Medical Journal, 2*, 291–297.

Triandis, H. C. (2001). Individualism-collectivism and personality. *Journal of Personality, 69*, 907–924.

Triandis, H. C., & Gelfand, M. J. (1998). Converging measurement of horizontal and vertical individualism and collectivism. *Journal of Personality and Social Psychology, 74*, 118–128.

Triebwasser, J., Chemerinski, E., Roussos, P., & Siever, L. J. (2012). Schizoid personality disorder. *Journal of Personality Disorders, 26*, 919–926.

Triebwasser, J., Chemerinski, E., Roussos, P., & Siever, L. J. (2013). Paranoid personality disorder. *Journal of Personality Disorders, 27*, 795–805.

Trull, T. J., & Durrett, C. A. (2005). Categorical and dimensional models of personality disorder. *Annual Review of Clinical Psychology, 1*, 355–380.

Wang, W., Du, W., Wang, Y., Livesley, W. J., & Jang, K. L. (2004). The relationship between the Zuckerman–Kuhlman personality questionnaire and traits delineating personality pathology. *Personality and Individual Differences, 36*, 155–162.

Wang, Y., Zhu, X., Cai, L., Wang, Q., Wang, M., Yi, J., & Yao, S. (2013). Screening cluster A and cluster B personality disorders in Chinese high school students. *BMC Psychiatry, 13*, 116.

Wang, D., Li, S., & Hu, M. (2017). Comparisons of the influence of raising people's identity on mental health between two-parents family children and single parent family children by propensity score matching. *Journal of Hygiene Research, 46*, 709–716.

Widiger, T. A., & Simonsen, E. (2005). Alternative dimensional models of personality disorder: Finding a common ground. *Journal of Personality Disorders, 19*, 110–130.

World Health Organization. (2017). *International classification of diseases* (11th beta Ed.). Retrieved October 12, 2018, from http://www.who.int/classifications/icd/revision/en

Wright, A. G., Thomas, K. M., Hopwood, C. J., Markon, K. E., Pincus, A. L., & Krueger, R. F. (2012). The hierarchical structure of DSM-5 pathological personality traits. *Journal of Abnormal Psychology, 121*, 951.

Wu, L. T., Blazer, D. G., Gersing, K. R., Burchett, B., Swartz, M. S., Mannelli, P., & Workgroup, N. A. (2013). Comorbid substance use disorders with other Axis I and II mental disorders among treatment-seeking Asian Americans, Native Hawaiians/Pacific Islanders, and mixed-race people. *Journal of Psychiatric Research, 47*, 1940–1948.

Yang, J., McCrae, R. R., Costa, P. T., Jr., Yao, S., Dai, X., Cai, T., & Gao, B. (2000). The cross-cultural generalizability of Axis-II constructs: An evaluation of two personality disorder assessment instruments in the People's Republic of China. *Journal of Personality Disorders, 14*, 249–263.

Zhang, T., Chow, A., Wang, L., Dai, Y., & Xiao, Z. (2012). Role of childhood traumatic experience in personality disorders in China. *Comprehensive Psychiatry, 53*, 829–836.

Personality Traits in Contemporary China: A Lexical Approach

Xu Shao, Hao Chai, and Wei Wang

1 Introduction

When it comes to the study of personality, there are two interdependent and inter-related aspects, disordered and normal personality trait. We have illustrated the relationships between personality disorders and Chinese culture in Chapter "Cultural Contribution to Personality Disorders in China". As a logical continuation, we will look into what the relationships between normal personality traits and the Chinese culture are. There are several definitions of personality up to date. For instance, personality is an individual's characteristic pattern of thought, emotion, and behavior, together with the psychological mechanisms behind those patterns (Funder 1997). Other scholars believe that personality is a set of habitual behaviors, cognitions and emotion patterns influenced by both biological and environmental factors (Triandis and Suh 2002; Corr and Matthews 2009).

Despite the disparity among the several definitions, personality trait does indeed exhibit the differences between individuals, and it can be evaluated by self- or peer-reported questionnaires (McCrae 2004). Enough evidence has shown that the normal personality traits can be measured by a five-factor structure (Costa and Widiger 1994; Goldberg and Rosolack 1994), one example of which is the Big-Five model, the Revised NEO Personality Inventory (NEO-PI-R; Costa and McCrae 1994).

Personality cannot be shaped without a background culture, i.e., the powerful environment factor. Of course, different cultural contexts play different roles in this process. There are two important domains regarding the cross-cultural comparison

X. Shao · W. Wang (✉)
Department of Clinical Psychology and Psychiatry/School of Public Health, Zhejiang University College of Medicine, Hangzhou, China
e-mail: drwangwei@zju.edu.cn

H. Chai
Department of Psychology, College of Education, Zhejiang University of Technology, Hangzhou, China

© Springer Nature Singapore Pte Ltd. 2019   93
W. Wang (ed.), *Chinese Perspectives on Cultural Psychiatry*,
https://doi.org/10.1007/978-981-13-3537-2_6

studies in psychology: an "emic" concept, which is defined as what is native or indigenous to a specific culture and may not make sense in other cultures; and an "etic" concept, which is defined as what is cross-culturally universal and applicable. Comparisons among different cultures have revealed that the emic-component contribution to personality is exclusive to a specific culture, while the etic-component exists in all kinds (Church 1987). For instance, Gençöz and Öncül (2012) developed a 45-item instrument with strong psychometric properties called Basic Personality Traits Inventory to measure basic personality traits in the Turkish culture. Alongside with the same five personality factors as described by NEO-PI-R, investigators revealed a unique sixth factor, "Negative Valence", that is, "one's negative self-attributions". The "Negative Valence" might be considered as an emic-component in the Turkish culture. There is another trait measure instrument, the alternative five-factor model of the Zuckerman-Kuhlman Personality Questionnaire (ZKPQ), which describes the Impulsive Sensation Seeking, Neuroticism-Anxiety, Aggression-Hostility, Activity, and Sociability. ZKPQ has been tested out cross-culturally in six countries including China, Germany, Italy, Spain, Switzerland, and the United States (Rossier et al. 2007).

Empirical evidence shows that the five-factor model (see Chapter "Personality Traits Characterized by the Adjectives in A Dream of Red Mansions" for an example) is the most commonly used structure to describe personality and it has won relatively great popularity across different cultures (Costa et al. 2001; Yamagata et al. 2006), despite that there is difficulty in constructing in illiterate and indigenous society (Gurven et al. 2013). Evidence is still cumulative to support the universality of the five-factor model, and culture uniqueness of trait structure also needs more demonstration (Church 2016).

Due to that all significant personality attributes are rooted in languages (Saucier and Goldberg 2001), the psycho-lexical method (also in Chapter "Personality Traits Characterized by the Adjectives in A Dream of Red Mansions") has been employed to measure personality, thus offering a short and novel path to explore personality traits (John et al. 1988; Whitmore et al. 2004). Nonetheless, this method has encountered repetitive criticism for several reasons, such as that the adjectives are too simple to explain complex but important traits, or they have ambiguous meanings to describe some specific constructs. Despite this, there is no doubt that the study of personality structure with the psycho-lexical method is productive (Ashton and Lee 2005; de Raad and Barelds 2008) and it has become a classic and traditional methodology up to date. Consistently, the psycho-lexical method has displayed a five-factor model of personality in Dutch (de Raad 1992; Muris et al. 2005), English (Peabody 1987), German (Angleitner et al. 1990), Italian (Caprara and Perugini 1994), Russian (Shmelyov and Pokhil'ko 1993), Croatian (Mlačić and Ostendorf 2005), Hong Kong Chinese, Japanese, and Filipino (Bond 1979; Yang and Bond 1990), Polish (Szarota 1996), Argentine (Ledesma et al. 2011), Flemish (van den Broeck et al. 2014) and other cultures.

Besides focusing on the five-factor model, researchers are interested in other personality structures. One study in Persian samples confirmed three kinds of model of statistic robustness: respectively two-factor model labeled as Agreeableness, and

Success and Motivation; three-factor model as Morality, Positive versus Negative Emotionality, and Achievement; and four-factor model as Morality, Positive versus Negative Emotionality, Achievement, and Affection (Farahani et al. 2016). Investigators identified two-factor solution of Communion and Agency, as well as three-factor solution of Affiliation, Dynamism and Order (de Raad et al. 2014) in studies of Romanian context (Burtăverde and de Raad 2017). Another study in Lithuanian culture presented a two-factor model (Dynamism and Social Propriety) and substantiated a three-factor model (Dynamism, Affiliation and Order) (Livaniene and de Raad 2017). A six-factor model of personality based on lexicon in another study has been put forward, former five of which are parallel to the five-factor model, while the sixth, Honesty-Humility, also partly covers Agreeableness (Ashton and Lee 2007; Lee and Ashton 2008).

Though Western models of personality traits have depicted a vivid picture of etic cross-cultural personality traits and scientific methodologies, more emic intra-cultural elements in the Chinese context are supposed to be counted (Cheung et al. 2011). In order to examine the applicability of the Temperament and Character Inventory (TCI, Cloninger et al. 1994) in China, a similar three-factor structure for character domains was discovered (Chen et al. 2013). The character might still be categorized into self-directedness, cooperativeness and self-transcendence as in TCI, but purposefulness and responsibility, which were originally subcategorized into self-directedness, now belonged to cooperativeness in the Chinese version due to their high factor loadings on this target factor. Several groups of researcher carried out studies of personality-relevant Chinese adjectives in China. Using 60 adjectives about creativity, Rudowicz and Yue (2002) found five factors, that is, Innovative or Dynamic, Intellectual abilities, Social style, Obedience or Social acceptance, Discipline or Dutifulness. Using 410 adjectives picked out carefully, Wang and Cui (2004) discovered seven factors, including Talents, Ways of Life, Extraversion, Kindness, Emotionality, Human Relations, and Behavioral Styles. In another work, 3159 personality descriptors, adjectives and nouns both included, were chosen from the Contemporary Chinese Dictionary and ranked on the basis of frequency (Zhou et al. 2009). In this study, 413 terms of most frequently used ones were employed to undergo self-ratings and peer-ratings in two Chinese samples. An emic Chinese personality structure of seven factors was then identified, namely Extraversion, Conscientiousness/Diligence, Negative Valence or Noxious Violativeness, Unselfishness, Emotional Volatility, Intellect/ Positive Valence, and Dependency/Fragility.

Although there are some discrepancies among studies conducted in China as mentioned above, there is still suitability for the five-factor model. Apparently the first factor covers Emotionality; the second Social style, and Extraversion; the third Discipline or Dutifulness, and Behavioral Styles; the fourth Obedience or Social acceptance, Kindness, and part of Human Relations; the fifth Intellectual abilities, Talents, and part of Ways of Life. In Chapter "Personality Traits Characterized by the Adjectives in A Dream of Red Mansions", we have already tested the personality structure by picking out the adjectival personality descriptors in a novel, A Dream of Red Mansions, which is a famous representative of Chinese culture. Now, we would like to test the model in another Chinese sample, to check whether the classic model fits in the contemporary China, and to look for any possible culture-specific factor in the model.

Nonetheless, there are some shortcomings in previous Chinese psycho-lexical studies on personality descriptors, such as the vocabulary pools used were not large enough to cover more lexicons, and the participants were not equally distributed in China. Therefore, in the current study, we selected a larger dataset of adjectives in two Chinese dictionaries. We recruited participants from 29 provinces or cities, who were university students in the four areas of China. We aimed to detect whether there was an "emic" contribution to personality by means of Chinese adjectives. Our second purpose was to choose some adjectives with highest loadings on the target personality trait so as to develop a short edition of personality rating scales.

2 Study 1: Adjective Selection for Self-Rating Scales

2.1 Participants

Seven contributors of this book (including three co-authors of this chapter; four women and three men all majoring in psychology or psychiatry) acted as judges. Six of us picked out over 6000 adjectives describing personality using The Modern Chinese Dictionary and Its Supplements (Beijing, The Commercial Publishing House, 1998) and A Chinese-English Dictionary, Revised Edition (Beijing, Foreign Language Teaching and Research Press, 1995). All synonyms were aggregated and the awkward, less-frequently used or slang adjectives were excluded. With no new words added, the rest 650 adjectives were regarded as exhaustive. Finally, these words were examined and approved by the senior author of this chapter.

Six hundred university students (398 women, mean age 19.3 years with 1.1 S.D., range 17–23 years; 202 men, mean age 19.6 years with 1.3 S.D., range 17–25 years) were asked to rate themselves in terms of the 650 adjectives. They were not paid for their cooperation. Free from somatic or psychiatric illnesses, all participants were studying in the Eastern (Hangzhou), Western (Taiyuan), Southern (Haikou) and Northern (Haerbin) parts of China, majoring in the Arts, Education, Foreign Languages, Mechanics, or Medicine.

They finished the self-rating scales in evening classes or other quiet rooms, using the Likert type scales: (1) very unlike me, (2) moderately unlike me, (3) somewhat like and unlike me, (4) moderately like me, and (5) very like me.

2.2 Statistics

The rating answers to the 650 adjectives by 600 participants were analyzed to Principal Component Analysis. The factor loadings underwent orthogonal rotation with the varimax normalized method.

Table 1 Factor analysis results of the personality-relevant 650 Chinese adjectives

Factor	Eigenvalue	Explained variance
I (Intelligent)	42.40	28.94
II (Emotional)	20.37	20.72
III (Conscientious)	14.21	20.50
IV (Unsocial)	10.04	12.54
V (Agreeable)	6.90	11.22

After Yu et al. (2009)

2.3 Results

Altogether, 20 factors with eigenvalues larger than 1.0 were extracted, with the first five most prominent. A level-off showed up clearly from the sixth factor on. The first five factors made up 31.31% of the total variance, while none of the rest over 1.78%. The eigenvalues and the variance explained by the factors are shown in Table 1. Therefore, a five-factor solution was performed. Respectively, the five factors were named as "Intelligent", "Emotional", "Conscientious", "Unsocial" and "Agreeable".

After the varimax normalized rotation, the top 20 adjectives with highest loadings on the target factor and cross-loading below 0.40 on other non-target factors were attained (Table 2). In total, 100 adjectives were picked out to create a short edition of self-rating scales, that is, the Chinese Adjective Descriptors of Personality (CADP).

3 Study 2: Test of Chinese Adjective Descriptors of Personality

The developed CADP was tested out among the adult university students (older than 18 years) in the Eastern (Hangzhou), Western (Taiyuan), Southern (Haikou) and Northern (Haerbin) parts of China.

3.1 Participants

Seven hundred and twenty university students (465 women, mean age 19.6 years with 1.1 S.D., range 18–23 years; 255 men, mean age 19.9 years with 1.1 S.D., range 18–23 years) were asked to rate themselves in relation to 100 adjectives. Again, they were not paid for their collaboration. Free from somatic or psychiatric illnesses; all participants were majoring in Arts, Education, Foreign Languages, Mechanics, Modern Medicine, or Traditional Chinese Medicine.

Table 2 Top 20 highest loading adjectives

Chinese	English Translation	Loading
I. Intelligent		
有才能的	Competent	0.72
学识渊博的	Knowledgeable	0.72
才思敏捷的	Creative in writing	0.72
天赋高的	Naturally gifted	0.71
才智出众的	Outstanding in wisdom	0.71
多才多艺的	Versatile	0.71
有才智的	Endowed	0.71
才华横溢的	Full of talents	0.70
有才干的	Talented or capable	0.70
有才华的	Artistically gifted	0.69
有文才的	Literary-talented	0.69
有才略的	Sagacious	0.68
有才气的	Artistically talented	0.68
博学的	Erudite	0.68
智慧的	Bright	0.68
有才识的	Insightful	0.67
文思敏捷的	Good at writing	0.67
智力高的	Highly intelligent	0.67
足智多谋的	Wise and resourceful	0.66
敏感的	Sensible	0.66
II. Emotional		
性子躁的	Hot-tempered	0.64
暴躁的	Irascible	0.64
脾气大的	Temperamental	0.60
烈性的	Explosive	0.59
爱发脾气的	Stormy	0.59
急躁的	Fidgety	0.58
性急的	Impatient	0.57
冲动的	Impulsive	0.57
莽撞的	Foolhardy	0.56
脾气坏的	Quick-tempered	0.56
急性子的	Impetuous	0.55
易怒的	Irritable	0.55
火暴的	Fierce	0.54
毛躁的	Hasty	0.53
牛脾气的	Bullheaded	0.52
直性子的	Straightforward	0.52
快人快语的	Straight-talking	0.51
马虎的	Careless	0.49
多言的	Garrulous	0.49
心直口快的	Outspoken	0.46

(continued)

Table 2 (continued)

Chinese	English Translation	Loading
III. Conscientious		
脚踏实地的	Down-to-earth	0.63
有毅力的	Of willpower	0.62
坚韧不拔的	Firm and dauntless	0.61
意志坚定的	Determined	0.61
勤劳的	Diligent	0.60
耐劳的	Able to endure heavy work	0.59
坚毅的	Resolute	0.59
吃苦耐劳的	Able to endure hardships	0.58
刚毅的	Firm	0.57
勤俭的	Thrifty	0.56
持之以恒的	Tireless	0.56
顽强的	Steadfast	0.56
不屈不挠的	Tenacious	0.54
孜孜不倦的	Assiduous	0.53
自强不息的	Constantly effortful	0.51
有意志力的	Having strong willpower	0.51
刚强的	Strong-minded	0.49
有恒心的	Persevering	0.49
严格的	Strict	0.49
锲而不舍的	Persistent	0.47
IV. Unsociable		
孤僻的	Unsociable and eccentric	0.64
思想迟钝的	Obtuse	0.62
死板的	Inflexible	0.62
蠢笨的	Stupid and clumsy	0.61
愚笨的	Foolish	0.60
呆板的	Stiff and awkward	0.59
刻薄的	Mean	0.59
孤傲的	Aloof and arrogant	0.59
古板的	Old-fashioned and inflexible	0.59
低能的	Imbecile	0.59
愚蠢的	Stupid	0.59
粗鲁的	Rude	0.58
怯懦的	Cowardly	0.58
无能的	Incompetent	0.58
呆笨的	Dull	0.57
苛刻的	Overcritical	0.56
不中用的	Useless	0.56
迟钝的	Sluggish	0.56
清高的	Aloof and overconfident	0.55
气量狭小的	Narrow-minded	0.55

(continued)

Table 2 (continued)

Chinese	English Translation	Loading
V. Agreeable		
宽厚的	Lenient	0.65
朴实的	Plain and honest	0.64
忠厚的	Honest and tolerant	0.63
心肠好的	Kindhearted	0.62
和善的	Amiable	0.62
淳朴的	Naïve	0.62
忠诚的	Loyal	0.62
忠实的	Faithful	0.62
朴厚的	Simple and lenient	0.61
温存的	Attentive	0.54
忠顺的	Loyal and obedient	0.54
心肠软的	Softhearted	0.52
顺从的	Obedient	0.51
柔顺的	Docile	0.51
随顺的	Casual and obliging	0.50
温顺的	Meek and docile	0.47
脾气好的	Good-natured	0.47
贤惠的	(Of a woman) virtuous	0.46
文静的	Gentle and quiet	0.46
温柔的	Gentle and soft	0.45

After Yu et al. (2009)

They finished the self-rating scales in evening classes or other quiet rooms on-site, with the Likert type scales: (1) very unlike me, (2) moderately unlike me, (3) somewhat like and unlike me, (4) moderately like me, (5) very like me.

3.2 Statistics

The collected answers were submitted to Principal Component Analysis. The factor loadings underwent orthogonal rotation with the varimax normalized methods. The internal reliability (Cronbach's alpha) of each scale was calculated using the Reliability and Item Analysis. The gender differences on the mean individual scale scores were examined by two-way ANOVA and Duncan's multiple new range test. Pearson's rank correlation test was employed in search of potential relations within the scale scores and between them and participant's age. A p value less than 0.05 was taken as significant.

3.3   Results

Totally 15 factors with eigenvalues larger than 1.0 were obtained, with the first five most prominent, and with a clearly leveling-off from the sixth factor on. The first five made up 19.89, 9.66, 7.00, 5.48 and 4.18% of the total variance respectively (altogether 46.22%), and none of the rest over 2% of the total variance. The loadings of each item on the five factors are presented in Table 3. The respective Cronbach's alphas were satisfactory according to 20 items for each factor.

In general, loadings on the target factors were acceptable. The target loadings were positive, except for those on "Unsocial". However, there were some cross-loadings higher than 0.30. For example, one item (Rude) targeted at "Unsocial" was loaded 0.39 on "Emotional". Six items targeted at "Agreeable" (Honest and tolerant, 0.39; Naïve, 0.41; Simple and lenient, 0.41; Plain and honest, 0.47; Faithful, 0.42; Loyal, 0.41) were loaded highly on "Conscientious", one item (Kindhearted, 0.35) was loaded on "Unsocial" in an opposite way, and another item (Casual and obliging, −0.47) was also loaded on "Emotional" factor (Table 3).

Men scored on the five scales similar to woman (Fig. 1). The scales were significantly correlated with each other except that between "Emotional" and "Agreeable". "Conscientious" was correlated with "Intelligent" (r = 0.45) and with "Agreeable" (r = 0.42) moderately (Table 4). With the five scales referred to as repeated measures, two-ANOVA did not detect any gender differences (main effect, F (1, 718) = 0.54, p = 0.46). The participant's age was significantly, but weakly, correlated with "Conscientious" (n = 720, r = 0.13, p < 0.001) only. There were no other meaningful correlations in the study.

4   Discussion

Analyzing the 650 personality-relevant Chinese adjectives in study 1, we have discovered a five-factor model of personality traits, namely "Intelligent", "Emotional", "Conscientious", "Unsocial", and "Agreeable". Using the 100-adjective CADP in study 2, the five-factor model was again confirmed. Most intercorrelations of CADP scales were significant, especially those between "Conscientious" and "Intelligent" or "Agreeable". Therefore, our report is in line with the adjective method performed in other languages. In addition, no gender differences on the five CADP scales were detected, which is consistent with results of other researchers (Guenole and Chernyshenko 2005; Gomez 2006).

The first Chinese personality factor, named as "Intelligent", standing for the talented, competent, and creative traits, partly covers Openness to Experiences (Costa and McCrae 1994), Intellectual Abilities (Rudowicz and Yue 2002), and Capacity (Wang and Cui 2004). In line with the proposal that intelligence (or Openness to Experiences) is a trait dimension affecting almost every aspect of the personal life (Costa and McCrae 1994), participants in our study tended to value intelligence as

Table 3 Individual adjective loadings on the five CADP factors

Chinese	English translation	I	II	Factor III	IV	V
		α: 0.95	α: 0.91	α: 0.95	α: 0.91	α: 0.89
才华横溢的	Full of talents	**0.76**	−0.03	0.10	0.03	−0.02
才思敏捷的	Creative in writing	**0.75**	−0.01	0.15	0.17	0.00
有才能的	Competent	**0.75**	−0.01	0.18	0.22	0.04
学识渊博的	Knowledgeable	**0.74**	−0.03	0.15	0.05	0.01
有才华的	Artistically gifted	**0.73**	−0.02	0.16	0.02	0.07
有才智的	Endowed	**0.73**	0.00	0.18	0.21	0.05
天赋高的	Naturally gifted	**0.73**	0.04	0.06	0.03	0.00
才智出众的	Outstanding in wisdom	**0.73**	0.01	0.20	0.06	−0.03
有文才的	Literary-talented	**0.72**	−0.10	0.12	0.04	0.08
有才干的	Talented or capable	**0.71**	0.01	0.18	0.04	0.08
有才气的	Artistically talented	**0.71**	0.05	0.19	0.15	0.04
有才识的	Insightful	**0.70**	−0.06	0.22	0.14	0.05
智力高的	Highly intelligent	**0.69**	0.02	0.17	0.19	0.00
多才多艺的	Versatile	**0.69**	0.00	0.04	0.04	0.00
博学的	Erudite	**0.69**	−0.09	0.15	0.00	0.03
有才略的	Sagacious	**0.68**	−0.01	0.22	0.12	0.05
智慧的	Bright	**0.67**	−0.01	0.20	0.19	0.08
敏锐的	Sensible	**0.66**	−0.02	0.12	0.10	0.13
文思敏捷的	Good at writing	**0.66**	0.03	0.15	0.18	0.05
足智多谋的	Wise and resourceful	**0.63**	0.06	0.14	0.09	0.02
性子躁的	Hot-tempered	−0.07	**0.74**	−0.04	−0.21	−0.10
性急的	Impatient	−0.05	**0.70**	−0.09	−0.12	−0.08
急躁的	Fidgety	−0.05	**0.69**	−0.07	−0.09	−0.03
暴躁的	Irascible	−0.071	**0.68**	−0.01	−0.29	−0.20
易怒的	Irritable	0.00	**0.67**	−0.10	−0.15	−0.18

(continued)

Table 3 (continued)

Chinese	English translation	I	II	Factor III	IV	V
急性子的	Impetuous	−0.04	**0.66**	−0.01	0.07	−0.02
脾气大的	Temperamental	0.07	**0.66**	−0.04	−0.19	−0.19
爱发脾气的	Stormy	−0.02	**0.65**	−0.08	−0.23	−0.19
脾气坏的	Quick-tempered	−0.04	**0.63**	−0.06	−0.22	−0.26
烈性的	Explosive	0.06	**0.60**	0.07	−0.20	−0.07
冲动的	Impulsive	−0.08	**0.60**	−0.05	−0.14	0.05
火暴的	Fierce	−0.03	**0.59**	−0.09	−0.23	−0.23
牛脾气的	Bullheaded	0.00	**0.58**	−0.04	−0.24	−0.08
毛躁的	Hasty	−0.13	**0.57**	−0.15	−0.14	−0.05
莽撞的	Foolhardy	0.04	**0.52**	−0.19	−0.19	0.05
直性子的	Straightforward	0.00	**0.51**	0.08	0.18	0.04
心直口快的	Outspoken	0.19	**0.51**	0.05	0.25	0.16
快人快语的	Straight-talking	0.19	**0.48**	−0.02	0.15	0.10
马虎的	Careless	−0.10	**0.38**	−0.23	−0.12	0.03
多言的	Garrulous	0.17	**0.31**	−0.13	0.16	−0.01
坚忍不拔的	Firm and dauntless	**0.31**	−0.09	**0.71**	0.10	0.05
有毅力的	Of willpower	0.25	0.03	**0.70**	0.07	0.06
顽强的	Steadfast	0.20	−0.07	**0.70**	0.18	0.02
持之以恒的	Tireless	0.22	−0.24	**0.69**	0.05	0.03
意志坚定的	Determined	0.22	−0.08	**0.69**	0.17	0.01
锲而不舍的	Persistent	0.17	−0.13	**0.68**	0.03	0.00
有恒心的	Persevering	0.19	−0.11	**0.68**	0.00	0.00
有意志力的	Having strong willpower	0.23	−0.15	**0.68**	0.13	0.07
自强不息的	Constantly effortful	0.29	−0.05	**0.68**	0.13	0.04
不屈不挠的	Tenacious	0.24	−0.07	**0.68**	0.17	0.09
刚毅的	Firm	0.26	0.12	**0.66**	0.09	0.07

(continued)

Table 3 (continued)

Chinese	English translation	I	II	Factor III	IV	V
孜孜不倦的	Assiduous	0.19	−0.17	**0.65**	0.05	0.08
坚毅的	Resolute	0.25	−0.02	**0.64**	0.09	0.09
严格的	Strict	0.18	−0.01	**0.62**	0.00	0.08
吃苦耐劳的	Able to endure hardships	0.03	−0.05	**0.60**	0.04	0.17
脚踏实地的	Down-to-earth	0.01	−0.11	**0.59**	0.10	0.23
耐劳的	Able to endure heavy work	0.07	−0.09	**0.55**	0.12	0.22
勤劳的	Diligent	0.02	−0.08	**0.55**	0.15	0.26
勤俭的	Thrifty	−0.01	−0.14	**0.53**	0.02	0.15
刚强的	Strong-minded	0.27	0.15	**0.53**	0.09	0.11
蠢笨的	Stupid and clumsy	−0.17	0.07	−0.06	**−0.71**	−0.06
呆板的	Stiff and awkward	−0.11	0.06	−0.16	**−0.68**	0.05
愚笨的	Foolish	−0.15	0.04	−0.01	**−0.67**	−0.04
愚蠢的	Stupid	−0.19	0.05	−0.04	**−0.67**	0.00
思想迟钝的	Obtuse	−0.18	0.06	−0.06	**−0.67**	0.08
呆笨的	Dull	−0.17	0.08	−0.05	**−0.65**	0.00
低能的	Imbecile	−0.11	0.07	−0.05	**−0.65**	0.00
死板的	Inflexible	−0.19	0.10	−0.12	**−0.65**	0.05
无能的	Incompetent	−0.20	0.10	−0.03	**−0.64**	0.03
迟钝的	Sluggish	−0.22	0.03	−0.08	**−0.63**	0.05
不中用的	Useless	−0.15	0.06	−0.10	**−0.61**	0.02
怯懦的	Cowardly	−0.09	0.05	−0.20	**−0.61**	0.08
古板的	Old-fashioned and inflexible	−0.12	0.07	−0.12	**−0.61**	0.01
孤僻的	Unsociable and eccentric	−0.04	0.14	−0.04	**−0.58**	−0.01
刻薄的	Mean	0.04	0.21	−0.14	**−0.53**	−0.20
苛刻的	Overcritical	0.13	0.23	−0.15	**−0.47**	−0.16
气量狭小的	Narrow-minded	−0.12	0.21	−0.20	**−0.46**	−0.07
粗鲁的	Rude	0.01	**0.39**	−0.16	**−0.42**	−0.21
孤傲的	Aloof and arrogant	0.21	0.25	−0.08	**−0.40**	−0.17
清高的	Aloof and overconfident	0.29	0.20	0.00	**−0.40**	−0.11
温柔的	Gentle and soft	0.05	−0.24	0.03	−0.04	**0.63**
温顺的	Meek and docile	0.05	−0.22	0.01	−0.15	**0.62**
柔顺的	Docile	0.09	−0.13	0.10	−0.08	**0.61**
忠顺的	Loyal and obedient	0.06	−0.19	0.01	−0.11	**0.61**
心肠软的	Softhearted	−0.12	0.14	0.03	0.14	**0.58**
温存的	Attentive	0.14	−0.20	0.02	−0.06	**0.57**
和善的	Amiable	0.04	−0.11	0.16	0.25	**0.57**

(continued)

Table 3 (continued)

Chinese	English translation	I	II	Factor III	IV	V
宽厚的	Lenient	−0.04	−0.02	**0.34**	0.21	**0.57**
忠厚的	Honest and tolerant	−0.06	0.02	**0.39**	0.12	**0.56**
淳朴的	Naïve	−0.01	0.04	**0.41**	0.13	**0.54**
朴厚的	Simple and lenient	0.01	−0.02	**0.41**	0.14	**0.53**
心肠好的	Kindhearted	0.06	0.06	0.23	**0.35**	**0.51**
朴实的	Plain and honest	−0.03	−0.02	**0.47**	0.12	**0.51**
顺从的	Obedient	0.05	−0.01	−0.20	**−0.36**	**0.50**
忠实的	Faithful	0.05	0.10	**0.42**	0.22	**0.50**
忠诚的	Loyal	−0.01	0.10	**0.41**	0.21	**0.50**
贤惠的	(of a woman) Virtuous	0.10	−0.06	0.14	−0.02	**0.49**
随顺的	Casual and obliging	0.10	**−0.47**	0.06	0.05	**0.48**
脾气好的	Good-natured	0.06	0.02	−0.05	−0.21	**0.48**
文静的	Gentle and quiet	0.06	−0.23	0.19	−0.11	**0.42**
	Eigenvalue	19.89	9.66	7.00	5.48	4.18
	Explained variance	11.59	8.43	10.55	8.90	6.75

After Yu et al. (2009)
20 items for each factor and cross-loadings higher than 0.30 were in bold

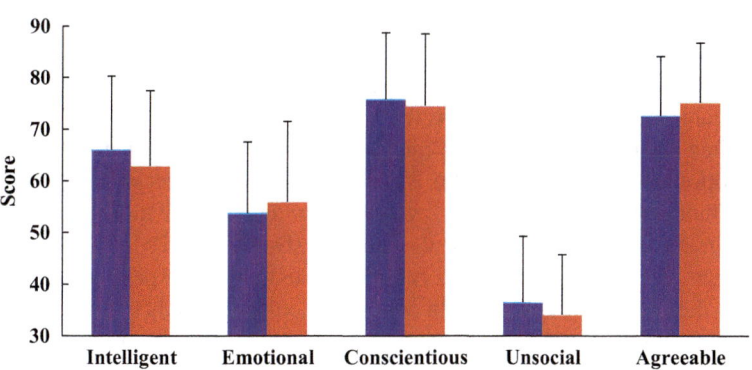

Fig. 1 Scale scores (mean ± S.D.) of the five CADP scales in men (violet bars, n = 255) and women (red bars, n = 465). (After Yu et al. 2009)

Table 4 Intercorrelation of the CADP five scales

	Intelligent	Emotional	Conscientious	Unsocial
Emotional	−0.06			
Conscientious	0.45	0.22		
Unsocial	−0.28	0.37	−0.33	
Agreeable	0.16	−0.28	0.42	−0.16

After Yu et al. (2009)

an essential aspect of personality (made up 19.89% of the total variance). One meta-analytical finding showed that more cognitively personality traits, rather than more emotionally ones, were largely associated with personal values (Parks-Leduc et al. 2015). This is in line with our result that Intelligent, more of individual cognition than of emotion, is the most important personality descriptor from Chinese perspective. Moreover, in contemporary China, people tend to value a person by his vocational development. For instance, a student with high academic grades may be considered as a good role model, who is worthwhile to learn from, and a man with high job title may be defined as a successful person. This kind of assessment system motivates people to pursue actual benefits in their position, and a person with high intelligence has potential competence over others to achieve what is called success. Therefore, "Intelligent" is brought up at first when it comes to describing one's personality traits.

The second factor "Emotional", which stands for temperamental, straightforward, and impatient traits, partly covers Neuroticism (Costa and McCrae 1994) or Emotionality (Wang and Cui 2004). Despite that Chinese people were once regarded as more reserved in emotion (Song 1985), results in our study showed that our participants might put emotion in an essential position and believe that the emotional aspect constituted personality. This phenomenon is in line with the results from the questionnaires. Considering the similarity between Emotional in our model and Neuroticism in the Big-Five, the high percentage of total variance explained by Emotional in our study is in accordance with the previous report that Chinese adolescents reported higher levels of neuroticism in a Big-Five personality inventory than European counterparts (Reese et al. 2014). Emotional experience also varies across different cultures. East Asians valued low-arousal positive emotions such as feeling calm more while Western Americans valued high-arousal ones such as feeling excited (Tsai 2007). Besides, Chinese experienced much lower-intensity negative emotions than Americans and Australians did (Eid and Diener 2001). In another study, Chinese men reported lower levels of emotion and were more prone to disengagement strategies about emotional regulation (Davis et al. 2012). Cultural norms of emotion expression might play a role in how individuals experience the emotion and how they regulate afterwards. In collectivist culture, people try to modify themselves and avoid impact on others so as to blend in their in-group (Lim 2016). Eastern culture requires people to adjust to others (Markus and Kitayama 1991), in which cases, low arousal emotions function better (Tsai et al. 2006). Consequently, Chinese people might put "Emotional" in a relatively important place as to the personality description, because low arousal emotion experience and emotional regulation are really unique and critical to the collectivist community.

The third factor "Conscientious", standing for diligent, steadfast, and persistent capacities, corresponds to Discipline or Dutifulness (Rudowicz and Yue 2002), and Ways of Life (Wang and Cui 2004). This is in accordance with modern personality theory that human potential and will are an important outgrowth of the human trait (Avrill 1997). Previous study found that people with conscientiousness retained more impact where individual-oriented tasks were preferred (Anderson et al. 2008). Further in a meta-analytic review, conscientiousness was found to be a consistent predictive factor for leadership effectiveness, which gives us some knowledge of the importance of this character and that it is worthwhile to cultivate this trait (Derue et al. 2011). In the Chinese tradition, both parents and teachers attach great importance to cultivating self-discipline and responsibility in the young, and link them with moral reality (Yang 1990). In workplace, perceptions of corporate social responsibility were found to be more positively related to employee's affective commitment in Collectivism (Mueller et al. 2012). Besides, Collectivism could also lead to sorts of appreciable team-oriented outcomes, including greater concern for others, in-group favoritism, conflict avoidance, and helping and cooperative behaviors (Taras et al. 2010). Another study showed that team follower collectivism was positively to their affective commitment to the organization (Chen et al. 2011). Putting also these solid evidence into account, we might conclude that in a collectivist culture like China, people are motivated to maintain conscientiousness in interpersonal relationship and in workplace.

The fourth factor "Unsocial", standing for stupid, dull or inflexible characters, corresponds partly to the negative poles of Extraversion (Costa and McCrae 1994), Social Life (Rudowicz and Yue 2002) or Extraversion (Wang and Cui 2004). Chinese students discerned unsocial behaviors and avoided using them to depict themselves. In tradition, the Chinese social system is relatively rigid and defensive, and independence was discouraged (Dunn et al. 1988). Conversely, in this day and age, when a peer is required to assess an individual, he or she would add an opinion of whether the person acts well in the social and cultural contexts. This is in accordance with another finding in a Chinese university student sample that self-esteem was positively correlated with impression management enhancement, one aspect of socially desirable responding (Li et al. 2015), which means individuals tend to see themselves as possessing positive personalities in the social environment. From cultural perspective, collectivist cultures have many kinds, among which one cardinal distinction lies between vertical and horizontal collectivist cultures. Vertical collectivist culture, where China belongs, is typical of traditionalist, emphasis of in-group cohesion, respect for in-group norms, and the directives of authorities. Therefore, people in this type of culture are heavily influenced by the behaviors and thoughts of the in-group which they are in, and behave themselves to conform to the community (Triandis and Suh 2002). In the contemporary China, people might tend to avoid being "unsocial" and try to socialize in a way that best suits the in-group.

The fifth factor "Agreeable", standing for gentle, docile or obedient aspects, corresponds partly to Agreeableness (Costa and McCrae 1994), Obedience or Social acceptance (Rudowicz and Yue 2002), and Kindness in Human Relations (Wang and Cui 2004). When it comes to virtue, both empathy and serenity are taken into consideration (Cawley et al. 2000). This is also the case in China, as obedience, quiet and patience are frequently stressed in the primary schools (Song 1985; Yang 1990). In addition, studies of Chinese organizational behavior uncovered that employees were chosen mainly based on the applicants' obedience to current employers (Redding and Wong 1986; Cross and Markus 1999). Nowadays in China, job-seeking behavior and the problems frequently encountered during the process would feedback the cognition of self-training, leading to the construction of personality traits. Being agreeable is a vital element of employer-employee relationship in modern society. One study concealed that employee's level of agreeableness moderated the impact of a leader's emotional exhibition, further affecting the team performance (Van Kleef et al. 2010). Another investigator had assessed personality traits of 190 health care managers and leadership behaviors of them by different raters, including colleagues, supervisors, subordinates and themselves, and found out that agreeableness predicted employee-oriented leadership behaviors for external raters, and change-oriented ones for managers themselves (Bergman et al. 2014). These findings indirectly revealed the importance of the fifth factor "Agreeable", since this factor overlaps with "Agreeableness" in the Big-Five used in the two studies above. At the same time, it is noteworthy that advocacy of "Agreeable" can be found in classic Confucian virtues, such as *Rén* (benevolence), *Ai* (affection), *Xin* (trustworthiness), *He* (harmony), *Ping* (peace), and *Li* (propriety) (Shek et al. 2013; also see Chapter "Hierarchical Needs and Psychological Disorders in China").

To sum up, the five-factor structures of personality in China were confirmed via the lexical method, and these basic structures were similar to the "etic" statement-questionnaire results. However, the unique part lies in that Intelligent is the most critical factor in Chinese context. The fact we did not found emic-component contribution to personality might be due to that people in collectivist culture have the tendency to describe personality less in conceptual trait terms and more in concrete behaviors in situational contexts (Valchev et al. 2013). In this study, a collectivist group showed fewer traits and more contextualization, while an individualist group showed the opposite. Church (2000) also presented the differences between collectivist and individualist cultures that people in the former culture focus more on contexts than on internal process when predicting the behavior of others. Besides, one rudimentary idea of classical Chinese cosmology was the notion of ceaseless transformation and flux. In this case, the whole world, individuals included, is best conceptualized as in process or transition, continually dynamic and adapting to context. The Confucian tradition is strongly embedded in concrete context and particularistic in its orientation (Giordano 2014). Therefore, Chinese people may prefer to describe personality by putting the person into specified circumstances or scenarios, instead of by depicting the person with abstract words in a rigid way. That is probably another reason of the absence of emic-component in Chinese personality descriptions.

Although personality traits differ among individuals, many of them function as a whole when a person is faced with challenges (McCrae and Costa 1996). People also think this way in a Chinese family and in society, since self-discipline, motivation, obedience, and social adaptation are always stressed and connected together, and these qualities are critical to assess a person's ability or vocational success (Song 1985; Yang 1990). This helps to illustrate the finding in our study that "Conscientious" was moderately correlated with "Intelligent" and "Agreeable". For example, 7 out of 20 adjectives on "Agreeable" were loaded highly on "Conscientious".

Besides, our model confirmed the finding that Extraversion, Agreeableness, and Conscientiousness of the Big-Five are typical traits that constitute a three-factor structure with fully cross-cultural replicability (de Raad et al. 2010), since we have "Conscientious" as the third factor, "Agreeable" the fifth, and "Unsocial", the fourth factor, which partly overlaps with the negative pole of Extraversion. Further research put forward the concept of three-factor "pan-cultural" personality structure, comprising Dynamsim, Affiliation, and Order (de Raad et al. 2014). Dynamsim connotates extroversion, vitality, activeness, and enterprise. Affiliation means fitting in an entity striving for unity within, such as being helpful and sympathetic. Order refers to being organized and controlled intellect. The shared coring of the pan-cultural structure is clearly contained in our Chinese version of personality factors. Using nine languages of multiple provenances, Chinese included, to avoid overrepresentation of Western culture, participants from rural and urban areas to increase samples' typicality, and English as a *lingua franca* to offset any bias towards one single language studied, other researchers found the cross-cultural ubiquity of two factors, Social Self-Regulation (propriety, socialization, community, solidarity) and Dynamism (activity, potency, ascendancy) (Saucier et al. 2014). Social Self-Regulation is overlapped with Agreeable and Dynamism the negative pole of Unsocial in our study.

According to another five-factor model proposed by McAdams and Pals (2006), a comprehensive understanding of personality includes: (1) Human Nature, which provides the general design for psychological individuality; (2) Dispositional Traits, broad individual differences across situations and over time; (3) Characteristic Adaptations, additional specific individual differences contextualized in time, situations and social roles; (4) Integrative Life Narratives, internalized and evolving life stories one constructs to establish self-identity; (5) Culture, embedded in which traits, adaptations and life narratives develop. What incites our interest is the role culture plays in shaping the whole personality. Dispositional traits are part of personality analogously displayed across cultures, while characteristic adaptations and life narratives are outcomes of cultural specificity (Timothy 2010). In our case, core meanings of the five factors are alike to those globally used personality structures, which show the universality of the dispositional traits in Chinese culture. Despite this, Chinese people have developed their personality traits distinctive from Western people. Conservativeness and mediocracy are philosophy of life learned from Confucian culture and carried on along the way since ancient times. The *Junzi* serves as an exemplar of the relational self that conforms to the ideal of optimal personal functioning and becomes well adept in collaborative and contextually attuned behavior within Chinese culture (Giordano 2014). As a consequence, the essence of personality underneath Chinese people may resemble that of their Western counterparts, but the Chinese cultural context guides people to form values and beliefs and identify who they are in a different manner. Evidence for the universality is instructive to analyze certain facets of personality, while evidence for variability is helpful to understand how contextual elements influence aspects of personality (Heine and Buchtel 2009).

Considering the adjective checklist has been used as a basic measure in clinical researches (Leohlin et al. 1998; Craig and Olson 2001), the CADP might also be trialed out in China. Moreover, we might administer a comparative study of CADP and questionnaires measuring disordered personality, to find out whether Chinese adjective descriptors are linked to personality dysfunctions. By doing so, the interrelationship between disordered and normal personality traits in Chinese culture might be established.

References

Anderson, C., Spataro, S. E., & Flynn, F. J. (2008). Personality and organizational culture as determinants of influence. *Journal of Applied Psychology, 93*, 702–710.

Angleitner, A., Ostendorf, F., & John, O. P. (1990). Towards a taxonomy of personality descriptors in German: A psycho-lexical study. *European Journal of Personality, 4*, 89–118.

Ashton, M. C., & Lee, K. (2005). A defense of the lexical approach to the study of personality structure. *European Journal of Personality, 19*, 5–24.

Ashton, M. C., & Lee, K. (2007). Empirical, theoretical, and practical advantages of the HEXACO model of personality structure. *Personality and Social Psychology Review, 11*, 150–166.

Avrill, J. R. (1997). The emotions: An integrative approach. In R. Hogan, J. A. Johnson, & S. R. Briggs (Eds.), *Handbook of personality psychology* (pp. 513–541). San Diego: Academic Press.

Bergman, D., Lornudd, C., Sjöberg, L., & Von Thiele Schwarz, U. (2014). Leader personality and 360-degree assessments of leader behavior. *Scandinavian Journal of Psychology, 55*, 389–397.

Bond, M. H. (1979). Dimensions used in perceiving peers: Cross-cultural comparisons of Hong Kong, Japanese, American and Filipino university students. *Internal Journal of Psychology, 14*, 47–56.

Burtăverde, V., & de Raad, B. (2017). Taxonomy and structure of the Romanian personality lexicon: Romanian personality structure. *International Journal of Psychology*. https://doi.org/10.1002/ijop.12464.

Caprara, G. V., & Perugini, M. (1994). Personality described by adjectives: The generalizability of the Big Five to the Italian lexical context. *European Journal of Personality, 8*, 357–369.

Cawley, M. J., III, Martin, J. E., & Johnson, J. A. (2000). A virtues approach to personality. *Personality and Individual Differences, 28*, 997–1013.

Chen, G. M., Sharma, P. N., Edinger, S. K., Shapiro, D. L., & Farh, J. L. (2011). Motivating and demotivating forces in teams: Cross-level influences of empowering leadership and relationship conflict. *Journal of Applied Psychology, 96*, 541–557.

Chen, Z., Lu, X., & Kitamura, T. (2013). The factor structure of the Chinese version of the Temperament and Character Inventory: Factorial robustness and association with age and gender. *Comprehensive Psychiatry, 54*, 292–300.

Cheung, F. M., van de Vijver, F. J., & Leong, F. T. (2011). Toward a new approach to the study of personality in culture. *American Psychologist, 66*, 593–603.

Church, A. T. (1987). Personality research in a non-Western culture: The Philippines. *Psychological Bulletin, 102*, 272–292.

Church, A. T. (2000). Culture and personality: Toward an integrated cultural trait psychology. *Journal of Personality, 68*, 651–703.

Church, A. T. (2016). Personality traits across cultures. *Current Opinion in Psychology, 8*, 22–30.

Cloninger, C. R., Przybeck, T. R., Svrakic, D. M., & Wetzel, R. D. (1994). *The temperament and character inventory (TCI): A guide to its development and use*. Missouri: Center for Psychobiology of Personality, Washington University.

Corr, P. J., & Matthews, G. (Eds.). (2009). *The Cambridge handbook of personality psychology*. Cambridge: Cambridge University Press.

Costa, P. T., Jr., & McCrae, R. R. (1994). *NEO Personality Inventory-Revised (NEO-PI-R) manual*. Odessa: Psychological Assessment Resources.

Costa, P. T., Jr., & Widiger, T. A. (1994). *Personality disorder and the five-factor model of personality*. Washington: American Psychological Association.

Costa, P. T., Jr., Terracciano, A., & McCrae, R. R. (2001). Gender differences in personality traits across cultures: Robust and surprising findings. *Journal of Personality and Social Psychology, 81*, 322–331.

Craig, R. J., & Olson, R. E. (2001). Adjectival descriptions of personality disorders: A convergent validity study of the MCMI-III. *Journal of Personality Assessment, 77*, 259–271.

Cross, S. E., & Markus, H. R. (1999). The cultural constitution of personality. In L. Pervin & O. John (Eds.), *Handbook of personality* (Vol. 2, pp. 376–396). New York: Guilford.

Davis, E., Greenberger, E., Charles, S., Chen, C., Zhao, L., & Dong, Q. (2012). Emotion experience and regulation in China and the United States: How do culture and gender shape emotion responding? *International Journal of Psychology, 47*, 230–239.

de Raad, B. (1992). The replicability of the big five personality dimensions in three word-classes of the Dutch language. *European Journal of Personality, 6*, 15–29.

de Raad, B., & Barelds, D. P. (2008). A new taxonomy of Dutch personality traits based on a comprehensive and unrestricted list of descriptors. *Journal of Personality and Social Psychology, 94*, 347–364.

de Raad, B., Barelds, D. P. H., Levert, E., Ostendorf, F., Mlačić, B., di Blas, L., Hřebíčková, M., Szirmák, Z., Szarota, P., Perugini, M., Church, A. T., & Katigbak, M. S. (2010). Only three factors of personality description are fully replicable across languages: A comparison of 14 trait taxonomies. *Journal of Personality and Social Psychology, 98*, 160–173.

de Raad, B., Barelds, D. P., Timmerman, M. E., de Roover, K., Mlačić, B., & Church, A. T. (2014). Towards a pan-cultural personality structure: Input from 11 psycholexical studies. *European Journal of Personality, 28*, 497–510.

Derue, D. S., Nahrgang, J. D., Wellman, N., & Humphrey, S. E. (2011). Trait and behavioral theories of leadership: An integration and meta-analytic test of their relative validity. *Personnel Psychology, 64*, 7–52.

Dunn, J. A., Zhang, X. Y., & Ripple, R. E. (1988). Comparative study of Chinese and American performance on divergent thinking tasks. *New Horizons, 29*, 7–20.

Eid, M., & Diener, E. (2001). Norms for experiencing emotions in different cultures: Inter- and intra-national differences. *Journal of Personality and Social Psychology, 81*, 869–885.

Farahani, M. N., de Raad, B., Farzad, V., & Fotoohie, M. (2016). Taxonomy and structure of Persian personality-descriptive trait terms. *International Journal of Psychology, 51*, 139–149.

Funder, D. C. (1997). *The personality puzzle*. New York: W W Norton and Co.

Gençöz, T., & Öncül, Ö. (2012). Examination of personality characteristics in a Turkish sample: Development of basic personality traits inventory. *Journal of General Psychology, 139*, 194–216.

Giordano, P. J. (2014). Personality as continuous stochastic process: What western personality theory can learn from classical confucianism. *Integrative Psychological and Behavioral Science, 48*, 111–128.

Goldberg, L. R., & Rosolack, T. K. (1994). The Big-Five structure as an integrated framework: An empirical comparison with Eysenck's P-E-N model. In C. F. Halverson, G. A. Kohnstamm, & R. P. Martin (Eds.), *The developing structure of temperament and personality from infancy to adulthood* (pp. 7–35). New York: Erlbaum.

Gomez, R. (2006). Gender invariance of the five-factor model of personality among adolescents: A mean and covariance structure analysis approach. *Personality and Individual Differences, 41*, 755–765.

Guenole, N., & Chernyshenko, O. S. (2005). The stability of Goldberg's Big Five IPIP personality markers in New Zealand: A dimensionality, bias, and criterion validity. *New Zealand Journal of Psychology, 34*, 86–96.

Gurven, M., von Rueden, C., Massenkoff, M., Kaplan, H., & Vie, M. L. (2013). How universal is the big five? Testing the five-factor model of personality variation among forager-farmers in the Bolivian Amazon. *Journal of Personality and Social Psychology, 104*, 354–370.

Heine, S. J., & Buchtel, E. E. (2009). Personality: The universal and the culturally specific. *Annual Reviews of Psychology, 60*, 369–394.

John, O. P., Angleitner, A., & Ostendorf, F. (1988). The lexical approach to personality: A historical review of trait taxonomic research. *European Journal of Personality, 2*, 171–203.

Ledesma, R. D., Sánchez, R., & Díaz-Lázaro, C. M. (2011). Adjective checklist to assess the big five personality factors in the Argentine population. *Journal of Personality Assessment, 93*, 46–55.

Lee, K., & Ashton, M. C. (2008). The HEXACO personality factors in the indigenous personality lexicons of English and 11 other languages. *Journal of Personality, 76*, 1001–1054.

Leohlin, J. C., McCrae, R. R., Costa, P. T., Jr., & John, O. P. (1998). Heritabilities of common and measure specific components of the Big Five personality factors. *Journal of Research in Personality, 32*, 431–453.

Li, F., Li, Y., & Wang, Y. (2015). Socially desirable responding in Chinese university students: Denial and enhancement? *Psychological Reports, 116*, 409–421.

Lim, N. (2016). Cultural differences in emotion: Differences in emotional arousal level between the East and the West. *Integrative Medicine Research, 5*, 105–109.

Livaniene, V., & de Raad, B. (2017). The factor structure of Lithuanian personality-descriptive adjectives of the highest frequency of use. *International Journal of Psychology, 52*, 453–462.

Markus, H. R., & Kitayama, S. (1991). Culture and the self: Implications for cognition, emotion, and motivation. *Psychological Review, 98*, 224–253.

McAdams, D. P., & Pals, J. L. (2006). A new Big Five: Fundamental principles for an integrative science of personality. *American Psychologist, 61*, 204–217.

McCrae, R. R. (2004). Human nature and culture: A trait perspective. *Journal of Research in Personality, 38*, 3–14.

McCrae, R. R., & Costa, P. T., Jr. (1996). Toward a new generation of personality theories: Theoretical contexts for the five-factor model. In S. Wiggins (Ed.), *The five-factor model of personality: Theoretical perspectives* (pp. 51–87). New York: Guilford.

Mlačić, B., & Ostendorf, F. (2005). Taxonomy and structure of Croatian personality-descriptive adjectives. *European Journal of Personality, 19*, 117–152.

Mueller, K., Hattrup, K., Spiess, S. O., & Lin-Hi, N. (2012). The effects of corporate social responsibility on employees' affective commitment: A cross-cultural investigation. *Journal of Applied Psychology, 97*, 1186–1200.

Muris, P., Meesters, C., & Diederen, R. (2005). Psychometric properties of the Big Five Questionnaire for Children (BFQ-C) in a Dutch sample of young adolescents. *Personality and Individual Differences, 38*, 1757–1769.

Parks-Leduc, L., Feldman, G., & Bardi, A. (2015). Personality traits and personal values: A meta-analysis. *Personality and Social Psychology Review, 19*, 3–29.

Peabody, D. (1987). Selecting representative trait adjectives. *Journal of Personality and Social Psychology, 52*(1), 59–71.

Redding, G., & Wong, G. Y. Y. (1986). The psychology of Chinese organizational behavior. In M. H. Bond (Ed.), *The psychology of the Chinese people* (pp. 267–295). London: Oxford University Press.

Reese, E., Chen, Y., McAnally, H. M., Myftari, E., Neha, T., Wang, Q., & Jack, F. (2014). Narratives and traits in personality development among New Zealand Māori, Chinese, and European adolescents. *Journal of Adolescence, 37*, 727–737.

Rossier, J., Aluja, A., García, L. F., Angleitner, A., de Pascalis, V., Wang, W., Kuhlman, M., & Zuckerman, M. (2007). The cross-cultural generalizability of Zuckerman's alternative five-factor model of personality. *Journal of Personality Assessment, 89*, 188–196.

Rudowicz, E., & Yue, X. (2002). Compatibility of Chinese and creative personalities. *Creativity Research Journal, 14*, 387–394.

Saucier, G., & Goldberg, L. R. (2001). Lexical studies of indigenous personality factors: Premises, products, and prospects. *Journal of Personality, 69*, 847–879.

Saucier, G., Thalmayer, A. G., Payne, D. L., Carlson, R., Sanogo, L., Ole-Kotikash, L., Church, A. T., Katigbak, M. S., Somer, O., Szarota, P., Szirmak, Z., & Zhou, X. (2014). A basic bivariate structure of personality attributes evident across nine languages. *Journal of Personality, 82*, 1–14.

Shek, D. T., Yu, L., & Fu, X. (2013). Confucian virtues and Chinese adolescent development: A conceptual review. *International Journal of Adolescent Medicine and Health, 25*, 335–344.

Shmelyov, A. G., & Pokhil'ko, V. I. (1993). A taxonomy-oriented study of Russian personality-trait names. *European Journal of Personality, 7*, 1–17.

Song, W. (1985). Analysis of results of administration of the MMPI to normal Chinese subjects. *Acta Psychologica Sinica, 17*, 346–355.

Szarota, P. (1996). Taxonomy of the Polish personality-descriptive adjectives of the highest frequency of use. *Polish Psychological Bulletin, 27*, 343–351.

Taras, V., Kirkman, B. L., & Steel, P. (2010). Examining the impact of culture's consequences: A three-decade, multilevel, meta-analytic review of Hofstede's cultural value dimensions. *Journal of Applied Psychology, 95*, 405–439.

Timothy, C. A. (2010). Current perspectives in the study of personality across cultures. *Perspectives on Psychological Science, 5*, 441–449.

Triandis, H. C., & Suh, E. M. (2002). Cultural influences on personality. *Annual Review of Psychology, 53*, 133–160.

Tsai, J. L. (2007). Ideal affect: Cultural causes and behavioral consequences. *Perspectives on Psychological Science, 2*, 242–259.

Tsai, J. L., Knutson, B., & Fung, H. H. (2006). Cultural variation in affect valuation. *Journal of Personality and Social Psychology, 90*, 288–307.

Valchev, V. H., van de Vijver, F. J., Nel, J. A., Rothmann, S., & Meiring, D. (2013). The use of traits and contextual information in free personality descriptions across ethnocultural groups in South Africa. *Journal of Personality and Social Psychology, 104*, 1077–1091.

van den Broeck, J., Bastiaansen, L., Rossi, G., Dierckx, E., Mikolajczak-Degrauwe, K., & Hofmans, J. (2014). Factorial validity of the personality adjective checklist in a Dutch-speaking sample. *Journal of Personality Assessment, 96*, 245–251.

van Kleef, G. A., Homan, A. C., Beersma, B., & van Knippenberg, D. (2010). On angry leaders and agreeable followers: How leaders' emotions and followers' personalities shape motivation and team performance. *Psychological Science, 21*, 1827–1834.

Wang, D. & Cui, H. (2004). Reliabilities and validities of the Chinese Personality Scale (QZPS). *Acta Psychologica Sinica (China), 36*, 347–358 (in Chinese).

Whitmore, J. M., Shore, W. J., & Smith, P. H. (2004). Partial knowledge of word meanings: Thematic and taxonomic representations. *Journal of Psycholinguistic Research, 33*, 137–164.

Yamagata, S., Suzuki, A., Ando, J., Ono, Y., Kijima, N., Yoshimura, K., Ostendorf, F., Angleitner, A., Riemann, R., Spinath, F. M., Livesley, W. J., & Jang, K. L. (2006). Is the genetic structure of human personality universal? A cross-cultural twin study from North America, Europe, and Asia. *Journal of Personality and Social Psychology, 90*, 987–998.

Yang, K. S. (1990). Chinese personality and its change. In M. H. Bond (Ed.), *The psychology of the Chinese people* (pp. 106–170). Hong Kong: Oxford University Press.

Yang, K. S., & Bond, M. H. (1990). Exploring implicit personality theories with indigenous or imported constructs: The Chinese case. *Journal of Personality and Social Psychology, 58*, 1087–1095.

Yu, S., Wei, L., He, W., Chai, H., Wang, D., Chen, W., & Wang, W. (2009). Description of personality traits by Chinese adjectives: A trial on university students. *Psychology of Language and Communication, 13*, 5–20.

Zhou, X., Saucier, G., Gao, D., & Liu, J. (2009). The factor structure of Chinese personality terms. *Journal of Personality, 77*, 363–400.

Personality Disorders Predicted by the Chinese Adjective Descriptors of Personality

Guorong Ma, Hongying Fan, and Wei Wang

1 Introduction

As Kluckhohn (Kluckhohn 1954) says, "Culture is to society what memory is to individuals", some scholars define culture as the part of the environment made by humans. It is the set of meanings that a group in a time and place come to adopt or develop, and these meanings facilitate smooth social coordination, clarify group boundaries, and provide a space for innovation (Geertz 1974; Markus et al. 1996; Oyserman 2011; Packer and Cole 2016). Put in a simple way, culture refers to the beliefs, values, and behaviors that together form an individual's way of life. Barkow et al. (1992) distinguished three kinds of culture: metaculture, evoked culture, and epidemiological culture. They argue that the psychology underlies culture and society, and there are biological determinants underly psychology. The biology that has been common to all humans as a species distinguishable from other species, results in a "metaculture" that corresponds to panhuman mental contents and organization. Biology in different ecologies results in "evoked culture" (for example, hot climate leads to light clothing), which reflects domain-specific mechanisms that are triggered by local circumstances, and leads to within-group similarities and between-groups differences. Finally, a useful idea (e.g., how to make a tool) is adopted by more and more people and becomes an element of culture (Campbell 1965), resulting in "epidemiological culture" (Triandis and Suh 2002).

Culture and personality are to a large extent connected with each other. According to the model of culture and personality by Church (2000), traits exist in all cultures, but account for behavior less in collectivist than in individualist cultures. Situational determinants of behavior are important universally, but more so in collectivist than in individualist cultures. Cognitive consistency among psychological processes and

G. Ma · H. Fan · W. Wang (✉)
Department of Clinical Psychology and Psychiatry/School of Public Health, Zhejiang University College of Medicine, Hangzhou, China
e-mail: drwangwei@zju.edu.cn

© Springer Nature Singapore Pte Ltd. 2019
W. Wang (ed.), *Chinese Perspectives on Cultural Psychiatry*,
https://doi.org/10.1007/978-981-13-3537-2_7

between psychological processes and behavior occurs universally, but is less important in collectivistic than in individualistic cultures. Psychiatrists have also witnessed the effects of culture and environment on the individual (Bains 2005). There is evidence that the psychiatric disorder patients display some clinical or epidemiological differences all over the world including China. For instance, Chinese adolescents had lowest score on average across six scales of somatic symptoms, depression, interpersonal relationships, powerlessness, impulsiveness and eating disorders, indicating that their state of mental health was the better than adolescents from Japan and Korea, but analysis of individual subscales revealed that they have experienced more depression than students from the two countries (Houri et al. 2012). Chinese elders have the lowest standardized prevalence of sleep complaints amongst six developing countries, including Cuba, the Dominican Republic, Peru, Venezuela, Mexico, China, India, and Puerto Rico (Mazzotti et al. 2012). Chinese patients with major depressive disorder had lower suicidality tendency than their counterparts in South Korea (Maniam and Chan 2013; Lim et al. 2014; Armitage et al. 2015). Further, Chinese bipolar disorder patients had a remarkably lower comorbidity of alcohol problems than the Western bipolar patients did (Tsai et al. 1997). Moreover, the prevalence of personality disorders in China was lower than that in the USA but higher than that in Western Europe (Huang et al. 2009).

One might suspect that all the aforementioned differences are associated either with the uniqueness of the Chinese culture, or with the personality trait differences. The Chinese Adjective Descriptors of Personality (CADP, see Chap. "Personality Traits in Contemporary China: A Lexical Approach") may help us answer the question. The normal traits of Intelligent, Emotional, Conscientious, Unsocial and Agreeable measured in CADP are comparable to the traits of the Big-Five model of personality, namely the Openness to Experience, Neuroticism, Conscientiousness, Extraversion, and Agreeableness. Because it was developed on the base of the Chinese culture, CADP might be more suitable for measuring the personality-related psychiatric disorders in China. de Fruyt et al. (2013) examined the relationships between two measures proposed to describe personality pathology, that is the Revised NEO Personality Inventory and the Personality Inventory for DSM-5 (American Psychiatric Association 2013), and found that general and maladaptive traits are subsumed under an umbrella of five to six major dimensions that can be interpreted from the perspective of the Big-Five Model or the Personality Psychopathology Five. Traits relating to intelligence are associated with mania in patients with bipolar I disorder, and partly concurred with the findings of the Big-Five personality traits in affective disorders (see Chap. "Predicting Affective States of Bipolar Disorder by the Chinese Adjective Descriptors of Personality"). For instance, using the NEO Personality Inventory and the Revised NEO Personality Inventory, it was reported that bipolar patients scored significantly higher on the Positive Emotion facet (subscale) of Extraversion than patients with unipolar depression (Michael et al. 1997). Similar findings were from Coulston et al. (2013), who examined differences between euthymic bipolar disorder and unipolar patients with respect to the inter-relationship between personality, coping style, and clinical outcomes. They found that compared to unipolar patients, bipolar disorder patients reported significantly higher scores on levels of extraversion, adaptive coping, self-esteem, and lower scores on trait anxiety and fear of negative evaluation. Moreover, extraversion was correlated positively with self-esteem, adaptive coping styles, and negatively with trait anxiety and fear of negative evaluation. Trait anxiety and fear of negative evaluation correlated positively with each other, and both correlated negatively with self-esteem and adaptive coping styles. Finally, self-esteem was correlated positively with adaptive coping styles.

On the other hand, empirical evidence has established the relationships between normal and disordered personality traits, for instance, between the normal personality traits measured through the Big-Five Model such as the Revised NEO Personality Inventory (Costa Jr and McCrae 1992; Jang and Livesley 1999) and the clinically defined personality disorders in the general and clinical populations (Kotov et al. 2010; Saulsman and Page 2004; Samuel and Widiger 2008). Huang et al. (2011) reported that the traits measured by the Zuckerman-Kuhlman Personality Questionnaire (ZKPQ, Zuckerman et al. 1993), a questionnaire measuring normal personality traits, were associated with the personality disorder functioning styles measured by the Parker Personality Measure (PERM, Parker and Hadzi-Pavlovic 2001). It is also reported that both normal personality and personality disorders were highly stable across the life span, and patients in therapy experienced no more personality change than did nonpatients (Ferguson 2010). One might wonder whether the CADP normal traits are associated with the disordered personality in Chinese healthy volunteers as well as in personality disorder patients.

A large body of literature describes the relationship between normal personality models, such as the Big-Five Model (e.g., Costa Jr and Widiger 2002), and abnormal personality (Larstone et al. 2002; Warner et al. 2004; for meta-analytic reviews, see Saulsman and Page 2004; Samuel and Widiger 2008). It has been suggested that the abnormal personalities are the extremes of normal personality variation (O'Connor and Dyce 2001; Miller et al. 2001; O'Connor 2005). Numerous results indicated that personality-descriptive models such as the Big-Five Model could capture substantial variance of personality pathology in adults (Costa Jr and Widiger 2002) and adolescents (de Clercq and de Fruyt 2003; Mervielde et al. 2005). For instance, to evaluate the relationships of the Big-Five model of the personality to personality disorders, 144 patients with personality disorders were asked to complete the NEO Five-Factor Inventory, an abbreviated version of the NEO Personality Inventory. Results indicated that the majority of the personality disorders can be differentiated using the Big-Five Model (Morey et al. 2000). Correlating the NEO Personality Inventory with the MMPI personality disorder scales and the Millon Clinical Multiaxial Inventory in adult volunteers, Costa Jr and McCrae (1990) reported that Openness to Experience was significantly correlated with the obsessive-compulsive, narcissistic, and antisocial personality disorders. Other findings revealed that Extraversion is highly consistent with the schizotypal, narcissistic, antisocial, avoidant, and passive-aggressive personality disorders (Widiger and Trull 1992); Conscientiousness is associated with the borderline, antisocial, obsessive-compulsive (Costa Jr and McCrae 1990), and passive-aggressive (Wiggins and Pincus 1989) personality disorders; Neuroticism is correlated with the paranoid, schizotypal, antisocial, borderline, narcissistic, and obsessive-compulsive personality disorders (Costa Jr and McCrae 1990); Agreeableness is associated with the antisocial, narcissistic, and dependent personality disorders (Widiger and Trull 1992; Costa Jr and McCrae 1992).

Based on these aforementioned findings, we therefore hypothesized that (1) CADP Intelligent is correlated with the PERM Paranoid, Schizotypal, Antisocial, Narcissistic, and Obsessive-Compulsive personality disorder functioning styles; (2) CADP Emotional with PERM Paranoid, Schizotypal, Antisocial, Borderline, Narcissistic, and Obsessive-Compulsive styles; (3) CADP Conscientious with PERM Borderline, Antisocial, Obsessive-Compulsive and Passive-Aggressive style; (4) CADP Unsocial with PERM Schizotypal, Narcissistic, Antisocial, Avoidant, and Passive-Aggressive styles; (5) CADP Agreeable with PERM Antisocial, Narcissistic, and Dependent styles; and (6) these correlations would be more pronounced in personality disorder patients. To prove these hypotheses, we therefore invited both healthy volunteers and personality disorder patients to undergo tests of CADP and PERM.

2 Methods

2.1 Participants

One hundred and ten healthy volunteers (60 women, 50 men; mean age, 20.78 years ±1.24 S.D., age range, 18–24 years) and 55 patients with personality disorders (30 women and 25 men; mean age, 20.82 ± 1.26, age range, 18–24) were invited to take part in the study. The healthy volunteers were not suffering or had suffered from any neurological or psychiatric problems through a brief interview, while the patients were diagnosed through the criteria of Diagnostic and Statistical Manual of Mental Disorders, Fifth Edition (American Psychiatric Association 2013). Among these patients, 6 patients were with the paranoid, 14 schizoid, 9 schizotypal, 3 antisocial, 5 borderline, 10 histrionic, 4 narcissistic, 6 avoidant, 9 dependent, 12 obsessive-compulsive and 11 passive-aggressive personality disorders. All participants were free from organic brain lesions according to recent magnetic resonance imaging or computed tomography scans, and were free from any antipsychotic drugs or alcohol for at least 72 h before taking the paper-pencil test. No age (t = −0.177, p = 0.86), gender (χ^2 = 0.000, p = 1.00) or education level (t = 0.47, p = 0.64) differences were found between the two groups.

2.2 Instruments

Participants were asked to complete the following questionnaires in a quiet room.

(A) The Chinese Adjective Descriptors of Personality (CADP), developed in Chap. "Personality Traits in Contemporary China: A Lexical Approach", with 100 Chinese adjectives, is designed to measure the personality traits such as the Intelligent, Emotional, Conscientious, Unsocial and Agreeable (20 adjectives each). Participants were asked to complete the rating items using the Likert type scales: 1-very unlike me, 2-moderately unlike me, 3-somewhat like and unlike me, 4-moderately like me, and 5-very like me. The internal alphas of each CADP factor in the two groups were satisfactory in the present study (see Results) as demonstrated in Chaps. "Personality Traits in Contemporary China: A Lexical Approach" and "Predicting Affective States of Bipolar Disorder by the Chinese Adjective Descriptors of Personality".

(B) The Parker Personality Measure (PERM, Parker and Hadzi-Pavlovic 2001), which measures 11 functioning styles of paranoid, schizoid, schizotypal, antisocial, borderline, histrionic, narcissistic, avoidant, dependent, obsessive-compulsive, and passive-aggressive personality disorders. Each PERM item has the same 5-point Likert scale as used in CADP measure. The internal alphas of each PERM scale in the two samples were satisfactory (Table 1) as reported previously (Wang et al. 2003; Huang et al. 2011).

(C) The Plutchik-van Praag Depression Inventory (PVP, Plutchik and van Praag 1987) contains 34 items; each item has a three-point scale (0, 1, 2), which corresponds to depressive tendencies. Participants have "possible depression" if they score between 20 and 25, or "depression" if they score higher than 25. The internal alpha of PVP was 0.93, which was also comparable to the previous report (Plutchik and van Praag 1987).

Table 1 Internal alphas and scale scores (Mean ± S.D.) of the Parker Personality Measure

	Healthy controls (n = 110)		Personality disorders (n = 55)		95% Confidence Interval
	Alpha	Score	Alpha	Score	
Paranoid	0.82	19.16 ± 6.06	0.76	28.31 ± 7.30*	−11.41 ~ −6.88
Schizoid	0.45	18.61 ± 3.78	0.54	22.89 ± 5.40*	−5.90 ~ −2.67
Schizotypal	0.67	9.15 ± 3.21	0.65	13.80 ± 4.44*	−5.98 ~ −3.31
Antisocial	0.74	17.56 ± 4.82	0.7	24.11 ± 6.39*	−8.49 ~ −4.60
Borderline	0.78	19.29 ± 5.59	0.78	28.96 ± 7.80*	−12.02 ~ −7.33
Histrionic	0.66	11.05 ± 3.34	0.5	16.09 ± 3.86*	−6.26 ~ −3.83
Narcissistic	0.78	14.69 ± 4.64	0.56	20.75 ± 4.96*	−7.65 ~ −4.46
Avoidant	0.8	23.30 ± 6.19	0.73	31.87 ± 7.02*	−10.79 ~ −6.36
Dependent	0.72	20.81 ± 5.22	0.75	27.98 ± 7.38*	−9.39 ~ −4.96
Obsessive-compulsive	0.6	16.17 ± 3.90	0.64	19.95 ± 4.32*	−5.15 ~ −2.40
Passive-aggressive	0.66	18.07 ± 4.58	0.78	24.64 ± 7.14*	−8.67 ~ −4.46

Note: *p < 0.05 vs. Healthy controls. After Fan et al. (2016)

2.3 Data Analyses and Statistics

Two-way ANOVA was applied to the five CADP trait or 11 PERM functioning style scores in the two groups (Group × Scale). Whenever a significant main effect was found, post-hoc analysis by the Student t test was employed to evaluate between-group differences. The Student t test was also employed to the mean PVP scores in the two groups. Inspired by a study (Schrijvers et al. 2010), we applied the multiple linear regression analysis (stepwise method) to search for the relationships between the five CADP traits and the 11 PERM scales, taking CADP traits as potential predictors for the PERM scales. A p value less than 0.05 was considered to be significant.

3 Results

The internal alphas of the five CADP traits were 0.97 for Intelligent, 0.92 for Emotional, 0.94 for Conscientious, 0.90 for Unsocial, and 0.92 for Agreeable in healthy controls; and in personality disorder patients the alphas were respectively, 0.96, 0.93, 0.93, 0.88, 0.85 for the same factors. The internal alphas of the 11 PERM functioning styles in both groups were also satisfactory (Table 1). The mean PVP score in personality disorder patients (16.60 ± 10.96 S.D.) was higher than that in healthy volunteers (7.70 ± 5.70 S.D., p < 0.001, 95% Confidence Interval (CI): −12.04 ~ −5.76).

Two-way ANOVA also detected significant differences of the five CADP traits in the two groups (group effect, F [1, 163] = 7.05, p = 0.009; mean square effect (MSE) = 1751.52; scale effect, F [4, 652] = 147.53, p < 0.001; MSE = 24350.80; and group × scale interaction effect, F [4, 652] = 18.53, p < 0.001; MSE = 3059.01). Post-hoc analysis revealed that personality disorders scored significantly higher than the controls did on the Emotional (p < 0.001, 95%CI: 16.50 ~ −5.83) and Unsocial (p < 0.001, 95%CI: −18.92 ~ −10.50) traits (Fig. 1).

Meanwhile, two-way ANOVA revealed significant differences of the 11 PERM styles between the two groups (group effect, F [1, 163] = 129.37, p < 0.001; MSE = 17027.84; scale effect, F [10, 1630] = 196.51, p < 0.001; MSE = 3413.80; and group × scale interaction effect, F [10, 1630] = 8.43, p < 0.001; MSE = 146.42). Post-hoc Student t test showed that personality disorder patients scored significantly higher than the healthy volunteers on all the personality disorder styles (all ps < 0.001; also see Table 1).

In healthy volunteers, PVP was significantly correlated with CADP Intelligent (r = −0.27, p = 0.005) and Unsocial (r = 0.24, p = 0.01) traits. It was also correlated with PERM Paranoid (r = 0.26, p = 0.006), Borderline (r = 0.27, p = 0.004), Dependent (r = 0.23, p = 0.015), and Obsessive-Compulsive (r = 0.25, p = 0.008) functioning styles. In personality disorder patients, PVP was significantly correlated with CADP Intelligent (r = −0.44, p = 0.001) trait, and PERM Borderline

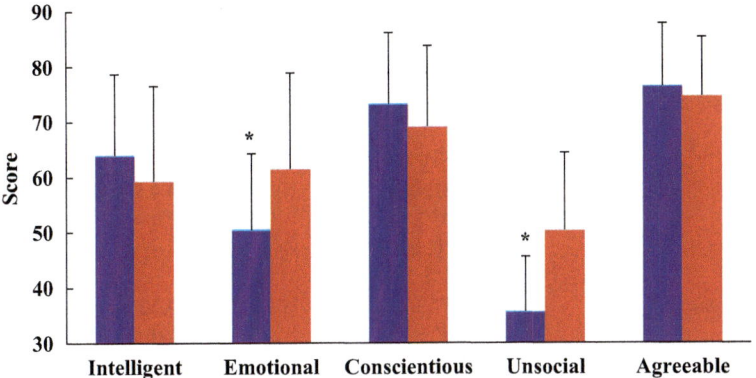

Fig. 1 A comparison of the scores in the Chinese Adjective Descriptors of Personality between healthy controls (violet bar; n = 110) and personality disorder patients (red bar; n = 55). *p < 0.05 vs. Healthy controls. (after Fan et al. 2016)

(r = 0.44, p = 0.001), Avoidant (r = 0.32, p = 0.02), and Dependent (r = 0.29, p = 0.03) functioning styles.

Considering the prediction of PERM functioning styles by CADP traits, the accounted variances (adjusted R^2 values) ranged from 0.06 to 0.40 in controls, and from 0.09 to 0.44 in personality disorder patients (Table 2). In personality disorder patients, most predictors of a given personality disorder functioning style were prominent (βs > 0.30) except for the trait of Agreeable; Intelligent predicted the Antisocial, Narcissistic, and Passive-Aggressive styles; Conscientious, the Obsessive-Compulsive and Passive-Aggressive (−) styles; Unsocial, the Schizotypal, Antisocial, Narcissistic, Avoidant, and Passive-Aggressive styles; Emotional, the Paranoid, Borderline, Histrionic, and Dependent styles. In controls, Unsocial (βs > 0.30) was the most prominent predictor of all the 11 PERM personality disorder styles. For instance, Unsocial predicted the Paranoid (β = 0.43), Schizotypal (0.43), Antisocial (0.51), Histrionic (0.42), Narcissistic (0.50), Avoidant (0.36), Dependent (0.47), Obsessive-Compulsive (0.39) and Passive-Aggressive (0.53) styles.

4 Discussion

We explored the potential predictability of the CADP traits to the personality disorder functioning styles in both personality disorder patients and healthy volunteers. The mean PVP score in personality disorder patients was higher than in healthy controls. Personality disorder patients scored significantly higher than the healthy volunteers did on the CADP Emotional and Unsocial traits and all 11 PERM functioning styles. PVP was significantly correlated with CADP Intelligent and Unsocial traits, and with PERM Paranoid, Borderline, Dependent, and Obsessive-Compulsive

Table 2 Stepwise multiple regressions predicting the Parker Personality Measure styles with the Chinese Adjective Descriptors of Personality traits in the healthy controls and the personality disorders

	Healthy controls (n = 110)		Personality disorders (n = 55)	
	Adjusted R^2	β (B, SE), predictors	Adjusted R^2	β (B, SE), predictors
Paranoid	0.18	**0.43 (0.31, 0.06) Unsocial****	0.39	**0.63 (0.32, 0.05) Emotional****
Schizoid	0.06	0.26 (0.20, 0.07) Unsocial**	–	–
Schizotypal	0.17	**0.43 (0.27, 0.05) Unsocial****	0.09	**0.32 (0.26, 0.10) Ensocial***
Antisocial	0.4	**0.51 (0.30, 0.05) Unsocial****	0.44	**0.51 (0.28, 0.07) Unsocial****
		−0.27 (−0.14, 0.05) Agreeable**		−0.22 (−0.16, 0.09) Agreeable
		0.39 (0.16, 0.04) Intelligent**		**0.48 (0.22, 0.06) Intelligent****
		−0.21 (−0.10, 0.05) Conscientious*		**−0.35 (−0.19, 0.07) Conscientious****
Borderline	0.3	0.29 (0.19, 0.06) Unsocial**	0.29	**0.55 (0.29, 0.06) Emotional****
		0.30 (0.14, 0.04) Emotional**		
		−0.22 (−0.10, 0.04) Intelligent*		
Histrionic	0.17	**0.42 (0.33, 0.07) Unsocial****	0.25	**0.52 (0.27, 0.06) Emotional****
Narcissistic	0.3	**0.50 (0.34, 0.06) Unsocial****	0.16	**0.43 (0.18, 0.06) Intelligent****
		0.35 (0.16, 0.04) Intelligent**		**0.34 (0.17, 0.07) Unsocial***
		−0.26 (−0.15, 0.05) Agreeable**		
Avoidant	0.12	**0.36 (0.28, 0.07) Unsocial****	0.15	**0.41 (0.25, 0.08) Unsocial****
Dependent	0.21	**0.47 (0.31, 0.06) Unsocial****	0.12	**0.37 (0.20, 0.07) Emotional****
Obsessive-compulsive	0.15	**0.39 (0.30, 0.07) Unsocial****	0.14	**0.39 (0.22, 0.07) Conscientious****
		0.26 (0.15, 0.05) Conscientious**		
Passive-aggressive	0.28	**0.53 (0.37, 0.06) Unsocial****	0.31	**0.43 (0.33, 0.09) Unsocial****
				0.67 (0.40, 0.09) Intelligent**
				−0.42 (−0.32, 0.10) Conscientious**

Note: *p < 0.05, **p < 0.01; βs valued larger than 0.30 were bolded for clarity; B and standardized error (SE) were unstandardized coefficients. After Fan et al. (2016)

functioning styles in healthy controls; while in personality disorder patients, it was significantly correlated with CADP Intelligent (−), and with PERM Borderline, Avoidant, and Dependent functioning styles. In personality disorder patients, four out five CADP predictors of personality disorder functioning style were prominent. These findings confirmed most of our hypotheses.

Patients scored significantly higher in PVP than the healthy volunteers did, which was in line with previous findings (Charney et al. 1981; Molinari and Marmion 1995; Depp and Jeste 2004). The PVP was also correlated with PERM Avoidant in the patients, which accorded with the high co-morbidity between avoidant personality disorder and major depression in clinics (Shea et al. 1987; Sanderson et al. 1994; Pepper et al. 1995). The correlation between PVP and CADP Unsocial in healthy volunteers, which agreed with the notion that the Unsocial represents the negative pole of extraversion (Costa and McCrae 1994) or Social Life (Rudowicz and Yue 2002), and extraversion negatively with depression (Cheng and Furnham 2003). In our healthy participants, PVP was also correlated with PERM Paranoid and Obsessive-Compulsive functioning styles. Indeed, major depression was frequently co-morbid with the paranoid and obsessive-compulsive personality disorders (Fava et al. 2002; Smulevich et al. 2012).

The Emotional and Unsocial scores were significantly elevated in personality disorder patients, which accorded with the finding that some personality disorders such as borderline, avoidant, and dependent types displayed higher neuroticism (Blais 1997), and that some personality disorders such as the narcissistic and histrionic types scored lower on extraversion (Saulsman and Page 2004).

Our results regarding prediction of PERM personality disorders by CADP traits were also quite interesting. Firstly, the Paranoid, Borderline, Histrionic, and Dependent personality disorders were strongly associated with the CADP Emotional trait in patients. In fact, neuroticism was consistently highly correlated with the paranoid, borderline, and dependent personality disorders in previous findings using, for example, NEO-PI-R or ZKPQ (Aluja et al. 2007a; b), and sometimes correlated with the histrionic personality disorder (Trobst et al. 2004). On the other hand, patients with paranoid, borderline, histrionic or dependent personality disorders have been shown to portray less emotional clarity, more difficulty in regulating emotional states, fewer emotional self-insights (Leible and Snell Jr 2004).

Secondly, the Schizotypal, Antisocial, Narcissistic, Avoidant, and Passive-Aggressive personality disorders were strongly associated with the CADP Unsocial trait in the patient group. Similarly, a relationship between extraversion (negative pole of the CADP Unsocial) and the schizotypal (−), antisocial, narcissistic and avoidant (−) personality disorders has been demonstrated in both healthy and patient samples (Trull 1992; Ball et al. 1997). Although an explicit explanation to the association between the Passive-Aggressive style and the Unsocial trait found in patients is still lacking, there are some evidences showing that avoidant (Aluja et al. 2007b) and passive-aggressive personality disorders were associated with neuroticism-anxiety (Aluja et al. 2007a). Moreover, the correlations between most facets of extraversion and the paranoid (−), dependent (−), and obsessive-compulsive (−) types were rather weak, which worked in concert with the current results, except histrionic (Aluja et al. 2007b). In clinics, the histrionic personality disorder, characterized by an excessive emotionality and attention seeking (American Psychiatric Association 2013), contrasted with the CADP Unsocial trait. The latter is characterized by the stupid, dull or inflexible behavior (see Chap. "Personality Traits in Contemporary China: A Lexical Approach").

Thirdly, the PERM Narcissistic, Antisocial, and Passive-Aggressive styles were strongly associated with the CDAP Intelligent trait in patients. In a previous study in healthy students, the PERM Narcissistic, Antisocial and Passive-Aggressive styles were co-loaded on a broad antisocial domain (Wang et al. 2003). Moreover, it has been revealed that the antisocial personality trait covers one part of the fierce and malicious traits, resembling the Machiavellian attitude (see Chap. "Adjectival Descriptors for Antisocial Personality Trait in Chinese Culture"). Machiavellian attitude, on the other hand, was correlated with the intelligence in western culture (Weinstock and Gharleghi 2013; Wilson et al. 1996).

Finally, the PERM Antisocial (−), Passive-Aggressive (−), and Obsessive-Compulsive styles were strongly associated with the Conscientious trait in patients. It has been shown that the conscientiousness was negatively correlated with the antisocial and passive-aggressive styles, and predicted workaholic characteristics (Lozano and Johnson 2001). On the other hand, the obsessive-compulsive personality disorder is linked with a maladaptive variant of normal-range conscientiousness (Samuel and Widiger 2011; Rector et al. 2002).

The current study design is only preliminary one and suffers from several design limitations. Firstly, subsample sizes of individual personality disorders were small and not equally distributed in number and age. A more extended recruitment of patients would make the current relationship clearer. Secondly, the internal reliability of the PERM Schizoid style was lower as in previous studies, which might also influence the current results. Thirdly, we did not include a group of non-Chinese people as controls. Nevertheless, our study has demonstrated that four out five CADP traits (except for Agreeable) were specifically associated with 10 out 11 personality disorder functioning styles (except for Schizoid), and the associations in patients were more specific and clearer. Therefore, our study indicated the validity of CADP for predicting personality disorder types, and warranted its application as an aid to diagnose personality disorders in China. In the next chapter, we will take as an example, the antisocial personality-related descriptions, for analyzing its trait domains in detail in Chinese context.

References

Aluja, A., Cuevas, L., García, L. F., & García, O. (2007a). Predictions of the MCMI-III personality disorders from NEO-PI-R domains and facets: Comparison between American and Spanish samples. *International Journal of Clinical and Health Psychology, 7*, 307–321.
Aluja, A., Cuevas, L., García, L. F., & García, O. (2007b). Zuckerman's personality model predicts MCMI-III personality disorders. *Personality and Individual Differences, 42*, 1311–1321.

American Psychiatric Association. (2013). *Diagnostic and statistical manual of mental disorder* (5th ed.). Washington, DC: American Psychiatric Association.

Armitage, C. J., Panagioti, M., Rahim, W. A., Rowe, R., & O'Connor, R. C. (2015). Completed suicides and self-harm in Malaysia: A systematic review. *General Hospital Psychiatry, 37*, 153–165.

Bains, J. (2005). Race, culture and psychiatry: A history of transcultural psychiatry. *History of Psychiatry, 16*, 139–154.

Ball, S. A., Tennen, H., Poling, J. C., Kranzler, H. R., & Rounsaville, B. J. (1997). Personality, temperament, and character dimensions and the DSM-IV personality disorders in substance abusers. *Journal of Abnormal Psychololgy, 106*, 545–553.

Barkow, G., Cosmides, L., & Tooby, J. (1992). *The adapted mind: Evolutionary psychology and the generation of culture*. New York: Oxford University Press.

Blais, M. A. (1997). Clinician ratings of the five-factor model of personality and the DSM-IV personality disorders. *Journal of Nervous and Mental Disease, 185*, 388–393.

Campbell, D. T. (1965). Variation and selective retention in socio-cultural evolution. In H. R. Barringer, G. Blanksten, & R. Mack (Eds.), *Social change in developing areas* (pp. 19–49). Cambridge: Schenkman.

Charney, D. S., Nelson, J. C., & Quinlan, D. M. (1981). Personality traits and disorder in depression. *American Journal of Psychiatry, 138*, 1601–1604.

Cheng, H., & Furnham, A. (2003). Personality, self-esteem, and demographic predictions of happiness and depression. *Personality and Individual Difference, 34*, 921–942.

Church, A. T. (2000). Culture and personality: Toward an integrated cultural trait psychology. *Journal of Personality, 68*, 651–703.

Costa, P. T., Jr., & McCrae, R. R. (1990). Personality disorders and the five-factor model of personality. *Journal of Personality Disorder, 4*, 362–371.

Costa, P. T., Jr., & McCrae, R. R. (1992). "Normal" personality assessment in clinical practice: The NEO Personality Inventory. *Psychological Assessment, 4*, 5–13.

Costa, P. T., Jr., & McCrae, R. R. (1994). *NEO Personality Inventory-Revised (NEO-PI-R) manual*. Odessa: Psychological Assessment Resources.

Costa, P. T., Jr., & Widiger, T. A. (2002). *Personality disorders and the five-factor model of personality*. Washington, DC: American Psychological Association.

Coulston, C. M., Bargh, D. M., Tanious, M., Cashman, E. L., Tufrey, K., Curran, G., Kuiper, S., Morgan, H., Lampe, L., & Malhi, G. S. (2013). Is coping well a matter of personality? A study of euthymic unipolar and bipolar patients. *Journal of Affective Disorders, 145*, 54–61.

de Clercq, B., & de Fruyt, F. (2003). Personality disorder symptoms in adolescence: A five-factor model perspective. *Journal of Personality Disorders, 17*, 269–292.

de Fruyt, F., de Clercq, B., de Bolle, M., Wille, B., Markon, K., & Krueger, R. F. (2013). General and maladaptive traits in a five-factor framework for DSM-5 in a university student sample. *Assessment, 20*, 295–307.

Depp, C. A., & Jeste, D. V. (2004). Bipolar disorder in older adults: A critical review. *Bipolar Disorders, 6*, 343–367.

Fan, H., Zhu, Q., Ma, G., Shen, C., Zhang, B., & Wang, W. (2016). Predicting personality disorder functioning styles by the Chinese Adjective Descriptors of Personality: A preliminary trial in healthy people and personality disorder patients. *BMC Psychiatry, 16*, 302.

Fava, M., Farabaugh, A. H., Sickinger, A. H., Wright, E., Alpert, J. E., Sonawalla, S., Nierenberg, A. A., & Worthington, J. J., III. (2002). Personality disorders and depression. *Psychological Medicine, 32*, 1049–1057.

Ferguson, C. J. (2010). A meta-analysis of normal and disordered personality across the life span. *Journal of Personality and Social Psychology, 98*, 659–667.

Geertz, C. (1974). "From the native's point of view": On the nature of anthropological understanding. *Bulletin of the American Academy of Arts and Sciences, 28*, 26–45.

Houri, D., Nam, E. W., Choe, E. H., Min, L. Z., & Matsumoto, K. (2012). The mental health of adolescent school children: A comparison among Japan, Korea, and China. *Global Health Promotion, 19*, 32–41.

Huang, Y., Kotov, R., de Girolamo, G., Preti, A., Angermeyer, M., Benjet, C., Demyttenaere, K., de Graaf, R., Gureje, O., Karam, A. N., Lee, S., Lépine, J. P., Matschinger, H., Posada-Villa, J., Suliman, S., Vilagut, G., & Kessler, R. C. (2009). DSM-IV personality disorders in the WHO World Mental Health Surveys. *British Journal of Psychiatry, 195*, 46–53.

Huang, J., He, W., Chen, W., Shen, M., & Wang, W. (2011). The Zuckerman-Kuhlman Personality Questionnaire predicts functioning styles of personality disorder: A trial in healthy subjects and personality-disorder patients. *Psychiatry Research, 186*, 320–325.

Jang, K. L., & Livesley, W. J. (1999). Why do measures of normal and disordered personality correlate? A study of genetic comorbidity. *Journal of Personality Disorders, 13*, 10–17.

Kluckhohn, C. (1954). Culture and behavior. In G. Lindzey (Ed.), *Handbook of social psychology (Chap. 2)* (pp. 921–976). Cambridge: Addison-Wesley.

Kotov, R., Gamez, W., Schmidt, F., & Watson, D. (2010). Linking "big" personality traits to anxiety, depressive, and substance use disorders: A meta-analysis. *Psychological Bulletin, 136*, 768–821.

Larstone, R. M., Jang, K. J., Livesley, W. J., Vernon, P. A., & Heike, W. (2002). The relationship between Eysenck's P-E-N model of personality, the five-factor model of personality, and traits delineating personality dysfunction. *Personality and Individual Differences, 33*, 25–37.

Leible, T. L., & Snell, W. E., Jr. (2004). Borderline personality disorder and multiple aspects of emotional intelligence. *Personality and Individual Difference, 37*, 393–404.

Lim, A. Y., Lee, A. R., Hatim, A., Tian-Mei, S., Liu, C. Y., Jeon, H. J., Udomratn, P., Bautista, D., Chan, E., Liu, S. I., Chua, H. C., & Hong, J. P. (2014). Clinical and sociodemographic correlates of suicidality in patients with major depressive disorder from six Asian countries. *BMC Psychiatry, 14*, 37.

Lozano, B. E., & Johnson, S. L. (2001). Can personality traits predict increases in manic and depressive symptoms. *Journal of Affective Disorders, 63*, 103–111.

Maniam, T., & Chan, L. F. (2013). Half a century of suicide studies-a plea for new directions in research and prevention. *Sains Malaysiana, 42*, 399–402.

Markus, H. R., Kitayama, S., & Heiman, R. (1996). Culture and "basic" psychological principles. In E. T. Higgins & A. W. Kruglanski (Eds.), *Social psychology: Handbook of basic principles* (pp. 857–913). New York: Guilford.

Mazzotti, D. R., Guindalini, C., Sosa, A. L., Ferri, C. P., & Tufik, S. (2012). Prevalence and correlates for sleep complaints in older adults in low and middle income countries: A 10/66 Dementia Research Group study. *Sleep Medicine, 13*, 697–702.

Mervielde, I., de Clercq, B., de Fruyt, F., & van Leeuwen, K. (2005). Temperament, personality, and developmental psychopathology as childhood antecedents of personality disorders. *Journal of Personality Disorders, 19*(2), 171–201.

Michael, B. R., Bindseil, K., Schuller, D. R., Rector, N. A., Trevor, Y. L., Cooke, R. G., Seeman, M., McCay, E. A., & Joffe, R. (1997). Relationship between the five-factor model of personality and unipolar, bipolar and schizophrenic patients. *Psychiatry Research, 70*, 83–94.

Miller, J. D., Lyman, D. R., Widiger, T. A., & Leukefeld, C. (2001). Personality disorders as extreme variants of common personality dimensions: Can the five factor model adequately represent psychopathy. *Journal of personality, 69*, 253–276.

Molinari, V., & Marmion, J. (1995). Relationship between affective disorders and Axis II diagnoses in geropsychiatric patients. *Journal of Geriatric Psychiatry and Neurology, 8*, 61–64.

Morey, L. C., Gunderson, J., Quigley, B. D., & Lyons, M. (2000). Dimensions and categories: The "big five" factors and the DSM personality disorders. *Assessment, 7*, 203–216.

O'Connor, B. P. (2005). A search for consensus on the dimensional structure of personality disorders. *Journal of Clinical Psychology, 61*, 323–345.

O'Connor, B. P., & Dyce, J. A. (2001). Rigid and extreme: A geometric representation of personality disorders in five-factor model space. *Journal of Personality and Social Psychology, 81*, 1119–1130.

Oyserman, D. (2011). Culture as situated cognition: Cultural mindsets, cultural fluency, and meaning making. *European Review of Social Psychology, 22*, 164–214.

Packer, M., & Cole, M. (2016). Culture in development. In M. H. Bornstein & M. E. Lamb (Eds.), *Social and personality development: An advanced textbook* (7th ed., pp. 67–124). New York: Psychology Press.

Parker, G., & Hadzi-Pavlovic, D. (2001). A question of style: Refining the dimensions of personality disorder style. *Journal of Personality Disorders, 15*, 300–318.

Pepper, C. M., Klein, D. N., Anderson, R. L., & Riso, L. P. (1995). DSM-III-R axis II comorbidity in dysthymia and major depression. *American Journal of Psychiatry, 152*, 239–247.

Plutchik, R., & van Praag, H. M. (1987). Interconvertability of five self-report measures of depression. *Psychiatry Research, 22*, 243–256.

Rector, N. A., Hood, K., Richter, M. A., & Michael Bagby, R. (2002). Obsessive-compulsive disorder and the five-factor model of personality: Distinction and overlap with major depressive disorder. *Behaviour Research and Therapy, 40*, 1205–1219.

Rudowicz, E., & Yue, X. (2002). Compatibility of Chinese and creative personalities. *Creativity Research Journal, 14*, 387–394.

Samuel, D. B., & Widiger, T. A. (2008). A meta-analytic review of the relationships between the five-factor model and DSM-IV-TR personality disorders: A facet level analysis. *Clinical Psychology Review, 28*, 1326–1342.

Samuel, D. B., & Widiger, T. A. (2011). Conscientiousness and obsessive-compulsive personality disorder. *Personality Disorders: Theory, Research, and Treatment, 2*, 161–174.

Sanderson, W. C., Wetzler, S., Beck, A. T., & Betz, F. (1994). Prevalence of personality disorders among patients with anxiety disorders. *Psychiatry Research, 51*, 167–174.

Saulsman, L. M., & Page, A. C. (2004). The five-factor model and personality disorder empirical literature: A meta-analytic review. *Clinical Psychology Review, 23*(8), 1055–1085.

Schrijvers, D. L., de Bruijn, E. R., Destoop, M., Hulstijn, W., & Sabbe, B. G. C. C. (2010). The impact of perfectionism and anxiety traits on action monitoring in major depressive disorder. *Journal of Neural Transmission, 117*, 869–880.

Shea, M. T., Glass, D. R., Pilkonis, P. A., Watkins, J., & Docherty, J. P. (1987). Frequency and implications of personality disorders in a sample of depressed outpatients. *Journal of Personality Disorders, 1*, 27–42.

Smulevich, A. B., Dubnitskaia, E. B., & Chitlova, V. V. (2012). Personality disorders and depression. *Zhurnal nevrologii i psikhiatrii imeni SS Korsakova, 112*, 4–11.

Triandis, H. C., & Suh, E. M. (2002). Cultural influences on personality. *Annual Review of Psychology, 53*, 133–160.

Trobst, K. K., Ayearst, L. E., & Salekin, R. T. (2004). Where is the personality in personality disorder assessment? A comparison across four sets of personality disorder scales. *Multivariate Behavioral Research, 39*, 231–271.

Trull, T. J. (1992). DSM-III-R personality disorders and the five-factor model of personality: An empirical comparison. *Journal of Abnormal Psychology, 101*, 553–560.

Tsai, S. Y., Chen, C. C., & Yeh, E. K. (1997). Alcohol problems and long-term psychosocial outcome in Chinese patients with bipolar disorder. *Journal of Affective Disorders, 46*, 143–150.

Wang, Q. (2016). How not to have nostalgia for the future: A reading of Lu Xun's "Hometown". *Frontiers of Literary Studies in China, 10*, 461–473.

Wang, W., Hu, L., Mu, L., Chen, D., Song, Q., Zhou, M., & He, C. (2003). Functioning styles of personality disorders and five-factor normal personality traits: A correlation study in Chinese students. *BMC Psychiatry, 3*, 11.

Warner, M. B., Morey, L. C., Finch, J. F., Gunderson, J. G., Skodol, A. E., Sanislow, C. A., Shea, M. T., McGlashan, T. H., & Grilo, C. M. (2004). The longitudinal relationship of personality traits and disorders. *Journal of Abnormal Psychology, 113*, 217–227.

Weinstock, M., & Gharleghi, M. (2013). Intelligent cities and the taxonomy of cognitive scales. *Architectural Design, 83*, 56–65.

Widiger, T. A., & Trull, T. J. (1992). Personality and psychopathology: An application of the five-factor model. *Journal of Personality, 60*, 363–393.

Wiggins, J. S., & Pincus, A. L. (1989). Conceptions of personality disorders and dimensions of personality. *Psychological Assessment, 1*, 305–316.

Wilson, D. S., Near, D., & Miller, R. R. (1996). Machiavellianism: A synthesis of the evolutionary and psychological literatures. *Psychological Bulletin, 119*, 285–299.

Zuckerman, M., Kuhlman, D. M., Joireman, J., Teta, P., & Kraft, M. (1993). A comparison of three structural models for personality: The Big Three, the Big Five, and the Alternative Five. *Journal of Personality and Social Psychology, 65*, 757–768.

Adjectival Descriptors for Antisocial Personality Trait in Chinese Culture

Chu Wang, Shaohua Yu, and Wei Wang

1 Introduction

In the previous two chapters, we have developed the Chinese Adjective Descriptors of Personality (CADP) to measure normal personality traits through Chinese adjectives, and used CADP traits successfully to predict personality disorder functioning styles in both healthy volunteers and personality disorder patients. We further question whether the Chinese adjectives could describe one type personality disorder by illustrating the related trait domains. The antisocial personality disorder might serve as an example for this purpose. The disorder is characterized by "a pervasive pattern of disregard for, and violation of, the rights of others that begins in childhood or early adolescence and continues into adulthood", and patients with antisocial personality disorder are generally prone to criminal, delinquent, or aggressive acts, and associated with low socioeconomic status and urban settings, often harm others and threaten the maintaining of the social stability and harmony (American Psychiatric Association 2013). As we have depicted in Chapter "Narrations of Personality Disorders in a Dream of Red Mansions", the antisocial personality disorder was prominent and well-described in the late imperial China, and explained with characters of A Dream of Red Mansions. It is also of great significance to illustrate antisocial personality disorder and its possible structure in the contemporary China.

On the other hand, the Diagnostic and Statistical Manual of Mental Disorders, Fifth Edition (DSM-5, American Psychiatric Association, 2013) presents a dimensional trait model of personality disorders in Section III. According to this model,

C. Wang · W. Wang (✉)
Department of Clinical Psychology and Psychiatry/School of Public Health, Zhejiang University College of Medicine, Hangzhou, China
e-mail: drwangwei@zju.edu.cn

S. Yu
Department of Psychiatry, The Second Affiliated Hospital, Zhejiang University College of Medicine, Hangzhou, China

© Springer Nature Singapore Pte Ltd. 2019
W. Wang (ed.), *Chinese Perspectives on Cultural Psychiatry*,
https://doi.org/10.1007/978-981-13-3537-2_8

personality disorders are partly characterized by 25 maladaptive traits contained in five broad domains, namely Negative Affectivity, Detachment, Antagonism, Disinhibition, and Psychoticism. These traits are considered as maladaptive variants of the five domains of the Big-Five Model and as similar to the domains of the Personality Psychopathology Five (American Psychiatric Association 2013). Several studies have shown that the traits of antisocial personality are characterized by manipulativeness, callousness, deceitfulness, hostility, risk taking, impulsivity and irresponsibility in DSM-5 (Swann et al. 2009; Lynam and Vachon 2012; Anderson et al. 2014). At the same time, the connection between antisocial personality and psychopathy is established in documentation (Verona et al. 2001; Crocker et al. 2005; Coid and Ullrich 2010; Shepherd et al. 2018). Traditionally, psychopathy was defined as a cluster of inferred personality traits and socially deviant behaviors. Hare (1991) put forward that psychopathy was based on interpersonal, affective, and behavioral, Cooke and Michie (2001) developed a three-factor model of psychopathy as arrogant and deceitful interpersonal style, deficient affective experience, and impulsive and irresponsible behavioral style. On the other hand, the development of the Psychopathy Checklist-Revised (PCL-R, Hare 1991, 2003) has provided a reliable and valid assessment for the psychopathology constructs. The antisocial personality disorder has been trialed to correlate with PCL-R measures, and four dimensions are clearly presented as Interpersonal, Affective, Antisocial and Lifestyle (Gacono 1998; Hare 2003; Morana et al. 2006; Shepherd et al. 2018).

Furthermore, there might be some features specific to a given language and culture when involving antisocial behavior or personality. For example, the Chinese society, where Confucian teachings have been considered as the philosophical basis for Collectivism, is often treated as the prototypical collectivistic culture (Wang and Liu 2010). People in this culture have higher collectivistic attitude compared to several other cultures (Tu et al. 2011; Hsu and Barker 2013). The collectivistic people often make decisions based on the group, recognize the extended family as equally or more important, see themselves as interdependent, value harmony, and seek to fit into their society (Hsu and Barker 2013). Referring to communication strategies, they are more likely to encourage, give credit, and tend to appeal to win-win solutions in conflict situations than people in individualist cultures (Wang and Liu 2010). Their behaviors are often self-effacing and modest, because modesty is considered to be important to maintain group cohesiveness in a collectivistic society (Lee et al. 1997). In Chinese culture, the modesty is likely owing to the Chinese traditional values (Lee et al. 2001). Such manners might be contrary to antisocial personality traits, such as aggressive, assaulting or self-centered (Ma et al. 1996; Li et al. 2010). Cross-cultural results have also shown that compared to Canadian adults, Chinese adults gave less positive ratings to confessing their misdeeds, because they thought that such confessions did not redeem the negativity of bad behaviors, although they believe that it was commendable (Fu et al. 2001). In addition to masculinity/femininity trait between gender which also identifies cultural differences (Hofstede 1980), there was some evidence showing that males gained more antisocial behaviors and features than females did (Leahy et al. 2010; Mobarake 2015).

Therefore, the study purpose of the current chapter was to measure the antisocial personality traits in Chinese culture. As reported by McCrae (2004), personality trait which shows differences between individuals can be measured through self- or peer-reported questionnaires. Among several approaches to measure personality structure, the lexical approach has proven to be valid and fairly widely accepted among studies exploring major dimensions of personality (Ashton and Lee 2005; also see Chapter "Personality Traits In Contemporary China: A Lexical Approach"). The approach postulates that all significant individual and cultural differences embody in natural languages (de Raad 2000; Saucier and Goldberg 2001; Cheung et al. 2011; Saucier 2018). The application of lexical approach to normal personality generated the Big-Five structure and demonstrated its universality and equivalence among multiple cultures (Whitmore et al. 2004; Ashton and Lee 2005; Piedmont and Aycock 2007; Church 2016). As the extension of normal personality, personality disorders encountered in clinics also can be characterized by natural language adjectival descriptors (Moran 1999; Cooke et al. 2012; American Psychiatric Association 2013). Lexical approach generally adopts descriptive adjectives or adjectival phrases from natural languages to describe the personality structure, such as from dictionaries (Mlačić and Ostendorf 2005; Burtaverde 2016, also see Chapter "Personality Traits In Contemporary China: A Lexical Approach") or from theoretical writings (Craig and Olson 2001, also see Chapters "Personality Traits Characterized by the Adjectives in a Dream of Red Mansions" and "Narrations of Personality Disorders in a Dream of Red Mansions"). We used a variant of these methods, analysis of Chinese dictionaries to explore in which way antisocial personality traits is manifested in the Chinese language. We have hypothesized that: (1) with the antisocial personality adjectives in Chinese language, we could derive three or four factors; (2) males scored significantly higher on these factors and there might be some correlations between these factors.

2   Study 1: Adjectival Descriptors Selection

2.1   Participants

In order to rate the adjectives representing antisocial personality traits (see below), we have invited 301 undergraduate students from Eastern (Hangzhou and Hefei), Western (Taiyuan), Southern (Haikou) and Northern (Harbin) regions of China (180 women, mean age 19.8 years ±1.3 SD, age range, 17–22 years; 121 men, mean age 20.1 ± 1.4, age range, 17–22) to participant in the study. Participants were majoring in Arts, Education, Foreign Languages, Mechanics, Modern Medicine, or Traditional Chinese Medicine. All participants were free from somatic or psychiatric illnesses and were drug or alcohol free for at least 72 h prior to the test.

2.2   Measures

"The Modern Chinese Dictionary and Its Supplements" (Beijing, The Commercial Publishing House 1998) and "A Chinese English Dictionary, Revised Edition" (Beijing, Foreign Language Teaching and Research Press 1995) were used to select the adjectives describing antisocial personality. Former studies (Angleitner et al. 1990; Saucier and Goldberg 2001) suggested that adjectives had to fit the stem sentence such as "He/She is [adjective] by nature," or "What kind of person is He/She? He/She is [adjective]." Seven contributors of this book (two women and five men; three Ph.D. holders, one M.Sc. holder, two Ph.D. candidates, and one M.Sc. candidate in psychology) including three coauthors of this chapter served as judges. The 80 antisocial personality adjectives identified by an experienced psychiatrist from the two dictionaries were then evaluated by six other judges. If more than three judges evaluated an adjective as infrequently used, it was eliminated. The remaining adjectives were then evaluated by all seven judges and by the authors before being listed to the word pool. All synonyms were aggregated and the adjectives were dropped until all judges and authors agreed that there was no awkward, less-frequently used, or slang adjective. The resulting 48 adjectives in the word pool were considered exhaustive, since no remaining words could be dropped and no new words could be added.

Participants were asked to rate the resulting 48 adjectives in a quiet room, using a five-point Likert rating scale: 1-very unlike me, 2-moderately unlike me, 3-somewhat like and unlike me, 4-moderately like me, and 5-very like me.

2.3   Statistical Analyses

Answers to the 48 adjectives were subjected to the principal component analysis. The factor loadings were rotated orthogonally using the varimax normalized methods.

2.4   Results

The principal component analysis yielded 12 eigenvalues greater than 1.0, and the scree test had suggested a three-factor solution. The eigenvalues of first five factors were 12.9, 3.1, 2.4, 1.7, and 1.6 respectively, with the first three factors altogether accounted for 38.2% of the total variance. None of the remaining components accounted for more than 3.5% of the variance.

After the varimax normalized methods, three factors were obtained. The first factor, labeled Intolerant, was defined by adjectives such as Intolerant (0.71), Oversensitive (0.67), and Paranoid (0.67). The second factor, labeled Assaulting, was defined by Belligerent (0.68), Assaulting (0.66), and Apt to struggle (0.59). The third factor, labeled Fierce and Malicious, was defined by high loadings of Cruel (0.67), Fierce and Malicious (0.67), Wily (0.63), and Cold-blooded (0.63). Based on the ten adjectives with the highest loadings on each factor, we developed a thirty-adjective inventory, the Chinese Adjectival Descriptors for Antisocial Personality Trait (CADAP) (Table 1).

3 Study 2: Testing of the Chinese Adjectival Descriptors for Antisocial Personality Trait

Since the numbers of adjectival descriptors were reduced, which might cause a change of the general matrix structure, the CADAP was administered to another group of university students in the four geographical regions of China.

3.1 Participants

From the same universities as in Study 1, we invited 448 undergraduate students (302 women, mean age 19.3 ± 1.1, age range, 17–23; 146 men, mean age 19.6 ± 1.4, age range, 15–25) to participate in this study. They were majoring in the same subjects as participants in Study 1. All participants were free from somatic or psychiatric illnesses and were asked to be drug or alcohol free for at least 72 h prior to the test.

3.2 Measures

Participants were asked to complete the Chinese Adjectival Descriptors for Antisocial Personality Trait (CADAP) in a quiet room, using a five-point Likert rating scale: 1-very unlike me, 2-moderately unlike me, 3-somewhat like and unlike me, 4-moderately like me, and 5-very like me.

3.3 Statistical Analyses

Answers to the CADAP items were subjected to the principal component analysis. The factor loadings were rotated orthogonally using the varimax normalized methods. Once factors and the related items were identified, their scores were calculated in each gender group. The internal reliabilities (the Cronbach alphas) for each factor

Table 1 Principal component analysis on the 48 adjectives in 301 students

Chinese adjective (English translation)	Factor I Intolerant	Factor II Assaulting	Factor III Fierce and Malicious
爱吵架的 Quarrelsome	0.46	0.16	0.33
爱打架的 Fighting	0.03	0.16	0.43
爱将人军的 Fond of cornering people	0.33	0.51	−0.07
霸道的 High-handed	0.38	0.21	0.49
暴戾的 Ruthless and tyrannical	0.35	0.13	0.59
猜疑的 Suspicious	0.57	0.08	−0.01
残酷的 Cruel	0.19	0.03	0.67
残忍的 Cold-blooded	0.21	0.07	0.63
粗鲁的 Rude	0.46	0.14	0.45
刁悍的 Cunning and fierce	0.18	0.30	0.54
刁滑的 Crafty	0.30	0.18	0.56
刁顽的 Cunning and stubborn	0.48	0.10	0.44
多疑的 Paranoid	0.67	0.22	0.06
反复无常的 Capricious	0.55	0.06	0.16
放荡不羁的 Wild and unconventional	−0.07	0.11	0.42
攻击性强的 Aggressive	0.07	0.57	0.42
乖僻的 Eccentric	0.52	0.09	0.17
诡计多端的 Tricky	0.04	0.32	0.44
好斗的 Belligerent	0.18	0.68	0.20
好胜的 Contending	0.15	0.57	−0.08

(continued)

Table 1 (continued)

Chinese adjective (English translation)	Factor I Intolerant	Factor II Assaulting	Factor III Fierce and Malicious
好战的 Bellicose	0.10	0.58	0.34
好争论的 Argumentative	0.18	0.55	−0.07
记仇的 Hatred-bearing	0.45	0.17	0.30
奸诈的 Wily	0.25	0.10	0.63
尖刻的 Caustic	0.50	0.17	0.24
狡猾的 Cunning	0.19	0.25	0.59
狡狯的 Sly	0.13	0.17	0.27
狡黠的 Astute	0.24	0.16	0.53
狡诈的 Fraudulent	0.01	0.14	0.56
进攻性的 Assaulting	0.14	0.66	0.23
苛刻的 Overcritical	0.49	0.09	0.36
刻薄的 Mean	0.40	0.11	0.51
蛮横的 Rude and unreasonable	0.30	0.16	0.33
泼妇似的 Shrewish	0.23	0.07	0.41
气量狭小的 Intolerant	0.71	0.03	0.10
善于斗争的 Apt at struggle	−0.01	0.59	0.31
善战的 Good at fighting	−0.08	0.58	0.32
嗜赌的 Gambling-thirsty	0.20	0.22	0.33
狭隘的 Narrow-minded	0.57	−0.06	0.14
心肠坏的 Malicious	0.23	0.09	0.47

(continued)

Table 1 (continued)

Chinese adjective (English translation)	Factor I Intolerant	Factor II Assaulting	Factor III Fierce and Malicious
心地狭窄的 Small-minded	0.65	−0.02	0.17
心毒的 Vicious	0.23	0.04	0.54
心眼窄的 Over-sensitive	0.67	0.10	0.20
凶暴的 Fierce and brutal	0.48	0.14	0.49
凶残的 Brutal	0.08	0.03	0.57
凶狠的 Fierce and malicious	0.27	−0.02	0.67
有心计的 Calculating	−0.07	0.50	0.20
专断的 Arbitrary	0.20	0.30	0.47
Eigenvalue	12.9	3.1	2.4
% of the total variance	26.9	6.4	4.9

After Yu et al. (2009)

were also calculated in all participants. The gender difference of individual factor scores was evaluated by two-way ANOVA (i.e., gender × factor score). Once a significant main effect was detected, the Student t test was employed as a means of post-hoc comparison. Moreover, the Pearson correlation test was used to search for possible relationships within three factors. A p value less than 0.05 was considered to be significant.

3.4 Results

The principal component analysis yielded seven eigenvalues greater than 1.0. The first five factors had eigenvalues of 7.5, 2.8, 2.0, 1.2, and 1.2, respectively, and the scree plot indicated a leveling-off after the fourth factor. None of the remaining factors accounted for more than 4.0% of the variance. The first three factors were similar to those identified in study 1, which accounting for 40.7% of the total variance (Table 2).

All the adjectives had loadings higher than 0.30 on their target factors. The internal alphas were 0.85, 0.81, and 0.81 for Fierce and Malicious, Assaulting, and Intolerant, respectively. Two-way ANOVA detected significant gender differences (group effect, F $(1, 446) = 4.99$, $p < 0.01$). The post-hoc Student t test showed that men scored significantly higher on Fierce and Malicious (14.9 ± 5.7 versus

Table 2 Principal component analysis on the 30 adjectives (the Chinese Adjectival Descriptors for Antisocial Personality Trait) in 448 students

Chinese adjective (English translation)	Factor I Fierce and Malicious	Factor II Assaulting	Factor III Intolerant
凶狠的 Fierce and malicious	**0.70**	0.12	0.17
狡猾的 Cunning	**0.67**	0.07	0.18
凶残的 Brutal	**0.66**	0.01	0.03
残忍的 Cold-blooded	**0.65**	0.12	0.24
奸诈的 Wily	**0.65**	0.13	0.19
残酷的 Cruel	**0.59**	0.12	0.16
心毒的 Vicious	**0.57**	0.04	0.15
狡诈的 Fraudulent	**0.56**	0.08	0.23
刁滑的 Crafty	**0.55**	0.20	0.19
暴戾的 Ruthless and tyrannical	**0.48**	0.20	0.26
进攻性的 Assaulting	0.22	**0.69**	0.09
攻击性强的 Aggressive	0.21	**0.69**	0.12
好战的 Bellicose	0.21	**0.69**	0.11
善于斗争的 Apt at struggle	0.29	**0.62**	−0.04
好胜的 Contending	−0.27	**0.62**	0.09
善战的 Good at fighting	0.24	**0.59**	0.00
好争论的 Argumentative	−0.06	**0.58**	−0.03
好斗的 Belligerent	0.06	**0.58**	0.13
爱将人军的 Fond of cornering people	0.12	**0.39**	0.21
有心计的 Calculating	0.34	**0.30**	0.08

(continued)

Table 2 (continued)

Chinese adjective (English translation)	Factor I Fierce and Malicious	Factor II Assaulting	Factor III Intolerant
气量狭小的 Intolerant	0.10	0.08	**0.75**
心眼窄的 Over-sensitive	0.15	0.08	**0.74**
多疑的 Paranoid	0.09	0.08	**0.68**
心地狭窄的 Small-minded	0.24	0.05	**0.63**
狭隘的 Narrow-minded	0.15	0.00	**0.62**
猜疑的 Suspicious	0.08	0.02	**0.58**
苛刻的 Overcritical	0.36	0.20	**0.46**
乖僻的 Eccentric	0.24	0.17	**0.40**
反复无常的 Capricious	0.20	0.04	**0.37**
尖刻的 Caustic	0.26	0.20	**0.36**
Eigenvalue	7.5	2.8	2.0
% of the total variance	24.8	9.2	6.7

After Yu et al. (2009)

13.9 ± 5.5, $p < 0.05$) and Assaulting (26.7 ± 7.2 versus 25.1 ± 7.2, $p < 0.05$) than women did. However, there was no gender difference on Intolerant (20.7 ± 6.5 versus 20.8 ± 6.8, $p > 0.05$). The Pearson correlation test revealed that the Fierce and Malicious factor was significant-positively correlated with Assaulting (n = 448, $r = 0.41$, $p < 0.05$) and Intolerant ($r = 0.56$, $p < 0.05$); Assaulting was also significantly correlated with Intolerant ($r = 0.33$, $p < 0.05$) (Fig. 1).

4   Discussion

Through analyzing the 48 antisocial personality-related Chinese adjectives in Study 1, we have clearly demonstrated a three-factor (scale) – structured questionnaire measuring antisocial personality traits in Chinese culture (CADAP). The three factors, namely Intolerant, Assaulting, and Fierce and Malicious, supported our first hypothesis. In Study 2, using the 30-adjective CADAP, the three-factor model was again confirmed with satisfactory internal reliabilities. Men scored significantly

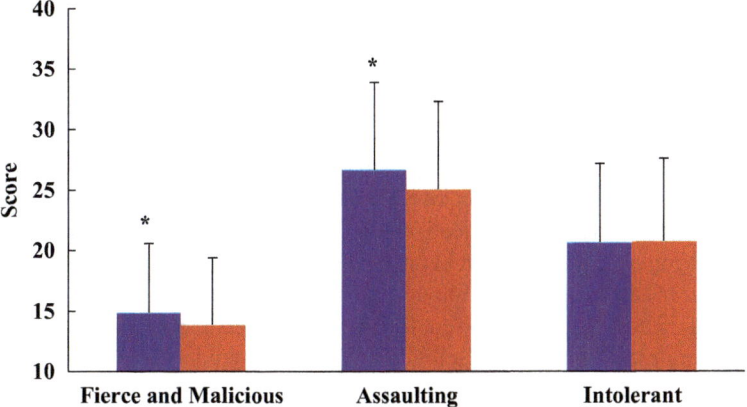

Fig. 1 Scale scores (mean ± S.D.) of the three CADAP factors in men (violet bars, n = 146) and women (red bars, n = 302). *, $p < 0.05$ vs. Women. (After Yu et al. 2009)

higher on Fierce and Malicious and Assaulting factors and the significant correlations between the three factors supported our second hypothesis.

The three-factor structure of CADAP showed some resemblance to the structures of Psychopathy (Hare and Neumann 2005). The Fierce and Malicious factor is comparable to the Affective factor (e.g., lack of remorse or guilt, shallow affect, callous/ lack of empathy, failure to accept responsibility for actions) in PCL-R; Assaulting to Antisocial (poor behavior controls, early behavior problems, juvenile delinquency, revocation of conditional release, criminal versatility), and Intolerant to Interpersonal (glib/superficial charm, grandiose self-worth, pathological lying, conning/manipulative). However, we did not detect a factor that could be comparable to the Lifestyle factor (stimulation seeking, impulsivity, irresponsible, parasitic orientation, lack of realistic goals). On the other hand, the four-factor PCL-R model can be used to explore the relationships between the emergence of early antisocial tendencies and development of other psychopathic personality features in previous longitudinal research (Hare and Neumann 2005). For example, traits such as callousness and impulsivity in psychopathy are predictors of future antisocial behavior (Vitacco et al. 2002; Frick et al. 2003).

The factor Fierce and Malicious conveying the emotion aspect of antisocial personality was corresponded partly to antisocial personality disorder in DSM-5 (American Psychiatric Association 2013). Adjectives including Cruel, Fierce and malicious, Brutal, Cold-blooded and Ruthless which indicated disregard for others, the unconcern for the feelings of others, and the lack of the capacity for empathy were in accordance with the Callousness traits representing lack of concern for feelings or problems of others and lack of guilt or remorse. Cunning, Wily, Fraudulent, and Crafty which conveying the expressions of lying, and frequent-using of aliases were comparable to Deceitfulness traits. This factor was also comparable to the Machiavellian attitude representing domineering, impersonal, suspicious, practical, cold, impersonal, exploitative and so on (Wilson et al. 1996), which was considered to be relevant with antisocial behaviors (Lau and Marsee 2013). Similarly, in Hungarian culture, adjectives like cunning, wily, and crafty were also found to be associated with antisocial behaviors in emotional aspect (Szirmák and de Raad 1994).

The Assaulting factor appeared to represent the aggressive component of antisocial personality disorder. Assaulting and Aggressive were the most prominent behavior characteristics of antisocial personality disorder and often used to evaluate antisocial personality traits. Adjectives under this factor were similar to Hostility trait conveying persistent or frequent angry feelings and Impulsivity trait conveying acting on a momentary basis without a plan or consideration of outcomes. Apt to struggle, Contending, and Good at fighting illustrated the trends to involve into power struggles. Bellicose and Belligerent showing a tendency to stir up problems, also reported by former study (Craig and Olson 2001). Individuals scoring high on this factor were also considered to be quarrelsome, which appeared to be related to findings of Italian (di Blas 2005) and Dutch (de Raad and Hoskens 1990; de Raad 1992) studies that traits such as Quarrelsome were negative features of the Agreeableness domain in the Big-Five model. People with Assaulting factor tended to damage relationships with others, which was opposite to collectivism culture.

The factor Intolerant including adjectives showing the relationships with others such as Small-minded, Narrow-minded, and Overcritical that implied the irresponsibility for mistakes and the tendency to blame others for personal failures. Oversensitive and Capricious loading in this factor expressed the instability of emotion, people with these traits might be unreliable and untrustworthy. These adjectives were also reported in former studies measuring normal personality traits in Turkish (Goldberg and Somer 2000) and Croatian cultures (Mlačić and Ostendorf 2005) in order to represent the negative features of Agreeableness domain. Adjectives including Paranoid and Suspicious were used to characterize the cognitive aspect of antisocial personality disorder, and were opposite to Agreeableness as well (Blackburn and Fawcett 1999; Shedler and Westen 2004). Tolerant, the antonym of Intolerant, was also found in Dutch (de Raad 1992), French (Boies et al. 2001), Italian (Caprara and Perugini 1994) and Turkey (Goldberg and Somer 2000) cultures, as the trait of Agreeableness domain. Tolerance is a virtue in relationship, "Be strict with yourself and lenient towards others" is also the important norm in Chinese culture.

The gender differences between Fierce and Malicious and Assaulting were in accordance with former studies demonstrated that males had more antisocial behaviors and criminal activities than females did (Heidensohn 1997; Barriga et al. 2001; Mobarake 2015). Generally speaking, males were less emotional than females (Campbell 2006). It might be due to the role of a strict father and a loving mother in Chinese traditional family. When faced with dangers, females were less able to cope with fear (Campbell 2006), leading to less violence. The reasons above could be used to explain that females had lower scale scores on Fierce and Malicious and Assaulting than males did. In addition, the inter-correlations between Fierce and Malicious, Assaulting, and Intolerant factors were in line with previous studies showing the significant correlation between the PCL-R dimensions (Hare and

Neumann 2006, 2008), and also in accordance with studies showing the dimensions in PCL-R were all associated with violence (Kennealy et al. 2010).

However, one might also bear in mind several limitations of the present study design. Firstly, our participants were college students, therefore, the results therefore might not be simply generalized to other age populations. Secondly, all data came from self-reports, which might be subject to recall bias or social desirability. Thirdly, adjectives referring to criminal activity were not included in CADAP. As suggested by former literature (Rossier et al. 2007), behaviors might be determined more by the social norms than traits in collectivistic environment. Consequently, people would rate themselves in a way fitting the Chinese collectivistic culture through expressing antisocial tendencies in the more internalizing way especially in criminal activities. Nevertheless, we have developed a three-factor-structured CADAP with satisfactory internal reliabilities, and found the gender differences and inter-correlations between these factors, which characterize the unique adjectival descriptors of antisocial personality in Chinese culture and might help to explore the influence of contemporary Chinese culture on antisocial personality disorder. Except for searching the cultural contributions on both normal and disordered personality traits in Chinese society, further studies in regard to antisocial personality disorder might be trialed in sorts of patients with psychological problems including personality and bipolar disorders.

References

American Psychiatric Association. (2013). *Diagnostic and statistical manual of mental disorder* (5th ed.). Washington, DC: American Psychiatric Association.

Anderson, J. L., Sellbom, M., Wygant, D. B., Salekin, R. T., & Krueger, R. F. (2014). Examining the associations between DSM-5 section III antisocial personality disorder traits and psychopathy in community and university samples. *Journal of Personality Disorders, 28*, 675–697.

Angleitner, A., Ostendorf, F., & John, O. P. (1990). Towards a taxonomy of personality descriptors in German: A psycho-lexical study. *European Journal of Personality, 4*, 89–118.

Ashton, M. C., & Lee, K. (2005). A defence of the lexical approach to the study of personality structure. *European Journal of Personality, 19*, 5–24.

Barriga, A. Q., Morrison, E. M., Liau, A. K., & Gibbs, J. C. (2001). Moral cognition: Explaining the gender difference in antisocial behavior. *Merrill-Palmer Quarterly, 47*, 532–562.

Blackburn, R., & Fawcett, D. (1999). The Antisocial Personality Questionnaire: An inventory for assessing personality deviation in offender populations. *European Journal of Psychological Assessment, 15*, 14–24.

Boies, K., Lee, K., Ashton, M. C., Pascal, S., & Nicol, A. A. M. (2001). The structure of the French personality lexicon. *European Journal of Personality, 15*, 277–295.

Burtaverde, V. (2016). The structure of personality in Romania. A lexical approach. *Romanian Journal of Experimental Applied Psychology, 7*, 265–267.

Campbell, A. (2006). Sex differences in direct aggression: What are the psychological mediators? *Aggression and Violent Behavior, 11*, 237–264.

Caprara, G. V., & Perugini, M. (1994). Personality described by adjectives: The generalizability of the Big Five to the Italian lexical context. *European Journal of Personality, 8*, 357–369.

Cheung, F. M., van de Vijver, F. J., & Leong, F. T. (2011). Toward a new approach to the study of personality in culture. *American Psychologist, 66*, 593–603.

Church, A. T. (2016). Personality traits across cultures. *Current Opinion in Psychology, 8*, 22–30.

Coid, J., & Ullrich, S. (2010). Antisocial personality disorder is on a continuum with psychopathy. *Comprehensive Psychiatry, 51*, 426–433.

Cooke, D. J., & Michie, C. (2001). Refining the construct of psychopathy: Towards a hierarchical model. *Psychological Assessment, 13*, 171–188.

Cooke, D. J., Hart, S. D., Logan, C., & Michie, C. (2012). Explicating the construct of psychopathy: Development and validation of a conceptual model, the comprehensive assessment of psychopathic personality (CAPP). *International Journal of Forensic Mental Health, 11*, 242–252.

Craig, R. J., & Olson, R. E. (2001). Adjectival descriptions of personality disorders: A convergent validity study of the MCMI-III. *Journal of Personality Assessment, 77*, 259–271.

Crocker, A. G., Mueser, K. T., Drake, R. E., Clark, R. E., McHugo, G. J., Ackerson, T. H., & Alterman, A. I. (2005). Antisocial personality, psychopathy, and violence in persons with dual disorders: A longitudinal analysis. *Criminal Justice and Behavior, 32*, 452–476.

de Raad, B. (1992). The replicability of the big five personality dimensions in three word-classes of the Dutch language. *European Journal of Personality, 6*, 15–29.

de Raad, B. (2000). *The Big Five Personality Factors: The psycholexical approach to personality.* Ashland: Hogrefe and Huber Publishers.

de Raad, B., & Hoskens, M. (1990). Personality-descriptive nouns. *European Journal of Personality, 4*, 131–146.

di Blas, L. (2005). Personality-relevant attribute-nouns: A taxonomic study in the Italian language. *European Journal of Personality, 19*, 537–557.

Frick, P. J., Cornell, A. H., Barry, C. T., Bodin, S. D., & Dane, H. E. (2003). Callous-unemotional traits and conduct problems in the prediction of conduct problem severity, aggression, and self-report of delinquency. *Journal of Abnormal Child Psychology, 31*, 457–470.

Fu, G., Lee, K., Cameron, C. A., & Xu, F. (2001). Chinese and Canadian adults' categorization and evaluation of lie- and truth-telling about prosocial and antisocial behaviors. *Journal of Cross-Cultural Psychology, 32*, 720–727.

Gacono, C. B. (1998). The use of the psychopathy checklist-revised (PCL-R) and rorschach in treatment planning with antisocial personality disordered patients. *International Journal of Offender Therapy and Comparative Criminology, 42*, 49–64.

Goldberg, L. R., & Somer, O. (2000). The hierarchical structure of common Turkish person-descriptive adjectives. *European Journal of Personality, 14*, 497–531.

Hare, R. D. (1991). *Manual for the Hare Psychopathy Checklist-Revised.* Toronto: Multi-Health Systems.

Hare, R. D. (2003). *The Hare Psychopathy Checklist-Revised* (2nd ed.). Toronto: Multi-Health Systems.

Hare, R. D., & Neumann, C. S. (2005). Structural models of psychopathy. *Current Psychiatry Reports, 7*, 57–64.

Hare, R. D., & Neumann, C. S. (2006). The PCL-R assessment of psychopathy: Development, structural properties, and new directions. In C. Patrick (Ed.), *Handbook of psychopathy* (pp. 58–90). New York: Guilford.

Hare, R. D., & Neumann, C. S. (2008). Psychopathy as a clinical and empirical construct. *Annual Review of Clinical Psychology, 4*, 217–246.

Heidensohn, F. (1997). Gender and crime. In M. Maguire, R. Morgan, & R. Reiner (Eds.), *The Oxford handbook of criminology* (2nd ed., pp. 761–798). Oxford: Oxford University Press.

Hofstede, G. (1980). *Culture's consequences: International differences in worked related values.* Beverly Hills: Sage.

Hsu, S. Y., & Barker, G. G. (2013). Individualism and collectivism in Chinese and American television advertising. *International Communication Gazette, 75*, 695–714.

Kennealy, P. J., Skeem, J. L., Walters, G. D., & Camp, J. (2010). Do core interpersonal and affective traits of PCL-R psychopathy interact with antisocial behavior and disinhibition to predict violence? *Psychological Assessment, 22*, 569–580.

Lau, K. S., & Marsee, M. A. (2013). Exploring narcissism, psychopathy, and Machiavellianism in youth: Examination of associations with antisocial behavior and aggression. *Journal of Child and Family Studies, 22*, 355–367.

Leahy, D., O'Neill, D., & Hammond, S. (2010). An examination of gender differences in antisocial personality. *Personality and Mental Health, 4*, 133–145.

Lee, K., Cameron, C. A., Xu, F., Fu, G., & Board, J. (1997). Chinese and Canadian children's evaluations of lying and truth telling: Similarities and differences in the context of pro-and antisocial behaviors. *Child Development, 68*, 924–934.

Lee, K., Xu, F., Fu, G., Cameron, C. A., & Chen, S. (2001). Taiwan and Mainland Chinese and Canadian children's categorization and evaluation of lie- and truth-telling: A modesty effect. *British Journal of Developmental Psychology, 19*, 525–542.

Li, Y., Wang, M., Wang, C., & Shi, J. (2010). Individualism, collectivism, and Chinese adolescents' aggression: Intracultural variations. *Aggressive Behavior, 36*, 187–194.

Lynam, D. R., & Vachon, D. D. (2012). Antisocial personality disorder in DSM-5: Missteps and missed opportunities. *Personality Disorders: Theory, Research, and Treatment, 3*, 483–495.

Ma, H. K., Shek, D. T., Cheung, P. C., & Lee, R. Y. (1996). The relation of prosocial and antisocial behavior to personality and peer relationships of Hong Kong Chinese adolescents. *Journal of Genetic Psychology, 157*, 255–266.

McCrae, R. R. (2004). Human nature and culture: A trait perspective. *Journal of Research in Personality, 38*, 3–14.

Mlačić, B., & Ostendorf, F. (2005). Taxonomy and structure of Croatian personality-descriptive adjectives. *European Journal of Personality, 19*, 117–152.

Mobarake, R. K. (2015). Age and gender difference in antisocial behavior among adolescents' school students. *Mediterranean Journal of Social Sciences, 6*, 194–200.

Moran, P. (1999). The epidemiology of antisocial personality disorder. *Social Psychiatry and Psychiatric Epidemiology, 34*, 231–242.

Morana, H. C. P., Câmara, F. P., & Arboleda-Flórez, J. (2006). Cluster analysis of a forensic population with antisocial personality disorder regarding PCL-R scores: Differentiation of two patterns of criminal profiles. *Forensic Science International, 164*, 98–101.

Piedmont, R. L., & Aycock, W. (2007). An historical analysis of the lexical emergence of the Big Five personality adjective descriptors. *Personality and Individual Differences, 42*, 1059–1068.

Rossier, J., Aluja, A., García, L. F., Angleitner, A., de Pascalis, V., Wang, W., Kuhlman, M., & Zuckerman, M. (2007). The cross-cultural generalizability of Zuckerman's alternative five-factor model of personality. *Journal of Personality Assessment, 89*, 188–196.

Saucier, G. (2018). Culture, morality and individual differences: Comparability and incomparability across species. *Philosophical transactions of the Royal Society of London. Series B, Biological Sciences, 373*. https://doi.org/10.1098/rstb.2017.0170.

Saucier, G., & Goldberg, L. R. (2001). Lexical studies of indigenous personality factors: Premises, products, and prospects. *Journal of Personality, 69*, 847–879.

Shedler, J., & Westen, D. (2004). Refining personality disorder diagnosis: Integrating science and practice. *American Journal of Psychiatry, 161*, 1350–1365.

Shepherd, S. M., Campbell, R. E., & Ogloff, J. R. (2018). Psychopathy, antisocial personality disorder, and reconviction in an Australian sample of forensic patients. *International Journal of Offender Therapy and Comparative Criminology, 62*, 609–628.

Swann, A. C., Lijffijt, M., Lane, S. D., Steinberg, J. L., & Moeller, F. G. (2009). Trait impulsivity and response inhibition in antisocial personality disorder. *Journal of Psychiatric Research, 43*, 1057–1063.

Szirmák, Z., & de Raad, B. (1994). Taxonomy and structure of Hungarian personality traits. *European Journal of Personality, 8*, 95–117.

Tu, Y. T., Lin, S. Y., & Chang, Y. Y. (2011). A cross-cultural comparison by individualism/collectivism among Brazil, Russia, India and China. *International Business Research, 4*, 175–182.

Verona, E., Patrick, C. J., & Joiner, T. E. (2001). Psychopathy, antisocial personality, and suicide risk. *Journal of Abnormal Psychology, 110*, 462–470.

Vitacco, M., Neumann, C. S., Robertson, A., & Durrant, S. (2002). Contributions of impulsivity and callousness in the assessment of adjudicated male adolescents: A prospective study. *Journal of Personality Assessment, 78,* 87–103.

Wang, G., & Liu, Z. B. (2010). What collective? Collectivism and relationalism from a Chinese perspective. *Chinese Journal of Communication, 3,* 42–63.

Whitmore, J. M., Shore, W. J., & Smith, P. H. (2004). Partial knowledge of word meanings: Thematic and taxonomic representations. *Journal of Psycholinguistic Research, 33,* 137–164.

Wilson, D. S., Near, D., & Miller, R. R. (1996). Machiavellianism: A synthesis of the evolutionary and psychological literatures. *Psychological Bulletin, 119,* 285–299.

Yu, R., Yu, S., Liu, Y., Chen, W., Shen, M., Wang, D., & Wang, W. (2009). Adjectival descriptors for antisocial personality trait in Chinese university students. *Journal of Personality Disorders, 23,* 661–668.

Bipolar Disorders in Chinese Culture: From a Perspective of Harmony

Chanchan Shen, Yanli Jia, and Wei Wang

1 Cultural Influence on Bipolar Disorder

In previous chapters, we have discussed the disordered personality traits in Chinese culture, especially antisocial personality traits which cover three dimensions: Intolerant, Assaulting, and Fierce and Malicious. Under the cultural context where there is highly emphasizing on harmony, antisocial personality trait/disorder causes serious psychosocial problems. Therefore, any chaos harmful to the relationship harmony is to blame, which includes the one caused by bipolar disorder. In the perspective of Chinese culture, the manic phase is ascribed to be the characteristic of bipolar disorder, while depressive phase is more likely to be presented with somatic symptoms, thus the depressive state is paid less attention by patients themselves and their relatives.

In the current chapter, we would like to show how Chinese culture fashions the manifestations of bipolar disorder in the perspective of harmony, which is different from what is described in the Western world. In the first section, we will review the present definition and characteristic of bipolar disorder under the perspective of Western psychiatry, and later review the relationship between social culture and health/disease, including bipolar disorder. In the second section, we will present the features of Chinese culture closely relating to the theory of Traditional Chinese Medicine (TCM) and Confucianism, both of which are linked with harmony. The TCM system holds itself the concepts of disease and health in Chinese, while the Confucianism sets social norms for individuals, thus influences the attribution, presentation, and help-seeking behaviors of Chinese patients, especially those with psychological disorders. In the third section, we will focus on the impacts of these two components (TCM and Confucianism) on bipolar disorder, in terms of personal

C. Shen · Y. Jia · W. Wang (✉)
Department of Clinical Psychology and Psychiatry/School of Public Health, Zhejiang University College of Medicine, Hangzhou, China
e-mail: drwangwei@zju.edu.cn

© Springer Nature Singapore Pte Ltd. 2019
W. Wang (ed.), *Chinese Perspectives on Cultural Psychiatry*,
https://doi.org/10.1007/978-981-13-3537-2_9

beliefs, attribution, and behavior. In the fourth section, we will illustrate the current status of bipolar disorder and its influencing factors in China which might provide some suggestions for future research and clinical work.

1.1   Western Orientation of Bipolar Disorder

Bipolar disorder is defined by Western psychiatrists as significantly abnormal fluctuations of mood and energy/activity, characterized by recurrent mania or hypomania, and depression, and it has two major types, bipolar I (BD I) and II (BD II), which present different clinical symptoms. According to the two internationally recognized diagnostic instruments, i.e., the Diagnostic and Statistical Manual of Mental Disorders, Fifth Edition (DSM-5, American Psychiatric Association 2013) and the International Classification of Diseases (ICD-11 beta version, World Health Organization 2017), a manic (or hypomanic) episode is characterized as a distinct period with abnormally, persistently elevated, expansive, or irritable mood and persistently increased energy, accompanied by a cluster of excessive biological and psychological symptoms; while core symptoms of a major depressive episode are depressed mood and loss of interest or pleasure, with somatic and psychological changes that significant damage individual function. The diagnostic instruments, which are dominated by Anglo-Americans, are often translated and utilized in different cultures without cross-cultural validation, leaving little information on specific differences in the presentation of bipolar disorder across different cultures (American Psychiatric Association 2013).

The diagnostic criteria of bipolar disorder are originated from the modern Western society and moderate-high socioeconomic classes in developed countries. However, laypeople from both Western and Eastern cultures have low recognition rate of psychological illness, particularly bipolar disorder which is the least correctly labeled (Loo et al. 2012). In addition, there are definitely cultural variants in the understanding and expressing of the symptoms of bipolar disorder, thus leading to different attribution, presentation, communication, and coping strategies of these problems across cultures.

1.2   Cultural Influences on Bipolar Disorder

There is not much evidence showing that certain ethnic groups have a greater risk of developing bipolar disorder. According to the lifetime prevalence of bipolar disorder in various countries/areas of Americas, Europe, Asia, Lebanon and New Zealand, the prevalence of BD I and BD II ranges up to 1.1% (Merikangas et al. 2011). Under the influence of biologization of human mind, etiological studies have concluded that bipolar disorder is a polygenic and constitutional factors (Barnett and Smoller 2009; Chiao and Blizinsky 2010; Craddock and Sklar 1999; Mcguffin et al. 2003) that is somewhat far away from psychosocial origins (Etain et al. 2010; Johnson et al. 2008; Proudfoot et al. 2011). Moreover, in pathophysiological perspective, bipolar disorder is regarded as a disease of neuronal circuit dysfunction of emotion regulation (Strakowski et al. 2004, 2012).

Considering significant differences in the way emotions are experienced, expressed and regulated in different geographic areas (Davis et al. 2012; Grabell et al. 2015; Huwaë and Schaafsma 2016; Jack 2013), it is logically viable to postulate that the diagnostic assessment and clinical management of bipolar disorder are affected by cultural context (Kirmayer and Groleau 2001). A large sample epidemiological survey showed that the 12-month prevalence of bipolar disorder is lower for African American than for non-Hispanic whites after adjusting for sociodemographic characteristics (Gibbs et al. 2013). Moreover, the prevalence of BD I in different countries was correlated with cultural values (e.g., low Power Distance and high Individualism, low Long-Term Orientation and high Performance Orientation) (Johnson and Johnson 2014), supporting that the disorder was influenced to some extent by culture.

The ethnocultural aspects could affect the clinical presentation by shaping the individuals' patterns of emotional experience, expression and regulation. These aspects also affect the diagnosis which is based on patients' expression of symptoms with culturally acceptable manner, and on their help-seeking behaviors by meanings patients attach to the disorder (American Psychiatric Association 2013). However, there is little information on specific differences in the clinical features of bipolar disorder across different cultures, since diagnostic instruments are usually translated and applied in various cultures without transcultural validation (American Psychiatric Association 2013). In the case of depressive symptoms, the way a depressive individual expresses is definitely influenced by culture (Kirmayer and Groleau 2001; Kleinman 1978). For example, Chinese patients with depression disorder are more likely to report somatic symptoms, such as fatigue, pain and dizziness (Lee et al. 2007; Ryder et al. 2008; Yen et al. 2000), though they also report emotional distress when questioned further (Lin and Cheung 1999). When it comes to manic episode of bipolar disorder, the clinical features seem to be without significant cultural differences, but some manic symptoms show various cultural sensitivities (Egeland and Hostetter 1983). Some symptoms, such as psychomotor agitation and decreased need for sleep, are free from cultural influence, while the grandiosity and excessive involvement in activities are greatly complicated by cultural influences (Egeland and Hostetter 1983). Geographically, a low occurrence of flight of ideas and a relatively high proportion of patients presenting persecutory and self-blaming delusions were found in Indian manic patients (Sethi and Khanna 1993).

Abundant evidence from anthropological and ethnographic studies also indicates that people generally depend on culturally-derived metaphors to comprehend diseases, especially those abstracted maladies like psychological disorders (McMullen and Conway 1996; Sontag 1989). As the most typical example of Eastern culture, Chinese culture offers typical characteristics of bipolar disorder in collectivist culture. In order to have an idea of the attribution, presentation of bipolar disorder and people's understanding of the disease in the context of Chinese culture, we will first access to some knowledge about cultural factors influencing the ideas regarding health/well-being and disease in China, which include the perspective of harmony from both biological and social aspects.

2 Harmony in Chinese Culture and Health

Chinese culture is characterized as collectivistic (low Individualism) and hierarchical (high power distance) in its interpersonal orientation, with harmony highly valued and emphasized. The concept of harmony is a philosophical foundation of Chinese thoughts, including Confucianism, Moism (墨家) and Daoism, which further greatly influences the thinking and behavioral patterns of the Chinese people. From the perspective of ancient Chinese philosophy, harmony is dynamic equilibrium of "*Yin*" (阴) and "*Yang*" (阳), where "*Yin*" stands for female force, such as passivity and dark, whereas "*Yang*" stands for male force, such as activity and light. The opposite but inter-complementary "*Yin*" and "*Yang*" contains each other and together forms a changing unity of harmony, which is embedded in the traditional doctrine of the Chinese that "persons are an integral part of nature" (天人合一). From the medical point of view, harmony in Chinese adopts a holistic conceptualization of an individual and environment in the totality of body, mind, emotion, spirit and environment (Chan et al. 2000). Therefore, harmony is rich of connotation and consists of multiple dimensions, essentially including sustainable relationship between individual and natural (or biological harmony) as well as between individual and individual (or social harmony), which influences Chinese beliefs about the world, including conception of health.

2.1 Biological Harmony and Health

The cosmologic concepts of harmony construct the very basis of Chinese thoughts about the "biological" identity, which is greatly reflected in the TCM. The TCM is founded upon *Yin-Yang* equilibrium philosophy as well as the Five Elements Theory (五行学说), pointing out that individual health is characterized by the dynamic equilibrium internally and externally, with the external factors including social and biological aspects and the inner factors including biological and psychological aspects. According to the naive materialistic belief about world, the world is constituted with *Wu Xing* (五行, five basic elements), they are *Jin* (金, metal), *Mu* (木, wood), *Shui* (水, water), *Huo* (火, fire), and *Tu* (土, earth), elements that make up the whole body. There is mutual promotion and restraint between the five elements, reflecting that there are general relationships among matters. Such concepts have been absorbed by the TCM and are incorporated with the pathophysiology process of disease/health, resulting in Theory of viscera – visualization of Five Elements Theory. The theory explains that the liver, heart, spleen, lung and kidney, correspond to wood, fire, earth, metal and water, respectively. As the Theory of viscera clarifies, the five viscera generate five basic emotions which are joy, anger, sad, worry, and fear respectively. From holistic perspective of TCM, it is regarded that physical and emotional are indivisible but different aspects of the same human existence (Chan et al. 2000), in other words, there is an interrelationship between physical and emotional entities, with the physical/biological inner determining emotional/psychological inner, and emotional/psychological inner moderating physical/biological inner. In this way, the healthy status is regarded as the harmonious equilibrium of five viscera and five emotions with the effect of internal environment and external conditions. Therefore, a healthy person is one who achieves harmony of both physical and emotional aspects.

Different from Western biological orientation of medicine, the TCM attaches particular importance to social and psychological issues: the five basic emotions – joy, anger, sadness, worry and fear were derived from the five elements, and to the pathophysiology of disease. Similar to mutual generation and restriction of the five phases elements, five basic emotions promote and restrict each other, thus they can be used as tools to treat diseases. In *Huang Di Nei Jing* (黄帝内经, the Yellow Emperor's Internal Canon of Medicine) (Li and Li 2005), it is well illustrated that "anger impairs the liver, while sorrow dominates over anger" (怒伤肝, 悲胜怒), and "joy impairs the heart while fear dominates over joy" (喜伤心, 恐胜喜). In a well-known traditional story *Fan Jin Zhong Ju* (范进中举, Mr. Fan Chin Passing Civil Exam) (Yang 1973), the excessive joy of passing the provincial civil service examination causes Mr. Fan Jin to be crazy, and his father-in-law whom he is afraid of most, slapps him afterwards, resulting in the recovery of Fan Jin. Such a story illustrates that the excessive emotion causes individual disharmony, and another antagonistic strong emotion makes up for the unequilibrium to treat the disorder, which reflects one of the TCM principles. In addition to the emotion, social condition is also included in the physiopathology of disease, for example, cultivation of character is also put on the significant position when referring to the treatment of psychological disorders, especially under the influence of the harmony concept in social aspect. Some Chinese idioms reflect these clarifications, such as to "cultivate one's moral character" (修身养性). When there is a need to treat a disease, patients are often suggested that they should cultivate their minds (Lan et al. 2018). The TCM stresses the importance of social condition, and Chinese culture, especially the secular Confucian culture, has put this to an end.

2.2   Social Harmony and Health

The "social" identity is greatly influenced by the ancient Chinese social and cultural values about harmony, which is founded on the ground of the Confucianism. From the social and cultural perspective, harmony is regarded as equilibrium in the present of inherent diversity (while sustaining hierarchical relationship) and treated as a core value in collectivist Chinese culture (Chen 2000; Leung et al. 2002, 2011).

Plenty of Chinese common sayings are involves harmony with great importance, such as "Harmony is valuable" (和为贵), and "If the family lives in harmony, all affairs will prosper" (家和万事兴). In classical Confucian doctrines, harmony has rich connotations, essentially embracing disagreement and open debates (Leung et al. 2002). In the celebrated Confucian work, the Analects, there is a saying "The gentleman agrees with others without being an echo; the small man echoes without being in agreement" (君子和而不同, 小人同而不和). The intrinsic meaning of this quote is that *Junzi* (君子, gentleman) is able to maintain rapport even if they may hold different opinions; while *Xiao Ren* (小人, small man), a person with vile character, echo another's opinions but actually privately disagree, which is not in harmonious relationship. Harmony is particularly emphasized towards individual relationships or social relationships so that pursuit of harmony is able to promote equilibrium and the maintenance of hierarchical relationship in the context of collectivistic and hierarchical circumstance in Chinese culture (Chen 2000).

2.2.1 Collectivism Orientation, Hierarchical Structure and Harmony

One salient feature of Chinese culture, long considered collectivistic, is the "group" and "family" orientation (Faure and Fang 2008). Contrary to Individualism emphasizing the independence from groups, Collectivism emphasizes the interdependence of individuals. Therefore, the Chinese tend to value interdependence, family integrity, and cooperation (Triandis 1995). Culture values and beliefs about Collectivism of the Chinese inhibit the expressions of overt negative emotion or harmful behaviors in order to maintain interpersonal harmony (Bond 2004). With a collectivistic orientation, overt emotional expression may be considered a threat to interpersonal harmony and therefore is highly discouraged, whereas it may be seen as more acceptable means to achieve self-reliance in individualistic culture (Bond 2004; Triandis 1995). The collectivistic ideology interacts with hierarchical consciousness and assures the consolidation of hierarchical structure of ancient China.

There is no doubt that traditional Chinese society is with highly hierarchical structure of particularistic relationships, attaching great importance to seniority with power and prerogatives who possesses the ability to execute a strong control over the interaction and decision making in negotiating conflicts (Bond and Hwang 1986). For thousands of years, the hierarchical thoughts have influenced the thinking patterns and behavioral patterns of the generations of Chinese. According to the *San Gang* (三纲), "ruler guides subject, father guides son, and husband guides wife" in a harmonious society, that is, there are norms for everyone according to their different roles in different situations. In the feudal society, hierarchy emphasizes that everyone should fall into proper places and order to promote the stability of the society (Leung et al. 2002).

However, with various advanced thoughts communicated and developed, the history left obsession of hierarchy which is still firmly rooted in the innermost parts of modern Chinese, even in university students with advanced education, the historical records affect their thoughts and behaviors. Compared to individuals from Western

background, modern Chinese still tend to yield to authority when involved in conflict (Tyler et al. 2000; Yuan 2010). When coming across predicaments, the Chinese
are willing to refer to senior with more authority and power. For example, when
they are involved in difficulties associated with interrelationship, it is considered to
be appropriate to find a person with relatively high status and authority, such as
superior, father, husband, and older brother, to negotiate conflicts.

2.2.2 Confucius and Secular Harmony

Harmony is seen as the most important culture value in Chinese culture, however,
Confucian ideals of harmony are often appropriated by the ruling class, aiming to
consolidate social hierarchy and preserve their power (Leung et al. 2002). The
Chinese political history associated with Collectivism and hierarchy, provides an
explanation and helps to illuminate that East Asians exhibit a clear pattern of conflict avoidance (Leung et al. 2002). In addition, the secular harmony, highly compat-
ible with the Collectivism and hierarchy of ancient Chinese society, was constantly
consolidated by dominance hierarchies of successive dynasties.

The secular version of harmony advocated by the dominators asks the public to
achieve the harmony by compromise, such as to submit to the authority (or power),
to avoid the interpersonal conflict. In this way, harmony is regarded as an instrument
by dominator to control people – a particular stress on harmony in relationship prof-
iting those in power and resource since it legitimizes their authority. Even nowadays, such concept of harmony has been accepted by a large portion of general
population. While harmony consists of several components, among which lack of
conflict is often considered as indispensable from secular perspective (Chen et al.
2016; Chen 2000; Lam et al. 2012; Leung et al. 2002), and individuals have obligation to implement various strategies to avoid or reduce conflict, such as the self-
restraint and self-discipline, the indirect communication (Chen 2000; Man and
Bond 2005). Among these different methods, emotion suppression is considered as
a significant way to maintain and promote harmony in interdependent culture (Wei
et al. 2013). The Chinese suppress both positive and negative emotions more in
daily social interactions, and suppress positive emotions less in interaction with
close others (Huwaë and Schaafsma 2016). Much empirical evidence have shown
the restrained emotional expression in Chinese in terms of cognition and emotion
experience (Davis et al. 2012), and physiological response (Tsai and Levenson
1997) and behavioral aspect (Li et al. 2010).

The harmony defined in Chinese culture respects the emotional suppression,
rather than the "emotional harmony". Therefore, once involved in interpersonal
conflict, like other agencies in Collectivism culture, the Chinese suffer from higher
level of emotional distress (Tsai and Levenson 1997; Tsai et al. 2006). A cross-
cultural study indicated that Chinese adolescents, with less conflict with parents and
more parental warmth, showed stronger association between conflict with parent
and depressed mood than American adolescents did, but parental warmth and acceptance did not buffer the detrimental effects of negative life events on depressed

mood (Greenberger et al. 2000). When faced with conflict stress, vulnerable individuals encountering emotional distress mainly express their somatic symptoms (Ryder, et al. 2008; Yen et al. 2000; Zhang 1995), because they are trained to suppress emotional expression.

On the other hand, the emotional expression in Chinese is highly correlated with personality. The emotion restraint, thought as self-discipline, is highly praised (Bond 1993) and posed to the lower neuroticism, since Confucian tradition highly praised that strong emotional experience should be managed internally by personality cultivation rather than by explicit expression of emotion (Cheng et al. 2008).

2.3 Disease Being Defined as Disharmony

The Chinese philosophy of harmony fashions the construction of common sense. Unlike the western psychiatric perspective based on Cartesian mind-body dualism, the TCM originated from *Yin-Yang* equilibrium philosophy characterized diseases as both internal and external origins of dysfunction (Wu 1982). If both internal and external factors, functioning alone or in concert, contribute to the imbalance of *Yin-Yang*, they will lead to the diseased state (Luk and Bond 1992). Compared with Western cultures, the external factors, especially family-related issues (Greenberger et al. 2000), were more related with self-distress. Symptoms reflect the internal and external un-equilibrium, showing disturbances or disharmony of the functional systems that have emotional, somatic, and social influences. Therefore, people could place themselves anywhere along the dimensions of bodily, social, and environmental distress to stress those aspects of their sufferings so that they can be best understood and reactivated by others (Kirmayer and Groleau 2001).

In this sense, operating (or controlling) either internal or external factors could prevent or treat disease. As the harmony is highly respected in Chinese culture, it is everyone's responsibility to control him−/herself to avoid any conflict which is disruptive to harmony. Therefore, the disharmony reflects the disrespected character of an individual, i.e., inability of self-control, manifesting as an excessive emotional expression and conflict, especially the interpersonal conflict within family. Since culture plays a role in moderating the meaning and influences of life experiences, conformity with cultural ideologies of the individual might be just as important as any specific attributional pattern for the psychic economy; moreover, the sources of self-esteem lie not simply in the experience of success or failure or the achievement of personal goals but in the fulfillment of larger social and cultural ideals of personhood and morality (Shweder et al. 1997). Psychological patients in China are inclined to attribute environmental issues and their characters of self-discipline to their disorders, since self-harmony is touched by balance between internal and external interactions, which is greatly moderated by their self-discipline. In addition, psychological patients are easier to disclose their somatic symptoms because psychosocial distress indicates that the distress originates from inner factor and their negative traits to regulate the interior factors. The disclosure of psychosocial distress shoulders the burdens of disconformity with cultural expectance, which stigmatizes patients' personality and morals (Kleinman 1982). However, when patients who initially report only physical distress find it safe to express themselves, they can be expected to disclose the psychological and social dimensions of their distress (Kirmayer and Groleau 2001).

3   Bipolar Disorder in Chinese Cultural Context

As mentioned above, we have learned the importance of the TCM and secular harmony in the construction of ideas of health and disease in Chinese culture. Health is defined as *Yin-Yang* equilibrium and harmony on the physical, emotional and social aspects. As we have mentioned before, among all of the psychiatric disorders, bipolar disorder is one of most interesting problems characterized by extreme fluctuations of emotion and energy, with two striking phases of bipolar mania/ hypomania and bipolar depression. One might imagine that these two significantly different phases reflect the predominance of excessive *Yin* and *Yang* respectively.

3.1   Chinese Beliefs about Bipolar Disorder

The 12-month prevalence of BD I and BD II in metropolitan China was 0.1%, which was consistent with findings in other countries and societies (Lee et al. 2007). Although it seems that there are no abundant evidences showing the cultural variants of bipolar disorder, the value orientation of Collectivism influences the presentation and understanding of bipolar disorder symptoms, and also influences the understanding of etiology of the disorder on the cultural base that the management of emotion should be achieved through cultivation of personality. With the Chinese conventional values highlighting the importance of family, bipolar disorder is closely associated with family, especially when regarding clinical characteristics and treatments.

Concerning the etiology of bipolar disorder, Chinese people are inclined to ascribe bipolar disorder to stress, both internally and externally (Lan et al. 2018; Ng 2009). The Chinese young patients are likely to locate agency of bipolar disorder etiology within the characterological selfhood (Ng 2009), other than the "neurochemical selfhood" imagined by many patients in the USA (Rose 2003) who hold the belief that the genetic and neuropathological determinants underlie bipolar disorder. In Chinese patients with bipolar disorder, the personality described by Chinese adjectives is specifically related to the bipolar symptoms. Agreeable and Emotional traits, associated with emotional expression, are positively correlated with the depressive symptoms in BD I patients; whereas these traits negatively predict the hypomania symptoms in BD II patients (see Chapter "Predicting Affective States Of Bipolar Disorder By The Chinese Adjective Descriptors Of Personality").

In Chinese culture, people respect sages who are with the desirable personality traits such as self-cultivation, to restrict their emotional expression (Cheng et al. 2008). However, the predisposing character of bipolar disorder is often described as personal flaw, such as impatience and irritability on emotional aspect (Lan et al. 2018), and burdening excessive pressure and inability to manage their thoughts on cognitive aspect (Ng 2009). On the contrary, elder patients inclined to use external circumstances to explain the control over and responsibility for their illness (Ng 2009), for example, excessive responsibilities and financial stress. Nevertheless, the beliefs about bipolar disorder support the idea that it is multifactorial and influenced by both traditional culture and cultural change (Luk and Bond 1992). The cultural meanings of mania, including overexpressing negative emotion which is contradictory with Chinese values to self-control of emotion expression (Cheng et al. 2008), may lead to stigma in Chinese. One study has shown that when it comes to communication of bipolar disorder, Chinese patients moving to New Zealand found it difficult to disclose the illness to their Chinese friends than to Western people, since they experienced strong discrimination from people who share the same culture (Wang and Henning 2010). In return, the stigma and stereotype accompanying the disease also leads ordinary people to misunderstand the etiology and clinical presentation of bipolar disorders, also acting as barrier to recovery (Perlick et al. 2001). Again, as stated before, in Chinese culture, bipolar disorder reflects the fluctuation of two extreme representation of disharmony with intermittent "harmony". That is, manic episode is an exterior representation of disharmony, while depressive is an interior representation of disharmony.

3.2 Bipolar Disorder in Traditional Chinese Medicine

In *Huang Di Nei Jing*, psychological disorders were first formally described and classified as *Dian* (癲), *Kuang* (狂), and *Xian* (癇), resembling psychosis, mania and epilepsy respectively. Through the lens of the TCM, *Kuang Zheng* (狂症, Kuang Disease) which has been considered as bipolar mania in Western modern psychiatry, was demonstrated in *Huang Di Nei Jing* as "when mania begins, the patient feels sad at first, frequently forgetful, easy to flare into rage and often fearful, usually caused by excessive anxiety and hunger. When mania begins to attack, the patient sleeps little and does not feel hungry. He is proud of himself, personally feels that himself is intelligent and noble, and swears at others day and night" (Li and Li 2005). Such descriptions clearly show the legible clinical pictures of *Kuang Zheng*, including attribution and presentation. In line with psychobiological orientation of the TCM, the causal attribution of *Kuang Zheng* is disharmony of physical aspect and emotion, that is, excessive hunger and worry. Regarding the clinical symptoms of *Kuang Zheng*, the initial symptoms are something similar to depression, such as sadness, memory impairment, irritability and a sense of fear, while the typical symptoms are something similar to mania, such as sleeplessness, grandiosity of self, talkativeness that can escalate to psychosis. There is no doubt that the basic belief derived from the TCM pose influences on the Chinese people to explain, think and communicate what happens when presenting mania-like behaviors in self and others.

In addition, the Confucianism has put the concept of health into the psychosocial realm. Through the lens of secular Confucianism, laypeople define the distortions of interior mental status and exterior behavioral present as a psychological disorder. Therefore, with desirable tendency to appreciate emotional restrain to achieve harmony, excessive emotional expression was considered as destruction of harmony and repelled by the public, thus stigmatized the psychological disorder.

3.3   Clinical Features of Bipolar Disorder

3.3.1   Mania Episode

Under the influence of culture which recommends suppression of emotional expression, the Chinese are inclined to blame explicit manic behaviors more than depression, since the former is often thought as extreme emotion expression significantly destroying the interpersonal harmony, especially the family structure. Although most bipolar disorder patients and their family members define bipolar disorder as fluctuations between depression and elevated mood, such as irritability, anger, or agitation, they describe the main characteristics of the disorder mostly for its manic stage, such as "high peak" or "upsurge", with few referring to its depressive symptom (Lan et al. 2018).

According to several psychometric studies on the symptoms of (hypo)mania based on Mood Disorder Questionnaire and Hypomania Checklist, scholars stated that the symptoms are clustered into elevated mood overactivity (such as higher self-confidence, more energy, activity, sociability, and talkativeness, and less sleep) and irritable behavior (such as thoughts raced, irritability, easily distractedness, excessive foolish or risky actions) by factor analysis among Chinese patients (Wu et al. 2008; Chung et al. 2010; Lin et al. 2011). Although these questionnaires take no account of psychotic symptoms such as the lack of insight which also can be seen in manic episode, neither the diagnostic criteria which clearly depicts the core features of mania, including hyperthymic symptoms and destructive symptoms. The hyperthymic symptoms can be seen as positive or beneficial to individual, while the destructive symptoms are always seen as devastating to individual and his or her interpersonal relationships and are more likely to blame in a culture with Collectivistic orientation. In an in-depth interview research (Lan et al. 2018), 20 patients with BD I and 22 family members of these patients were enrolled, and their answers were analyzed based on the following basic themes: illness description, causal attribution, treatment-related issues and psychosocial issues. Besides considering the distinctive answers of participants, the authors have studied the family concerns and spiritual aspects of etiology and management of bipolar disorder. In accordance with the cultural value of emphasis on harmony, Chinese terms chosen to describe mania are mostly aggressive emotional-words which are harmful to interpersonal harmony, and the unrespectable personality traits which are linked with the inability to control individual's temper and emotion, such as "short-tempered or bad-tempered" and "impatient" (Lan et al. 2018). Of course, mania sometimes is described as a positive euphoric state (Wu et al. 2008; Chung et al. 2010; Lin et al. 2011). The symptoms of bipolar disorder, especially of BD I, are the extremes of emotional expression with loss of control, danger, and unpredictability (Cheung 1990; Mak and Chen 2010), resembling those of the *Kuang Zheng* in the TCM (presenting extroverted, aggressive, and excited behaviors, talkativeness, shouting, restlessness, and forceful physical movements; Jiang 2003). All these negative emotions and personality traits are associated with the problematic interpersonal-relationship, for instance the conflicts, especially the family struggles of the bipolar disorder patients. Meanwhile, the symptoms of manic patients and what their relatives acknowledge are mostly anger-related manifestations, such as irritability and impulsivity (Lan et al. 2018). However, the DSM-5 (American Psychiatric Association 2013) assigns a priority to elevated and expansive mood rather than irritable one, as the diagnosis of bipolar disorder requires more symptoms besides irritability.

Interestingly, no patients or their relatives reported the grandiosity or flight of ideas as the symptoms of mania (Lan et al. 2018), although these symptoms are also clustered into irritable behaviors together with the aggressive, excessive, and foolish risky-behaviors (Chung et al. 2010; Lin et al. 2011; Wu et al. 2008). Similar situations were also observed in other Eastern countries, such as India (Sethi and Khanna 1993). These clinical features seem to contradict with the harmony beliefs of the TCM, since the self-grandiose in the TCM is clearly described as a characteristic of *Kuang Zheng*. These symptoms are subjective experiences under manic phase, but patients interviewed are in relatively stable condition. The concealment of these symptoms might reflect the influences of social cultural context to some extent. They are inclined to hide such self-grandiose symptoms in order to win some respect after the disease, since the Confucius has educated these people to practice *Zhong Yong* (中庸, Doctrine of Mean).

3.3.2 Depressive Episode

The depressive episode is another salient presentation of bipolar disorder (American Psychiatric Association 2013), and bipolar patients experience depressive episodes much more than mania (Judd et al. 2003). Mania is considered to be relatively culture-independent by many researchers; nonetheless it is generally acknowledged that the experiences and expressions of depression are shaped by local cultural background and sociocultural norms (Lutz 1985). These conclusions are drawn based on the associations between culture and depression. Indeed, there is few researches who have focused on bipolar depression from the perspective of culture, even fewer of Chinese culture. In DSM-5 (American Psychiatric Association 2013), there is no comparative criteria highlighting the differences between bipolar depression and unipolar depression. However, compared to unipolar depression, bipolar depression presents more atypical symptoms (such as hypersomnia, hyperphagia, and leaden paralysis), earlier age of onset, more morning mood worsening, more hospitalizations, more improper functioning, more depressive episodes, and shorter depressive episodes (Mitchell et al. 2010), which are more severe and set greater challenge for management. In the discussion of depression and Chinese culture in this section, we will mention the literature regarding both bipolar depression and unipolar depression.

In DSM-5 (American Psychiatric Association 2013), depression is represented by a combination of various symptoms, essentially those of the psychological dimension, such as low mood, loss of interest, and impaired concentration, and equally those of the somatic dimension, such as sleep disturbance, pain, and lack of energy (Romera et al. 2008; Shafer 2010; Tylee and Gandhi 2005). In addition, using different assessments of depression, some scholars (e.g. Shafer 2010) found other dimensions such as interpersonal and psychomotor problems, which might be grouped in the pool of depressive symptoms. In clinics, especially during primary care, depression can be difficult to be recognized in patients reporting somatic complaints (Tylee and Gandhi 2005).

In fact, studies have shown strong evidence that Chinese depressive patients endorse more somatic symptoms (Kleinman 1978, 1982; Ryder et al. 2008; Yen et al. 2000; Parker et al. 2001). It is also well illustrasted that experience of psychological disorders is more likely to be expressed as somatized distress rather than psychological distress in Chinese and other East Asian cultures (Kleinman 2004). Many Chinese depressive patients do not report directly their psychological discomfort, such as sadness, but rather report feelings of boredom and inner pressure, or non-specific constitutional symptoms of pain and fatigue. For example, Cheung et al. (1981) have investigated the treatment-seeking of depressed patients at general clinics. Among all symptoms reported, the most common one is feelings of tirement and fatigability with a frequency of 90%, followed by feeling of pain with a frequency of 89%, and gastrointenstinal/cardiovascular symptoms with a frequency of 87%. Compared to physical disease, these somatic symptoms of depressed patients are more vague and diffuse. In addition, many of these patients also suffer from psychological distress, such as sadness, irritability and loss of interest, but they do not attach great importance to these presentations.

Another highly cited research is by Kleinman (1982), who also describes the phenomenology of somatization in depressed Chinese patients. In their 93 cases of depression, including unipolar depression and bipolar depression, physical symptoms of depression were obviously evident. For example, headaches, whether primary or secondary, were experienced by 90% of depressive patients, followed by insomnia of 78%, and by dizziness of 73%. In addition, other symptoms were common in patients with depression, such as pain (other than headaches), memory impairment, anxiety, weakness, loss of energy, feeling of swelling or fullness in head, neck or brain, and irritability. Taken together, the somatic symptoms in depression are mostly central nervous system related symptoms, which might reflect the biologicalization of psychological disorder, and that the psychological disorder is regarded as brain disorder in modern Western psychiatry.

As mentioned above, depressive symptoms possess both psychological and physical dimensions, and Chinese depressed patients are more likely to report the somatic symptoms than psychological distress. In addition, they pay little attention to sadness and may rationalize and camouflage their negative emotions (Cheung et al. 1981). However, when questioned further, they will describe their psychological dimension of depressive symptoms, such as anhedonia, dysphoria, hopelessness and loss of self-esteem, if they feel it is safe for self-disclosure (Kleinman 1982). This is an interesting phenomenon which reflects that culture shapes the clinical complaints of patients' psychological disorders, especially those of Chinese patients with depression. We have acknowledged that it is highly praised for achieving and maintaining harmony, including the physical, psychological and social harmonic structures in Chinese culture. With the integrated psychobiological orientation of the TCM, there are interactions between emotional (psychological) and physical components in human beings. An individual may put the disharmony in any of the dimensions, where the physical dimension causes least damage to the interpersonal harmony, and it is sensible to avert his/ her emotional unequilibrium to physical disharmony which is reflected on the somatic symptoms.

4 Future Implications

4.1 Issues in Current Treatment and Suggestions

Cultural issues affect individuals' help-seeking behaviors, because their thinking styles about psychological disorder are shaped by culture. Several large-scale epidemiological studies have shown that the rate of psychological patients seeking medical help is low, even in the most developed cities in China (Shen et al. 2006; Lee et al. 2009; Phillips et al. 2009; Yan et al. 2013). In a psychiatric epidemiological survey in metropolitan China (Shen et al. 2006), the investigators collected a sample of 2633 adults in Beijing and 2568 adults in Shanghai, based on the strictly stratified two-stage systematic selection Scheme. A structured diagnostic interview, the Chinese version of the World Health Organization Composite International Diagnostic Interview, was used to assess the psychiatric disorders including anxiety, mood, impulse-control, and substance use disorders and rated the severity of the disorders. The results showed that the estimated 12-month prevalence of any mood disorders is 2.2%, BD I and BD II is 0.1%, and major depressive disorder 2.0%. However, only 3.4% patients sought treatment within 12 months of the interview. The situation for bipolar disorder seems especially challenging, since it is a chronic disabling disease.

Management of bipolar disorder might require pharmacological or non-pharmacological interventions, regarding its acute phases of mania or depression and regarding the long-term therapy for recurrence prophylactic effects. Patients from different cultural backgrounds seek different help patterns, for example, Western patients tend to endorse professional help, while Eastern patients prefer self-help and social help (Loo et al. 2012). Out of the lack of public awareness about psychological disorders and the fear of stigmatization, the seeking-help rate of Chinese patients with psychological disorders is fairly low (Phillips et al. 2009). As part of professional help, drug treatment was considered as an effective therapy to stabilize the mood states of bipolar disorder as evidenced by various clinical evidences. However, in a variety of culture, non-adherence to psychotropic medications in psychiatric patients is pervasively severe, and approximately 31% of bipolar disorder patients did not take lithium or ceased their clinic-visiting (Putten 1975). There are numerous factors influencing psychotropic medication non-adherence (Gaw 2001), including therapeutic and side effects of medication, education, patients (e.g. health beliefs) and psychiatrist (e.g. countertransference) related issues, patient-doctor relationship factors and sociocultural aspects. The logistic attribution and ignorance of side-effect are specifically associated with non-adherence (Clatworthy et al. 2007), especially among Asian patients (Subramanian et al. 2017), which indicates that indigenous medicine and cultural context have special influences on drug compliance. For instance, bipolar disorder may be discredited and mania is thought as creativity and profit (Kyaga et al. 2011), people still want to look forward to being diagnosed as bipolar disorder (Chan and Sireling 2010), and these patients are unwilling to take lithium which would derive their periodic hypomania (Putten 1975).

Bipolar disorder is inclined to be considered as a disorder attributed to psychosocial etiology in Chinese culture, with functional consequences of disruptive family harmony. In the family-oriented culture, bipolar disorder causes great family distress and family conflict, which promote the help-seeking of suffering patients (Abekim et al. 2002). There are however, not very much research which have been conducted in China regarding the management of bipolar disorder. Compared with Western countries, there is striking unmet treatment of psychological disorder even in the most developed cities of China, where 80.2% patients with moderate and severe disorders receive no 12-month treatment (Shen et al. 2006). Under the influence of disorder resulting from unequilibrium between internal and external factors, the beliefs social-personal causes of psychological illness may directly lead to low rate of help-seeking (Chen and Mak 2008). Another main reason is the stereotype and stigma to patients with psychological disorder, for they are severely deviant from the cultural climate; in China, bipolar disorder is thought as mania with excessive emotion-expression infringing the doctrine of emotional restriction. In almost every religion in Chinese culture, the disease is considered due to negative unrespectable events, such as demonic possession and karma from prior lives originating from Daoism and Buddhism, respectively.

On the other hand, in China, the psychotropic medications are typically the mainstay of management of psychological problems including bipolar disorder, even with the understanding of psychosocial causes. In an interview of bipolar disorder patients in Taiwan, only 25% parents of patients support that psychiatric medication should be placed as the primary management (Lan et al. 2018), but most patients appreciate the importance of medication adherence (Wang and Henning 2010). However, the complexity and side effects of the medication regime were barriers to adherence (Wang and Henning 2010; Lan et al. 2018), such as the self-regulating of medication regime. In addition, there are lay health beliefs in Chinese that the Western medication is more effective and functions faster in many acute illnesses, while traditional Chinese medicine is better for chronic conditions with less side effects (Chan and Parker 2004), especially on the liver and kidney (Lan et al. 2018). Moreover, the Chinese hold more positive attitudes to the TCM, and consider it an effective complement to Western medicine for chronic or serious diseases (Chung 2014; Rochelle and Yim 2014), but the TCM may interact with current used psychotropic drugs (Chen et al. 2015). Even educated with the side effects of long-term lithium therapy, there is imperfect correspondence between Western biomedical and culturally acceptable side effect (Lee 1993), and doctor-patient relationship accounts more for the compliance of treatment (Lee et al. 1992; Wang and Henning 2010). Concerning the psychosocial orientation of bipolar disorder etiology, it would have various effects on the help-seeking behaviors in Chinese people. First, patients are reluctant to visit hospitals specializing in mental care, and they may be not willing to make a compromise to relieving manic/depressive symptoms with the cost of liver and kidney damage caused by Western medicine. Second, the great association between family and bipolar disorder to a large extent indicates that attention should be paid on the family related treatment issues. In this case, patients and their relatives seem to reach a consensus that there is a long-term family responsibility for caring (Lan et al. 2018), even though the bipolar disorder leads to a disruptive family harmony (Lan et al. 2018), causing significant distress to their family members (Wong et al. 2004). In return, family conflict contributes a lot to the help-seeking behaviors of patients (Abekim et al. 2002).

4.2 Inspirations from Chinese Culture

The *Yin* and *Yang* equilibrium offers holistic and paradoxical worldview and methodology that is significantly different from Western views. The diagnostic system of bipolar disorder is based on two systems, DSM (e.g., DSM-5, American Psychiatric Association 2013) and ICD (e.g., ICD-10, World Health Organization 1992) criteria. They are often directly translated and applied in different cultures without cross-cultural validation. There are some culture-sensitive symptoms such as grandiosity and flight of thoughts, which deserves more clinical attention and research. Meanwhile, in terms of diagnostic assessment, the self-disclosure of symptoms varies across ethnocultural groups, which requires a clinician's sensitivity to the expression of patients with different culture background.

Moreover, the harmony valued in Chinese culture may have some inspirations to the Western psychiatric medicine. The contemporary research indicates the disruption of neurotransmitter systems in bipolar disorder. Similar to Chinese harmony, the disharmony between excitatory and inhibitory neurotransmitter systems, neurotransmitters and receptors may contribute to bipolar disorder pathology. For example, there are indications of the increased mesencephalic, limbic and parietotemporoccipital serotonin and increased frontal dopamine underlie manic state, and of the decreased frontal and limbic serotonin, increased frontal and limbic acetylcholine and increased frontal dopamine underlie depressive state (Nikolaus et al. 2017).

Nevertheless, one should bear in mind that the disclosure of cultural characteristics may cause stereotype of that culture, since there is great diversity within a population and contemporary China is embracing a diversity of cultures. One should also be cautious of the danger of taking an exclusive perspective of Chinese harmony, ignoring multiple variations of the Chinese culture. The stereotypes of particular group, whether intentional or unintentional, are still deep-rooted and they interfere with the diagnosis and treatment of patients with psychological illness. The assessment of each patient should be based on specifically the personal background, especially under the influence of globalization where a broad international communication would interact with the native culture. Simultaneously, it remains to be further investigated what the alien culture brings to native culture and how they interact with each other leading to the influence on psychological illness and mental health service.

The culture models the characteristics of an individual, thus the personality trait of an individual with certain culture background may reflect the nature of that culture. In the following chapter, we would focus on the Chinese-featured personality and its association with bipolar disorder to investigate the relationship between bipolar disorder and Chinese culture from a new perspective.

References

Abekim, J., Takeuchi, D., & Hwang, W. C. (2002). Predictors of help seeking for emotional distress among Chinese Americans: Family matters. *Journal of Consulting and Clinical Psychology, 70*, 1186–1190.

American Psychiatric Association. (2013). *Diagnostic and statistical manual of mental disorder* (5th ed.). Washington, DC: American Psychiatric Association.

Barnett, J. H., & Smoller, J. W. (2009). The genetics of bipolar disorder. *Neuroscience, 164*, 331–343.

Bond, M. H. (1993). Emotions and their expression in Chinese culture. *Journal of Nonverbal Behavior, 17*, 245–262.

Bond, M. H. (2004). Culture and aggression – From context to coercion. *Personality and Social Psychology Review, 8*, 62–78.

Bond, M. H., & Hwang, K. (1986). The social psychology of Chinese people. *International Journal of Intercultural Relations, 11*, 212–214.

Chan, B., & Parker, G. (2004). Some recommendations to assess depression in Chinese people in Australasia. *Australian and New Zealand Journal of Psychiatry, 38*, 141–147.

Chan, D., & Sireling, L. (2010). 'I want to be bipolar'… a new phenomenon. *Psychiatrist, 34*, 103–105.

Chan, C., Ho, P. S., & Chow, E. (2000). A body-mind-spirit model in health: An Eastern approach. *Social Work in Health Care, 34*, 261–282.

Chen, G. M. (2000). The impact of harmony on Chinese conflict management. In G. M. Chen & R. Ma (Eds.), *Chinese conflict management and resolution* (pp. 3–17). Westport: Ablex.

Chen, S. X., & Mak, W. W. (2008). Seeking professional help: Etiology beliefs about mental illness across cultures. *Journal of Counseling Psychology, 55*, 442–450.

Chen, K. C., Lu, R., Iqbal, U., Hsu, K. C., Chen, B. L., Nguyen, P. A., Yang, H. C., Huang, C. W., Li, Y. C., Jian, W. S., & Tsai, S. H. (2015). Interactions between traditional Chinese medicine and western drugs in Taiwan: A population-based study. *Computer Methods and Programs in Biomedicine, 122*, 462–470.

Chen, C. C., Ünal, A. F., Leung, K., & Xin, K. R. (2016). Group harmony in the workplace: Conception, measurement, and validation. *Asia Pacific Journal of Management, 33*, 903–934.

Cheng, C., Lo, B., & Chio, H. (2008). The Tao (way) of Chinese coping. In M. H. Bond (Ed.), *The oxford handbook of Chinese psychology* (pp. 399–419). New York: Oxford University Press.

Cheung, F. M., Lau, B. W., & Waldmann, E. (1981). Somatization among Chinese depressives in general practice. *International Journal of Psychiatry in Medicine, 10*, 361–374.

Cheung, F. M. (1990). People against the mentally ill: Community opposition to residential treatment facilities. *Community Mental Health Journal, 26*(2), 205–212.

Chiao, J. Y., & Blizinsky, K. D. (2010). Culture-gene coevolution of individualism-collectivism and the serotonin transporter gene. *Proceedings of the Royal Society of London B: Biological Sciences, 277*, 529–537.

Chung, V. C. (2014). Views on traditional Chinese medicine amongst Chinese population: A systematic review of qualitative and quantitative studies. *Health Expectations, 17*, 622–636.

Chung, K. F., Tso, K. C., Cheung, E., & Wong, M. (2010). Validation of the Chinese version of the Mood Disorder Questionnaire in a psychiatric population in Hong Kong. *Psychiatry and Clinical Neurosciences, 62*, 464–471.

Clatworthy, J., Bowskill, R., Rank, T., Parham, R., & Horne, R. (2007). Adherence to medication in bipolar disorder: a qualitative study exploring the role of patients' beliefs about the condition and its treatment. *Bipolar Disorders, 9*, 656–664.

Craddock, N. J., & Sklar, P. (1999). Genetics of bipolar disorder. *Lancet, 381*, 1654–1662.

Davis, E., Greenberger, E., Charles, S., Chen, C., Zhao, L., & Dong, Q. (2012). Emotion experience and regulation in China and the United States: How do culture and gender shape emotion responding? *International Journal of Psychology, 47*, 230–239.

Egeland, J. A., & Hostetter, A. M. (1983). Amish Study, III: The impact of cultural factors on diagnosis of bipolar illness. *The American Journal of Psychiatry, 140*, 67–71.

Etain, B., Henry, C., Bellivier, F., Mathieu, F., & Leboyer, M. (2010). Beyond genetics: Childhood affective trauma in bipolar disorder. *Bipolar Disorders, 10*, 867–876.

Faure, G. O., & Fang, T. (2008). Changing Chinese values: Keeping up with paradoxes. *International Business Review, 17*, 194–207.

Gaw, A. (2001). *Concise guide to cross-cultural psychiatry*. Washington, DC: American Psychiatric Publishing.

Gibbs, T., Okuda, M., Oquendo, M., Lawson, W., Wang, S., Thomas, Y., & Blanco, C. (2013). Mental health of African Americans and Caribbean blacks in the United States: Results from the National Epidemiological Survey on Alcohol and Related Conditions. *American Journal of Public Health, 103*, 330–338.

Grabell, A. S., Olson, S. L., Miller, A. L., Kessler, D. A., Felt, B., Kaciroti, N., Wang, L., & Tardif, T. (2015). The impact of culture on physiological processes of emotion regulation: A comparison of US and Chinese preschoolers. *Developmental Science, 18*, 420–435.

Greenberger, E., Chen, C., Tally, S. R., & Qi, D. (2000). Family, peer, and individual correlates of depressive symptomatology among U.S. and Chinese adolescents. *Journal of Consulting and Clinical Psychology, 68*, 209–219.

Huwaë, S., & Schaafsma, J. (2016). Cross-cultural differences in emotion suppression in everyday interactions. *International Journal of Psychology, 53*, 176–183.

Jack, R. E. (2013). Culture and facial expressions of emotion. *Visual Cognition, 21*, 1248–1286.

Jiang, Y. P. (2003). The TCM diagnosis and treatment of bipolar disorder. *Acupuncture Today, 4*, 9.

Johnson, K. R., & Johnson, S. L. (2014). Cross-national prevalence and cultural correlates of bipolar I disorder. *Social Psychiatry and Psychiatric Epidemiology, 49*, 1111–1117.

Johnson, S., Cuellar, A., Ruggero, C., Winett-Perlman, C., Goodnick, P., White, R., & Miller, I. (2008). Life events as predictors of mania and depression in bipolar I disorder. *Journal of Abnormal Psychology, 117*, 268–277.

Judd, L. L., Schettler, P. J., Akiskal, H. S., Maser, J., Coryell, W., Solomon, D., Endicott, J., & Keller, M. (2003). Long-term symptomatic status of bipolar I vs. bipolar II disorders. *International Journal of Neuropsychopharmacology, 6*, 127–137.

Kirmayer, L. J., & Groleau, D. (2001). Affective disorders in cultural context. *Psychiatric Clinics of North America, 24*, 465–478.

Kleinman, A. (1978). Culture and depression. *Culture, Medicine and Psychiatry, 2*, 295–296.

Kleinman, A. (1982). Neurasthenia and depression: A study of somatization and culture in China. *Culture Medicine and Psychiatry, 6*, 117–190.

Kleinman, A. (2004). Culture and depression. *New England Journal of Medicine, 351*, 951–953.

Kyaga, S., Lichtenstein, P., Boman, M., Hultman, C., Långström, N., & Landén, M. (2011). Creativity and mental disorder: Family study of 300,000 people with severe mental disorder. *British Journal of Psychiatry, 199*, 373–379.

Lam, W. W., Fielding, R., Mcdowell, I., Johnston, J., Chan, S., Leung, G. M., & Lam, T. H. (2012). Perspectives on family health, happiness and harmony (3H) among Hong Kong Chinese people: A qualitative study. *Health Education Research, 27*, 767–779.

Lan, Y. C., Zelman, D. C., & Chao, W. T. (2018). Angry characters and frightened souls: Patients and family explanatory models of bipolar disorder in Taiwan. *Transcultural Psychiatry, 55*, 317–338.

Lee, S. B. (1993). Side effects of chronic lithium therapy in Hong Kong Chinese: An ethnopsychiatric perspective. *Culture Medicine and Psychiatry, 17*, 301–320.

Lee, S., Wing, Y. K., & Wong, K. C. (1992). Knowledge and compliance towards lithium therapy among Chinese psychiatric patients in Hong Kong. *Australian and New Zealand Journal of Psychiatry, 26*, 444–449.

Lee, D. T., Kleinman, J., & Kleinman, A. (2007). Rethinking depression: An ethnographic study of the experiences of depression among Chinese. *Harvard Review of Psychiatry, 15*, 1–8.

Lee, S., Tsang, A., Huang, Y. Q., He, Y. L., Liu, Z. R., Zhang, M. Y., Shen, Y. C., & Kessler, R. C. (2009). The epidemiology of depression in metropolitan China. *Psychological Medicine, 39*, 735–747.

Leung, K., Koch, P. T., & Lu, L. (2002). A dualistic model of harmony and its implications for conflict management in Asia. *Asia Pacific Journal of Management, 19*, 201–220.

Leung, K., Brew, F. P., Zhang, Z. X., & Zhang, Y. (2011). Harmony and conflict: A cross-cultural investigation in China and Australia. *Journal of Cross-Cultural Psychology, 42*, 795–816.

Li, Z., & Li, X. (2005). *Yellow Emperor's canon of medicine: Plain conversation*. Xi'an: Xi'an World Publishing Corporation (in Chinese).

Li, Y., Wang, M., Wang, C., & Shi, J. (2010). Individualism, collectivism, and Chinese adolescents' aggression: Intracultural variations. *Aggressive Behavior, 36*, 187–194.

Lin, K., & Cheung, F. (1999). Mental health issues for Asian Americans. *Psychiatric Services, 50*, 774–780.

Lin, C. J., Shiah, I. S., Chu, H., Tsai, P. S., Chen, C. H., Chang, Y. C., & Chou, K. R. (2011). Reliability and validity of the Chinese version of the Mood Disorder Questionnaire. *Archives of Psychiatric Nursing, 25*, 53–62.

Loo, P., Wong, S., & Furnham, A. (2012). Mental health literacy: A cross-cultural study from Britain, Hong Kong and Malaysia. *Asia-Pacific Psychiatry, 4*, 113–125.

Luk, C. L., & Bond, M. H. (1992). Chinese lay beliefs about the causes and cures of psychological problems. *Journal of Social and Clinical Psychology, 11*, 140–157.

Lutz, C. A. (1985). Depression and the translation of emotional worlds. In A. Kleinman & B. Good (Eds.), *Culture and depression: Studies in the anthropology and cross-cultural psychiatry of affect and disorder* (pp. 255–256). Berkeley: University of California Press.

Mak, W. W. S., & Chen, S. X. (2010). Illness behaviors among the Chinese. In M. H. Bond (Ed.), *The Oxford handbook of Chinese psychology* (pp. 421–439). New York: Oxford University Press.

Man, M. M., & Bond, M. H. (2005). A lexically derived measure of relationship concord in Chinese culture. *Journal of Psychology in Chinese Societies, 6*, 109–128.

Mcguffin, P., Rijsdijk, F., Andrew, M., Sham, P., Katz, R., & Cardno, A. (2003). The heritability of bipolar affective disorder and the genetic relationship to unipolar depression. *Archives of General Psychiatry, 60*, 497–502.

McMullen, L., & Conway, J. (1996). Conceptualizing the figurative expressions of psychotherapy clients. In J. S. Mio & A. N. Katz (Eds.), *Metaphor: Implications and applications* (pp. 59–71). Mahwah: Lawrence Erlbaum Associates.

Merikangas, K. R., Jin, R., He, J. P., He, J., Kessler, R. C., Lee, S., Sampson, N. A., Viana, M. C., Andrade, L. H., Hu, C., Karam, E. G., Ladea, M., Medina-Mora, M. E., Ono, Y., Posada-Villa, J., Sagar, R., Wells, J. E., & Zarkov, Z. (2011). Prevalence and correlates of bipolar spectrum disorder in the world mental health survey initiative. *Archives of General Psychiatry, 68*, 241–251.

Mitchell, P. B., Goodwin, G. M., Johnson, G. F., & Hirschfeld, R. M. (2010). Diagnostic guidelines for bipolar depression: A probabilistic approach. *Bipolar Disorders, 10*, 144–152.

Ng, E. (2009). Heartache of the state, enemy of the self: Bipolar disorder and cultural change in urban China. *Culture, Medicine and Psychiatry, 33*, 421–450.

Nikolaus, S., Müller, H. W., & Hautzel, H. (2017). Different patterns of dopaminergic and serotonergic dysfunction in manic, depressive and euthymic phases of bipolar disorder. *Nuklearmedizin, 56*, 191–200.

Parker, G., Cheah, Y. C., & Roy, K. (2001). Do the Chinese somatize depression? A cross-cultural study. *Social Psychiatry and Psychiatric Epidemiology, 36*, 287–293.

Perlick, D. A., Rosenheck, R. A., Clarkin, J. F., Sirey, J. A., Salahi, J., Struening, E. L., & Link, B. G. (2001). Stigma as a barrier to recovery: Adverse effects of perceived stigma on social adaptation of persons diagnosed with bipolar affective disorder. *Psychiatric Services, 52*, 1627–1632.

Phillips, M. R., Zhang, J., Shi, Q., Song, Z., Ding, Z., Pang, S., Li, X., Zhang, Y., & Wang, Z. (2009). Prevalence, treatment, and associated disability of mental disorders in four provinces in China during 2001–05: An epidemiological survey. *Lancet, 373*, 2041–2053.

Proudfoot, J., Doran, J., Manicavasagar, V., & Parker, G. (2011). The precipitants of manic/hypomanic episodes in the context of bipolar disorder: A review. *Journal of Affective Disorders, 133*, 381–387.

Putten, T. V. (1975). Why do patients with manic-depressive illness stop their lithium? *Comprehensive Psychiatry, 16*, 179–183.

Rochelle, T. L., & Yim, K. H. (2014). Factors associated with utilisation of traditional Chinese medicine among Hong Kong Chinese. *Psychology Health and Medicine, 19*, 453–462.

Romera, I., Delgado-Cohen, H., Perez, T., Caballero, L., & Gilaberte, I. (2008). Factor analysis of the Zung self-rating depression scale in a large sample of patients with major depressive disorder in primary care. *BMC Psychiatry, 8*, 4.

Rose, N. (2003). The neurochemical self and its anomalies. In R. Ericson & A. Doyle (Eds.), *Risk and morality* (pp. 407–437). Toronto: University of Toronto Press.

Ryder, A. G., Yang, J., Zhu, X., Yao, S., Yi, J., Heine, S. J., & Bagby, R. M. (2008). The cultural shaping of depression: Somatic symptoms in China, psychological symptoms in North America. *Journal of Abnormal Psychology, 117*, 300–313.

Sethi, S., & Khanna, R. (1993). Phenomenology of mania in eastern India. *Psychopathology, 26*, 274–278.

Shafer, A. B. (2010). Meta-analysis of the factor structures of four depression questionnaires: Beck, CES-D, Hamilton, and Zung. *Journal of Clinical Psychology, 62*, 123–146.

Shen, Y. C., Zhang, M. Y., Huang, Y. Q., He, Y. L., Liu, Z. R., Cheng, H., Tsang, A., Lee, S., & Kessler, R. C. (2006). Twelve-month prevalence, severity, and unmet need for treatment of mental disorders in metropolitan China. *Psychological Medicine, 36*, 257–267.

Shweder, R. A., Much, N. C., Mahapatra, M., & Park, L. (1997). The "big three"of morality (autonomy, community and divinity) and the "big three"explanations of suffering. In A. M. Brandt & P. Rozin (Eds.), *Morality and health* (pp. 119–169). Florence: Routledge.

Sontag, S. (1989). *AIDS and its metaphors*. New York: Farrar, Straus and Giroux.

Strakowski, S. M., Delbello, M. P., & Adler, C. M. (2004). The functional neuroanatomy of bipolar disorder: A review of neuroimaging findings. *Molecular Psychiatry, 10*, 105–116.

Strakowski, S. M., Adler, C. M., Almeida, J. R. C., Altshuler, L. L., Blumberg, H. P., Chang, K. D., DelBello, M. P., Frangou, S., McIntosh, A., Phillips, M. L., Sussmanh, J. E., & Townsend, J. D. (2012). The functional neuroanatomy of bipolar disorder: A consensus model. *Bipolar Disorders, 14*, 313–325.

Subramanian, K., Sarkar, S., & Kattimani, S. (2017). Bipolar disorder in Asia: Illness course and contributing factors. *Asian Journal of Psychiatry, 29*, 16–29.

Triandis, H. C. (1995). *Individualism and collectivism: New directions in social psychology*. Boulder: Westview Press.

Tsai, J. L., & Levenson, R. W. (1997). Cultural influences of emotional responding: Chinese American and European American dating couples during interpersonal conflict. *Journal of Cross-Cultural Psychology, 28*, 600–625.

Tsai, J. L., Levenson, R. W., & Mccoy, K. (2006). Cultural and temperamental variation in emotional response. *Emotion, 6*, 484–497.

Tylee, A., & Gandhi, P. (2005). The importance of somatic symptoms in depression in primary care. *Primary Care Companion to the Journal of clinical psychiatry, 7*, 167–176.

Tyler, T. R., Lind, E. A., & Huo, Y. J. (2000). Cultural values and authority relations: The psychology of conflict resolution across cultures. *Psychology, Public Policy, and Law, 6*, 1138–1163.

Wang, Y., & Henning, M. (2010). Bipolar disorder and medical adherence: A Chinese perspective. *Asian Journal of Psychiatry, 3*, 7–11.

Wei, M., Su, J. C., Carrera, S., Lin, S. P., & Yi, F. (2013). Suppression and interpersonal harmony: A cross-cultural comparison between Chinese and European Americans. *Journal of Counseling Psychology, 60*, 625–633.

Wong, D. F., Tsui, H. K., Pearson, V., Chen, E. Y., & Chiu, S. N. (2004). Family burdens, Chinese health beliefs, and the mental health of Chinese caregivers in Hong Kong. *Transcultural Psychiatry, 41*, 497–513.

World Health Organization. (1992). *The ICD-10 classification of mental and behavior disorders. Clinical descriptions and diagnostic guidelines*. Geneva: World Health Organization.

World Health Organization. (2017). *International classification of diseases* (11th beta Ed.). Retrieved October 12, 2018, from http://www.who.int/classifications/icd/revision/en

Wu, D. Y. (1982). Psychotherapy and emotion in traditional Chinese medicine. In A. J. Marsella & G. M. White (Eds.), *Cultural conceptions of mental health and therapy* (pp. 285–301). Dordrecht: Reidel.

Wu, Y. S., Angst, J., Ou, C. S., Chen, H. C., & Lu, R. B. (2008). Validation of the Chinese version of the Hypomania Checklist (HCL-32) as an instrument for detecting hypo(mania) in patients with mood disorders. *Journal of Affective Disorders, 106*, 133–143.

Yan, Z. Y., Gu, M. J., Zhong, B. L., Wang, C., Tang, H. L., Ling, Y. Q., Yu, X. W., & Li, M. Q. (2013). Prevalence, risk factors and recognition rates of depressive disorders among inpatients of tertiary general hospitals in Shanghai, China. *Journal of Psychosomatic Research, 75*, 65–71.

Yang, G. (1973). *The scholars*. Beijing: Foreign Languages Press.

Yen, S., Robins, C. J., & Lin, N. (2000). A cross-cultural comparison of depressive symptom manifestation: China and the United States. *Journal of Consulting and Clinical Psychology, 68*, 993–999.

Yuan, W. (2010). Conflict management among American and Chinese employees in multinational organizations in China. *Cross Cultural Management, 17*, 299–311.

Zhang, D. (1995). Depression and culture–A Chinese perspective. *Canadian Journal of Counselling, 29*, 227–233.

Predicting Affective States of Bipolar Disorder by the Chinese Adjective Descriptors of Personality

Bingren Zhang, Junpeng Zhu, and Wei Wang

1 Introduction

Bipolar I (BD I) and II (BD II) disorders exist extensively in the young population. They are severe and recurrent mood disorders accompanied by great morbidity, working as one of the main causes of world-wide disabilities (Cerimele et al. 2014). Although BD I and BD II are equal in prevalence across sexes, their clinical manifestations were different (Müller-Oerlinghausen et al. 2002). BD I has no less than one manic or mixed episodes, while BD II has a more chronic course mainly with major and minor depressive episodes and shorter inter-episodes. Furthermore, BD I has a higher prevalence of reckless activity, distractibility, psychomotor agitation, irritable mood and increased self-esteem (Serretti and Olgiati 2007), while BD II has more chronic depressive course (Judd et al. 2003), and is often over-activated in goal-directed tasks (Benazzi 2007). Besides, BD II has particularly elevated risk of suicide and poorer prognosis than BD I has (Phillips and Kupfer 2013; Cerimele et al. 2014).

In spite that the prevalence of bipolar disorder in China is comparable to that in Western societies (Merikangas et al. 2011), Chinese patients have some distinct characteristics, and learning more about these clinical features and their causes would be assistant in managing the patients in China and surrounding countries. Evidence has shown that generally, the comorbidity rate of alcohol dependence in Chinese bipolar disorder patients is lower than that in the Western patients (Tsai

B. Zhang · W. Wang (✉)
Department of Clinical Psychology and Psychiatry/School of Public Health, Zhejiang University College of Medicine, Hangzhou, China
e-mail: drwangwei@zju.edu.cn

J. Zhu
Department of Psychiatry, Zhejiang Provincial People's Hospital, Hangzhou, China

Department of Psychiatry, People's Hospital of Hangzhou Medical College, Hangzhou, China

© Springer Nature Singapore Pte Ltd. 2019   167
W. Wang (ed.), *Chinese Perspectives on Cultural Psychiatry*,
https://doi.org/10.1007/978-981-13-3537-2_10

et al. 1997). Furthermore, the comorbidity rate of diabetes in patients with bipolar disorder is higher in Taiwan (Chien et al. 2010). In Mainland China, concerning the cognitive aspects, younger bipolar disorder patients tended to attach importance to self-blame and individual responsibility for illness control (Ng 2009).

Several factors might contribute to the clinical distinctiveness of Chinese bipolar disorder. The first one might be the ways to express and control emotion in Chinese. The most important characteristic in Chinese culture is the high Collectivism along with power distance (Leung 2008), and Confucianism is its cornerstone (Bond and Pang 1991; Guo 1995). "Express joy or anger without form or color" is encouraged in Chinese culture to reach a balance (Krone and Morgan 2000; Tjosvold and Su 2007), i.e., to reinforce the positive effect for the negative, and the negative for the positive. Since childhood, the Chinese are told to control disruptive emotions, in order to keep harmonious social-interaction (Li et al. 2010). Bipolar disorder patients in China reflected greater concerns about irritability, anger, and family conflict than about other symptoms, contributing to stigma and family shame about the disease, and forcing the individuals with bipolar disorder to suppress emotional symptoms rather than to seek professional help (Lan et al. 2018). They used problem-focused, emotion-focused, and cultural coping methods to deal with their emotional problems and achieve their expected possible selves (Tse et al. 2014). When coping with emotional problems like depression, Chinese people tend to deny it or express it somatically, and prefer to use coping mechanisms like quiescence and stoicism, and the family or cultural support systems, instead of excessively "pathologize" aspects of human experience like the Western people do (Parker et al. 2001).

The second reason might be the differences in personality trait (Triandis and Suh 2002; Heine and Buchtel 2009). For example, Coulston et al. (2013) have found that bipolar disorder patients had elevated extraversion, adaptive coping and self-esteem, while decreased anxiety when it comes to the personality traits measured by the Big-Five Model or the Alternative Five-Factor Model. Bagby et al. (1997) have reported higher, but Stringer et al. (2014) reported lower openness to experience in bipolar disorders comparing with healthy individuals. In terms of the disorder subtypes, Saddichha and Schutz (2014) found both BD I and BD II patients were impulsive, while Dervic et al. (2015) have reported higher impulsivity in BD I rather than in BD II. Xu et al. (2015) and Yao et al. (2015) have found higher impulsive sensation seeking and borderline traits in BD I rather than in BD II respectively. On the other side, Kim et al. (2012) have reported that BD II patients had lower extraversion while higher neuroticism than BD I patients did.

So far, no study has explored the emic personality trait in Chinese culture that is linked with the bipolar disorder. A questionnaire based on the Chinese adjective pool has been developed and named the Chinese Adjective Descriptors of Personality (CADP, see Chapter "Personality Traits in Contemporary China: A Lexical Approach"), to measure five dimensions of Intelligent, Emotional, Conscientious, Unsocial and Agreeable. These dimensions are roughly corresponding to the personality domains of the Big-Five Model, namely Openness to experience, Neuroticism, Conscientiousness, Extraversion and Agreeableness. Interestingly, the factor Intelligent, which might be highly related but not equal to the Intelligence Quotient, turned to be the first among all personality dimensions. It differed from studies conducted in the Western society (Costa and McCrae 1997; Heine and Buchtel 2009). According to the social structural theory (White 1992; Lin 2001), in China it would be helpful to fit into society to have higher intelligence. Therefore, Chinese people tend to devote much attention and financial resources to child-education for intelligence assessing (Bush and Qiang 2000; Hui 2005). Unfortunately, their emotional expression or regulation problems sometimes display after an academic failure (Liu and Tein 2005).

Concerning the evidence on relationship between personality traits and affective disorders, besides the prominent traits of extraversion and neuroticism in bipolar disorders mentioned above (Bagby et al. 1997; Kim et al. 2012; Coulston et al. 2013), higher neuroticism was also found in unipolar depression (Jain, et al. 1999; Lozano and Johnson 2001). On the other side, there is a link between intelligence and mania (Maisel 2013), and between professional success, creativity and bipolar disorder (Jamison 1995). It is then presumable that the traits relating to intelligence are associated with mania in BD I patients, and traits concerning the emotional regulation are linked with depression in BD II patients.

In order to figure out whether in Chinese culture, the personality traits are related to the affective states (i.e., mania, hypomania, and depression) in the healthy volunteers and in patients with bipolar disorder, in the current study, we tested the Chinese versions of the CADP, the Mood Disorder Questionnaire (Hirschfeld et al. 2000), the Hypomanic Checklist-32 (Angst et al. 2005), and the Plutchik-van Praag Depression Inventory (Plutchik and van Praag 1987) in patients with BD I and BD II as well as in healthy volunteers.

2 Methods

2.1 Participants

We enrolled 216 healthy volunteers (92 men and 124 women; aged 20.42 years ± 1.23 S.D., ranged 17 ~ 24 years), 73 patients with bipolar I (BD I, 36 men and 37 women; aged 20.30 $\pm$ 1.31, ranged 17 ~ 24), and 35 bipolar II (BD II, 10 men and 25 women; aged 20.66 $\pm$ 1.06, ranged 18 ~ 23) in the current study, all the participants were Chinese Han youngsters and received nine-year compulsory education. No age (F [2, 321] = 0.99, MSE = 1.50, p = 0.37), education (F = 0.90, MSE = 1.01, p = 0.41), or gender (χ^2 = 4.16, p = 0.13) differences were found between-groups. After clinical interviews by two experienced psychiatrists, all the patients were diagnosed according to the DSM-5 (American Psychiatric Association 2013). Additionally, they suffered from no organic brain lesions according to magnetic resonance imaging or computed tomography scans and had to be free from antipsychotic drugs or alcohol for at least 72 h prior to testing. The healthy volunteers had no history of psychiatric or neurological abnormalities and were free from alcohol or drug use for at least 72 h prior to participating in the study. The demographic and clinical characteristics of patients, as well as of the healthy volunteers are illustrated in Table 1.

2.2 Questionnaires

Participants were asked to complete the following four questionnaires in a quiet room.

A. The Chinese Adjective Descriptors of Personality (CADP)

The CADP with 100 Chinese adjectives is designed to measure the personality traits such as the Intelligent, Emotional, Conscientious, Unsocial and Agreeable (20 adjectives each) (see Chapter "Personality Traits in Contemporary China: A Lexical Approach"). Participants were asked to complete the rating items using the Likert type scales: 1-very unlike me, 2-moderately unlike me, 3-somewhat like and unlike me, 4-moderately like me, and 5-very like me. Among all participants of the current study, its scale internal reliabilities were 0.96 for Intelligent, 0.93 for Emotional, 0.94 for Conscientious, 0.90 for Unsocial and 0.89 for Agreeable, respectively.

B. The Mood Disorder Questionnaire (MDQ)

Table 1 Clinical manifestations of patients with bipolar disorder type I (BD I, n = 73), and type II (BD II, n = 35)

	BD I	BD II
Mania attack (number range)	1–4	–
Hypomania attack (number range)	0–2	1–6
Depression attack (number range)	3–7	4–10
On-going mania (patient number)	12	0
On-going hypomania (patient number)	1	2
On-going depression (patient number)	30	27
On-going mixed states (mania/hypomania, and depression; patient number)	30	6
Disease duration (month; mean ± SD, range)	29.3 ± 7.4	31.2 ± 8.3
Medication (treatment)-naive (patient number)	50	17
Medicated with anxiolytics (alprazolam, clonazapam, or lorazepam; patient number)	4	5
Medicated with antidepressants (fluoxetine or sertraline; patient number)	15	16
Medicated with mood stabilizers (valproate or lithium; patient number)	9	8
Obsessive-compulsive disorder (patient number)	44	22
Sleep problem (difficulty falling into/ unrefreshing sleep; patient number)	41	24
Suicidal ideation (without attempt; patient number)	30	18

After Yu et al. (2015)

The MDQ consists of three parts, including 13 forced-choice (yes or no) questions to assess the presence of symptoms and behaviors related to mania or hypomania, one question to determine whether two or more symptoms have been experienced at the same time, and one question to determine the extent to which symptoms have caused functional impairment on a scale ranging from "no problems" to "serious problems" (Hirschfeld et al. 2000). The MDQ was comparable to other mania measures such as the Young Mania Rating Scale (Young et al. 1978). Among all participants of the current study, its scale internal reliability was 0.82.

C. The Hypomania Checklist-32 (HCL-32)

The HCL-32 is a self-assessment instrument comprising 32 items for detecting hypomanic symptoms (Angst et al. 2005). Individuals were instructed to answer the forced-choice (yes or no) questions about emotions, thoughts, or behaviors, and to answer questions regarding the duration, the impact of family, social and work life, or people's reactions. Among all participants of the current study, its scale internal reliability was 0.87.

D. The Plutchik-van Praag Depression Inventory (PVP)

The PVP contains 34 items (Plutchik and van Praag 1987). Each item has a three-point scale (0, 1, 2), which corresponds to depressive tendencies. Participants have "possible depression" if they score between 20 and 25, or "depression" if they score higher than 25. The PVP was comparable to other depression measures such as the Hamilton Depression Rating Scale (Hamilton 1967), and among all participants of the current study, its scale internal reliability was 0.92.

2.3   Statistical Analysis

Two-way ANOVA was applied to the mean scores of the five CADP scales in three groups of participants. One-way ANOVA was applied to the mean MDQ, HCL-32 and PVP scales in three groups of participants. Whenever a significant main effect was found, post-hoc analysis by the Dunnett test was employed to evaluate between-group differences. The Pearson correlation test was used to search for possible relations between MDQ, HCL-32, PVP and the five CADP scales. In addition, inspired by a study (Schrijvers, et al. 2010), we applied the multiple linear regression analysis (backward method) to confirm the relationships between the five CADP traits, MDQ, HCL-32 and PVP scales, taking CADP traits as potential predictors for the rest scales. A p value less than 0.05 was considered as significant. In the current study, we chose a conservative way to calculate the power statistic, by performing a post-hoc (instead of priori) analysis and employing the sample size (n = 35) of the smallest group. The power analysis for the two-way ANOVA produced an adequate power statistic of 86.28%.

3   Results

Two-way ANOVA has detected no significance of the mean scores of the five CADP traits among the three groups (group effect, F [2, 321] = 1.59, MSE = 341.04, p = 0.21) (Fig. 1). By contrast, one-way ANOVA has detected that the mean MDQ scores were significantly different among the three groups (F [2, 321] = 479.30, MSE = 1327.60, p < 0.001; the effect survived after controlling for PVP/ HCL-32), with BD I (p < 0.001; 95% confidence interval (CI): 6.38 ~ 7.46) and II (p < 0.001; 95% CI: 2.18 ~ 3.64) scored higher than healthy controls did, and BD I higher than BD II did (p < 0.001; 95% CI: 3.19 ~ 4.84). The mean HCL-32 scores were signifi-cantly different among the three groups (F [2, 321] = 188.79, MSE = 3308.48, p < 0.001; the effect survived after controlling for PVP/MDQ), with both BD I (p < 0.001; 95% CI: 9.20 ~ 11.93) and BD II (p < 0.001; 95% CI: 4.94 ~ 8.62) scored higher than healthy controls did, and BD I higher than BD II did (p < 0.001; 95% CI: 1.71 ~ 5.86). The mean PVP scores were also different among the three groups (F [2, 321] = 118.77, MSE = 6624.30, p < 0.001; the effect survived after controlling for MDQ/ HCL-32), with BD II higher than BD I (p < 0.001; 95% CI: 8.75 ~ 16.14) and healthy controls did (p < 0.001; 95% CI: 16.68 ~ 23.23), and BD I higher than healthy controls did (p < 0.001; 95% CI: 5.07 ~ 9.94) (Fig. 2).

When considering the relationships between the MDQ, HCL-32, PVP scales and personality traits, the Pearson correlation test had detected several significant cor-relations in the three groups. In BD I, MDQ was significantly correlated with Intelligent (n = 73, r = 0.25, p < 0.05), and PVP correlated with Emotional (r = 0.33, p < 0.001). In healthy controls, PVP was significantly correlated with Intelligent (n = 216, r = −0.22, p < 0.001) and Emotional (r = 0.21, p < 0.001). No significant correlations were found in BD II.

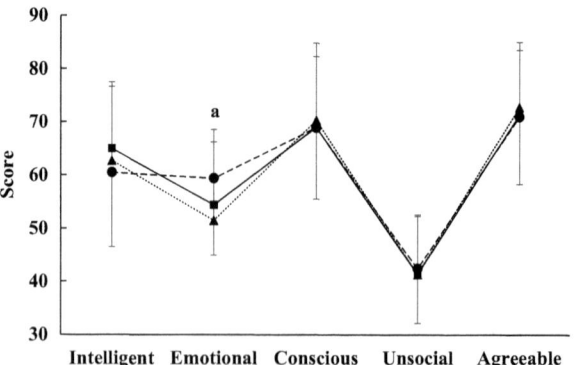

Fig. 1   Scores (mean ± S.D.) of the five scales of the Chinese Adjective Descriptors of Personality in the healthy volunteers (Controls, n = 216, closed triangle with dotted line) and patients with bipolar I (BD I, n = 73, closed square with thin line) and II (BD II, n = 35, closed circle with dashed line) disorders. a, p < 0.05 for BD II vs. Controls. (After Yu et al. 2015)

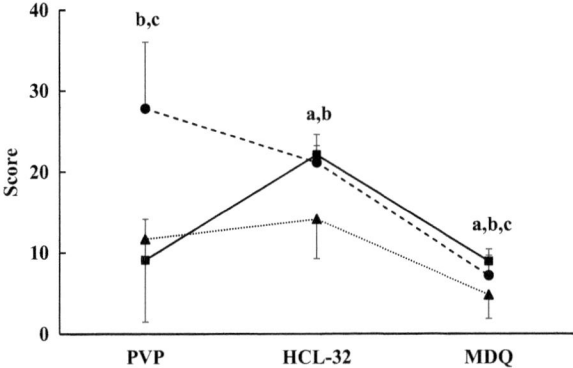

Fig. 2 Scores (mean ± S.D.) of the Mood Disorder Questionnaire (MDQ), the Hypomania Checklist-32 (HCL-32), the Plutchik-van Praag Depression Inventory (PVP) in the healthy volunteers (Controls, n = 216, closed triangle with dotted line) and patients with bipolar I (BD I, n = 73, closed square with thin line) and II (BD II, n = 35, closed circle with dashed line) disorder. (**a**) p < 0.05 for BD I vs. Controls; (**b**) p < 0.05 for BD II vs. Controls; (**c**) p < 0.05 for BD I vs. BD II. (After Yu et al. 2015)

Table 2 Backward multiple regression results of predicting the Mood Disorder Questionnaire (MDQ), the Hypomania Checklist-32 (HCL-32), and the Plutchik-van Praag Depression Inventory (PVP) by the Chinese Adjective Descriptors of Personality in the healthy volunteers (Controls, n = 216) and patients with bipolar I (BD I, n = 73) and II (BD II, n = 35) disorders

	Controls		BD I		BD II	
	aR^2	Beta, predictor	aR^2	Beta, predictor	aR^2	Beta, predictor
MDQ			0.05	**0.25 Intelligent**	0.10	**0.22 Intelligent**
						−0.24 Agreeable
						0.31 Unsocial
HCL-32			0.01	−0.15 Emotional	0.13	**−0.20 Intelligent**
						−0.31 Agreeable
						−0.26 Emotional
PVP	0.08	−0.16 Intelligent	0.15	**−0.24 Intelligent**		
		−0.10 Agreeable		**0.26 Agreeable**		
		0.17 Emotional		**0.34 Emotional**		

Note: Predictors with p < 0.05 were listed in the table; |beta| ≥ 0.20 were bolded for clarity; aR^2, adjusted R^2
After Yu et al. (2015)

Furthermore, some relationships between the MDQ, HCL-32 and PVP scales and personality traits were replicated by the backward multiple linear regression analysis. Although the adjusted R^2 values were relatively small (Table 2), there were some predictors in patient groups. In BD I, the CADP Intelligent trait (n = 73, beta = 0.25) predicted the MDQ; and the Intelligent (beta = −0.24), Agreeable (beta = 0.26), and Emotional (beta = 0.34) traits predicted the PVP. In BD II, the Intelligent (n = 35, beta = 0.22), Agreeable (beta = −0.24), and Unsocial (beta = 0.31) traits predicted the MDQ; and the Intelligent (beta = −0.20), Agreeable (beta = −0.31), and Emotional (beta = −0.26) traits predicted the HCL-32.

4 Discussion

In the current study, our results revealed that both BD I and BD II groups scored higher on the MDQ, HCL-32 and PVP, consistent with previous results (e.g., Zimmerman and Galione 2011; Leao and del Porto 2012). Additionally, BD I scored higher on the MDQ than BD II did, in accord with previous report (Isometsä et al. 2003). BD II got higher scores on the HCL-32 and PVP than BD I did, as documented before (Benazzi 2007). Moreover, we found relationships between personality traits and emotional scales in patient groups rather than in healthy controls, as those confirmed by the multiple linear regression analysis (Table 2). The associations found in patients partially confirmed our hypotheses on the one hand, partially in line with the findings of the Big-Five personality traits in bipolar patients on the other (Bagby et al. 1997; Jain et al. 1999; Lozano and Johnson 2001; Kim et al. 2012; Coulston et al. 2013).

In BD I group, the result that CADP Intelligent trait was significantly correlated with the MDQ score confirmed our second hypothesis and was consistent with the linkage between high intelligence, creativity and mood disorders (Jamison 1995; Maisel 2013). There might also be a Chinese culture contribution to the relationship. The Chinese conception of intelligence was significantly different from that of the Western society which defines it as the intellectual power of humans, which enable people to learn, form concepts, understand, and reason (Yang and Sternberg 1997; Serpell 2000). In general, the Chinese people recognize intelligence as the ability to empathize with and understand others, which is mainly related with individual's social roles and responsibilities (Serpell 2000). From the ancient philosophical perspective, Confucian thinks an intelligent person should devote his life to personality cultivation to embody benevolence and act according to what is right. As for Daoists, once an individual comprehends the *Dao*, i.e., the true greatness, and can put it into practice, he is intelligent (Yang and Sternberg 1997, also in Chapter "Societal Culture from Late Imperial to Contemporary China: As Indirectly Reflected in a Dream of Red Mansions"). It is then easier to understand that the Chinese respect intelligence to a large extent, and they take pride in being intelligent. This might be exactly the case in patients suffering from mania.

In BD I group, the CADP Intelligent trait was negatively correlated with the PVP. In fact, there is a tendency that intelligent people develop higher cognitive awareness so that more complex or multiple factors lead to their social success and lower risk of depression (Jorm 2001; Barnhill 2001). In our study we also found the correlation between Agreeable trait and PVP, similar with the previous results (Kahn et al. 1985; de Fruyt et al. 2006). Actually, an accumulation of complaining the excessive agreeableness may lead to depression (Castagnini and Berrios 2009; Weintraub 2012). However, in Chinese primary schools and organizations, the obedience, quietness and patience are usually stressed (Redding and Wong 1986; Yang 1990). In addition, our study demonstrated that the Emotional trait significantly predicted the PVP. In contrast with our first hypothesis, this association was found in BD I instead of BD II. It could be explained by the higher borderline trait in BD I (Yao et al. 2015), which is highly connected with depression (Levy et al. 2007), and the Emotional trait resembles borderline trait (see Chapter "Personality Traits in Contemporary China: A Lexical Approach"), therefore might lead to a higher depressive level.

In BD II group, the CADP Intelligent trait was associated with the MDQ such as that in BD I, which went beyond our second hypothesis, and suggested in Chinese culture, Intelligent trait has a specific influence on emotion control in bipolar patients. Moreover, the Agreeable trait was negatively associated with the MDQ, consistent with the negative relationship between agreeableness and the manic severity in bipolar disorders (Quilty et al. 2009; Kim et al. 2012; Quilty et al. 2013). We also found the correlation between the Unsocial trait and the MDQ, which fits into the findings that the Unsocial trait stands for a negative pole of Extraversion (see Chapter "Personality Traits in Contemporary China: A Lexical Approach"), and extraversion level was decreased in BD II patients (Kim et al. 2012).

The negative association found in BD II between the Intelligent trait and the HCL-32 was conflict with the positive correlation, found in both BD I and BD II groups, between the Intelligent trait and the MDQ. It might be explained by the theory that as human intelligence evolved, cognitions inhibiting the Behavioral Activation System, and activating Behavioral Inhibition System became amplified, resulting in intensified depressive inhibition, and resulted in a less prominent hypo-manic state (Bowins 2008). Moreover, the negative relationship between the Agreeable trait and the HCL-32 scale has similarity to that between the Agreeable trait and the MDQ, evidenced that BD II patients had less agreeableness or lower treatment-compliance in clinics (Látalová 2012). In contrast to one of our hypotheses, the Emotional trait was not positively associated with the PVP but negatively associated with the HCL-32 in BD II. Whether this correlation was influenced by Chinese culture remains unknown. Nevertheless, studies conducted in the Eastern countries supported this finding. For example, in a Japanese study (Sugaya et al. 2013), when comorbid with panic disorder, BD II patients who usually have higher HCL-32 score presented lower neuroticism than BD I patients, suggesting they are less emotional. In a Korean study (Kim et al. 2012), BD II scored lower on positive emotion than BD I did.

There are still some limitations in the present study design. Firstly, we did not employ other personality scales, such as the Minnesota Multiphasic Personality Inventory or the Eysenck Personality Questionnaire (Eysenck and Eysenck 1992; Ben-Porath and Tellegen 2011). Therefore, whether their personality traits are related to the affective states of bipolar disorder patients or to the affective states of the healthy people remains unanswered. Furthermore, because our participants were well-educated youngsters, the results might not be directly applied to other age populations. Thirdly, we just conducted the study in Chinese, and adding a control group of Western participants might be a wonderful choice. In addition, the prediction power (lower adjusted R^2 values) of personality traits to the affective states were weak because of the small sample sizes, which can be solved by employing a larger sample in the future.

Nevertheless, our results confirmed other studies showing that the Intelligent and Agreeable traits are emphasized in Chinese people (Chen 1994; Yang and Sternberg 1997), and indicated that the four CADP traits, namely Agreeable, Emotional, Unsocial, and Intelligent, make different contributions to the affective states in BD I and II disorders. From a limited aspect, our study might provide the culture-related evidence to study the expression or control of emotions in Chinese people, and in the next chapter we will summarize the relationship between family characteristics under Chinese culture and psychiatric disorders.

References

American Psychiatric Association. (2013). *Diagnostic and statistical manual of mental disorder* (5th ed.). Washington, DC: American Psychiatric Association.

Angst, J., Adolfsson, R., Benazzi, F., Gamma, A., Hantouche, E., Meyer, T. D., Skeppar, P., Vieta, E., & Scott, J. (2005). The HCL-32: Towards a self-assessment tool for hypomanic symptoms in outpatients. *Journal of Affective Disorders, 88*, 217–233.

Bagby, R. M., Bindseil, K. D., Schuller, D. R., Rector, N. A., Trevor, Y. L., Cooke, R. G., Seeman, M. V., McCay, E. A. T., & Joffe, R. (1997). Relationship between the five-factor model of personality and unipolar, bipolar and schizophrenic patients. *Psychiatry Research, 70*, 83–94.

Barnhill, G. P. (2001). Social attributions and depression in adolescents with Asperger syndrome. *Focus on Autism and Other Developmental Disabilities, 16*, 46–53.

Benazzi, F. (2007). Bipolar disorder-focus on bipolar II disorder and mixed depression. *Lancet, 369*, 935–945.

Ben-Porath, Y. S., & Tellegen, A. (2011). *MMPI-2RF: Manual for administration, scoring, and interpretation.* Minneapolis: University of Minnesota Press.

Bond, M. H., & Pang, M. K. (1991). Trusting to the Tao: Chinese values and the re-centering of psychology. *Bulletin of the Hong Kong Psychological Society, 26*(27), 5–27.

Bowins, B. (2008). Hypomania: A depressive inhibition override defense mechanism. *Journal of Affective Disorders, 109*, 221–232.

Bush, T., & Qiang, H. (2000). Leadership and culture in Chinese education. *Asia Pacific Journal of Education, 20*, 58–67.

Castagnini, A., & Berrios, G. E. (2009). Acute and transient psychotic disorders (ICD-10 F23): A review from a European perspective. *European Archives of Psychiatry and Clinical Neuroscience, 259*, 433–443.

Cerimele, J. M., Chwastiak, L. A., Dodson, S., Dodson, S., & Katon, W. J. (2014). The prevalence of bipolar disorder in general primary care samples: A systematic review. *General Hospital Psychiatry, 36*, 19–25.

Chen, M. J. (1994). Chinese and Australia concepts of intelligence. *Psychology and Developing Societies, 6*, 103–117.

Chien, I. C., Chang, K. C., Lin, C. H., Chou, Y. J., & Chou, P. (2010). Prevalence of diabetes in patients with bipolar disorder in Taiwan: A population-based national health insurance study. *General Hospital Psychiatry, 32*, 577–582.

Costa, P. T., Jr., & McCrae, R. R. (1997). Stability and change in personality assessment: The revised NEO personality inventory in the year 2000. *Journal of Personality Assessment, 68*, 86–94.

Coulston, C. M., Bargh, D. M., Tanious, M., Cashman, E. L., Tufrey, K., Curran, G., Kuiper, S., Morgan, H., Lampe, L., & Malhi, G. S. (2013). Is coping well a matter of personality? A study of euthymic unipolar and bipolar patients. *Journal of Affective Disorders, 145*, 54–61.

de Fruyt, F., van Leeuwen, K., Bagby, R. M., Rolland, J., & Rouillon, F. (2006). Assessing and interpreting personality change and continuity in patients treated for major depression. *Psychological Assessment, 8*, 71–80.

Dervic, K., Garcia-Amador, M., Sudol, K., Freed, P., Brent, D. A., Mann, J. J., Harkavy-Friedman, J. M., & Oquendo, M. A. (2015). Bipolar I and II versus unipolar depression: Clinical differences and impulsivity/aggression traits. *European Psychiatry, 30*, 106–113.

Eysenck, H. J., & Eysenck, S. B. G. (1992). *Manual of the Eysenck Personality Questionnaire-Revised.* San Diego: Education and Industrial Testing Service.

Guo, Z. (1995). Chinese Confucian culture and the medical ethical tradition. *Journal of Medical Ethics, 21*, 239–246.

Hamilton, M. (1967). Development of a rating scale for primary depressive illness. *British Journal of Social and Clinical Psychology, 6*, 278–296.

Heine, S. J., & Buchtel, E. E. (2009). Personality: The universal and the culturally specific. *Annual Review of Psychology, 60*, 369–394.

Hirschfeld, R. M. A., Williams, J. B. W., Spitzer, R. L., Calabrese, J. R., Flynn, L., Keck, P. E., Lewis, L., McElroy, S. L., Post, R. M., Rapport, D. J., Russell, J. M., Sachs, G. S., & Zajecka, J. (2000). Development and validation of a screening instrument for bipolar spectrum disorder: The Mood Disorder Questionnaire. *American Journal of Psychiatry, 157*, 1873–1875.

Hui, L. (2005). Chinese cultural schema of Education: Implications for communication between Chinese students and Australian educators. *Issues in Educational Research, 15*, 17–36.

Isometsä, E., Suominen, K., Mantere, O., Valtonen, H., Leppämäki, S., Pippingsköld, M., & Arvilommi, P. (2003). The Mood Disorder Questionnaire improves recognition of bipolar disorder in psychiatric care. *BMC Psychiatry, 3*, 8.

Jain, U., Blais, M. A., Otto, M. W., Hirshfeld, D. R., & Sachs, G. S. (1999). Five-factor personality traits in patients with seasonal depression: Treatment effects and comparisons with bipolar patients. *Journal of Affective Disorders, 55*, 51–54.

Jamison, K. R. (1995). Manic-depressive illness and creativity. *Scientific American, 272*(2), 62–67.

Jorm, A. F. (2001). History of depression as a risk factor for dementia: An updated review. *Australian and New Zealand Journal of Psychiatry, 35*, 776–781.

Judd, L. L., Akiskal, H. S., Schettler, P. J., Coryell, W., Maser, J., Rice, J. A., Solomon, D. A., & Keller, M. B. (2003). The comparative clinical phenotype and long term longitudinal episode course of bipolar I and II: A clinical spectrum or distinct disorders. *Journal of Affective Disorders, 73*, 19–32.

Kahn, J., Coyne, J. C., & Margolin, G. (1985). Depression and marital disagreement: The social construction of despair. *Journal of Social and Personal Relationships, 2*, 447–461.

Kim, B., Lim, J. H., Kim, S. Y., & Joo, Y. H. (2012). Comparative study of personality traits in patients with bipolar I and II disorder from the five-factor model perspective. *Psychiatry Investigation, 9*, 347–353.

Krone, K. J., & Morgan, J. M. (2000). Emotion metaphors in management: The Chinese. In S. Fineman (Ed.), *Emotion in organizations* (2nd ed., pp. 83–100). London: Sage.

Lan, Y. C., Zelman, D. C., & Chao, W. T. (2018). Angry characters and frightened souls: Patients and family explanatory models of bipolar disorder in Taiwan. *Transcultural Psychiatry, 55*, 317–338.

Látalová, K. (2012). Insight in bipolar disorder. *Psychiatric Quarterly, 83*, 293–310.

Leao, I. A., & del Porto, J. A. (2012). Cross validation with the mood disorder questionnaire (MDQ) of an instrument for the detection of hypomania in Brazil: The 32 items hypomania check-list, first revision (HCL-32-R1). *Journal of Affective Disorders, 140*, 215–221.

Leung, K. (2008). Chinese culture, modernization, and international business. *International Business Review, 17*, 184–187.

Levy, K. N., Edell, W. S., & McGlashan, T. H. (2007). Depressive experiences in inpatients with borderline personality disorder. *Psychiatric Quarterly, 78*, 129–143.

Li, Y., Wang, M., Wang, C., & Shi, J. (2010). Individualism, collectivism, and Chinese adolescents' aggression: Intracultural variations. *Aggressive Behavior, 36*, 187–194.

Lin, N. (2001). *Social capital: A theory of social structure and action*. New York: Cambridge University Press.

Liu, X., & Tein, J. (2005). Life events, psychopathology, and suicidal behavior in Chinese adolescents. *Journal of Affective Disorders, 86*, 195–203.

Lozano, B. E., & Johnson, S. L. (2001). Can personality traits predict increases in manic and depressive symptoms. *Journal of Affective Disorders, 63*, 103–111.

Maisel, E. (2013). *Why smart people hurt: A guide for the bright, the sensitive, and the creative*. Newburyport: Conari Press.

Merikangas, K. R., Jin, R., He, J. P., He, J., Kessler, R. C., Lee, S., Sampson, N. A., Viana, M. C., Andrade, L. H., Hu, C., Karam, E. G., Ladea, M., Medina-Mora, M. E., Ono, Y., Posada-Villa, J., Sagar, R., Wells, J. E., & Zarkov, Z. (2011). Prevalence and correlates of bipolar spectrum disorder in the world mental health survey initiative. *Archives of General Psychiatry, 68*, 241–251.

Müller-Oerlinghausen, B., Berghöfer, A., & Bauer, M. (2002). Bipolar disorder. *Lancet, 359*, 241–247.

Ng, E. (2009). Heartache of the state, enemy of the self: Bipolar disorder and cultural change in urban China. *Culture, Medicine and Psychiatry, 33*, 421–450.

Parker, G., Gladstone, G., & Chee, K. T. (2001). Depression in the Planet's largest ethnic group: The Chinese. *American Journal of Psychiatry, 158*, 857–864.

Phillips, M. L., & Kupfer, D. J. (2013). Bipolar disorder diagnosis: Challenges and future directions. *Lancet, 381*, 1663–1671.

Plutchik, R., & van Praag, H. M. (1987). Interconvertability of five self-report measures of depression. *Psychiatry Research, 22*, 243–256.

Quilty, L. C., Sellbom, M., Tackett, J. L., & Bagby, R. M. (2009). Personality trait preditors of bipolar disorder symptoms. *Psychiatry Research, 169*, 159–163.

Quilty, L. C., Pelletier, M., de Young, C. G., & Michael, B. R. (2013). Hierarchical personality traits and the distinction between unipolar and bipolar disorders. *Journal of Affective Disorders, 147*, 247–254.

Redding, G., & Wong, G. Y. Y. (1986). The psychology of Chinese organizational behavior. In M. H. Bond (Ed.), *The psychology of the Chinese people* (pp. 267–295). London: Oxford University Press.

Saddichha, S., & Schutz, C. (2014). Is impulsivity in remitted bipolar disorder a stable trait? A meta-analytic review. *Comprehensive Psychiatry, 55*, 1479–1484.

Schrijvers, D. L., de Bruijn, E. R., Destoop, M., Hulstijn, W., & Sabbe, B. G. C. C. (2010). The impact of perfectionism and anxiety traits on action monitoring in major depressive disorder. *Journal of Neural Transmission, 117*, 869–880.

Serpell, R. (2000). Intelligence and culture. In R. J. Sternberg (Ed.), *Handbook of intelligence* (pp. 549–578). Cambridge: Cambridge University Press.

Serretti, A., & Olgiati, P. (2007). Profiles of "manic" symptoms in bipolar I, bipolar II and major depressive disorders. *Journal of Affective Disorders, 84*, 159–166.

Stringer, D., Marshall, D., Pester, B., Baker, A., Langenecker, S. A., Angers, K., Frazier, N., Archer, C., Kamali, M., McInnis, M., & Ryan, K. A. (2014). Openness predicts cognitive functioning in bipolar disorder. *Journal of Affective Disorders, 168*, 51–57.

Sugaya, N., Yoshida, E., Yasuda, S., Tochigi, M., Takei, K., Otani, T., Otowa, T., Minato, T., Umekage, T., Konishi, Y., Sakano, Y., Chen, J., Nomura, S., Okazaki, Y., Kaiya, H., Sasaki, T., & Tanii, H. (2013). Prevalence of bipolar disorder in panic disorder patients in the Japanese population. *Journal of Affective Disorders, 147*, 411–415.

Tjosvold, D., & Su, F. (2007). Managing anger and annoyance in organizations in China: The role of constructive controversy. *Group and Organization Management, 32*, 260–289.

Triandis, H. C., & Suh, E. M. (2002). Cultural influences on personality. *Annual Review of Psychology, 53*, 133–160.

Tsai, S. Y., Chen, C. C., & Yeh, E. K. (1997). Alcohol problems and long-term psychosocial outcome in Chinese patients with bipolar disorder. *Journal of Affective Disorders, 46*, 143–150.

Tse, S., Yuen, Y. M., & Suto, M. (2014). Expected possible selves and coping skills among young and middle-aged adults with bipolar disorder. *East Asian Arch Psychiatry, 24*, 117–124.

Weintraub, M. (2012). Prosocial personality and cognitive buffers for partners of manic individuals. *Undergraduate Journal of Psychology at Berkeley, 5*, 20–28.

White, H. C. (1992). *Identity and control: A structural theory of social action*. Princeton: Princeton University Press.

Xu, S., Gao, Q., Ma, L., Fan, H., Mao, H., Liu, J., & Wang, W. (2015). The Zuckerman-Kuhlman Personality Questionnaire in bipolar I and II disorders: A preliminary report. *Psychiatry Research, 226*, 357–360.

Yang, K. S. (1990). Chinese personality and its change. In M. H. Bond (Ed.), *The psychology of the Chinese people* (pp. 106–170). Hong Kong: Oxford University Press.

Yang, S. Y., & Sternberg, R. J. (1997). Conceptions of intelligence in ancient Chinese philosophy. *Journal of Theoretical and Philosophical Psychology, 17*, 101–119.

Yao, J., Xu, Y., Qin, Y., Liu, J., Shen, Y., Wang, W., & Chen, W. (2015). Relationship between personality disorder functioning styles and the emotional states in bipolar I and II disorders. *PLoS One, 10*, e0117353.

Young, R. C., Biggs, J. T., Ziegler, V. E., & Meyer, D. A. (1978). A rating scale for mania: Reliability, validity and sensitivity. *British Journal of Psychiatry, 133*, 429–435.

Yu, E., Li, H., Fan, H., Gao, Q., Tan, Y., Lou, J., Zhang, J., & Wang, W. (2015). Relationship between Chinese adjective descriptors of personality and emotional symptoms in young Chinese patients with bipolar disorders. *Journal of International Medical Research, 43*, 790–801.

Zimmerman, M., & Galione, J. N. (2011). Screening for bipolar disorder with the Mood Disorder Questionnaire: A review. *Harvard Review of Psychiatry, 19*, 219–228.

Chinese Family Contributions to Psychological Disorders

Hongying Fan, You Xu, and Wei Wang

1 Introduction

The relationship between Chinese culture and psychological disorders (Chapter "Hierarchical Needs and Psychological Disorders in China") is frequently presented in family, the center of our life activities and the social system. Personality and bipolar disorders also have their family factor contributions (Chapters "Narrations of Personality Disorders in A Dream of Red Mansions", "Personality Traits in Contemporary China: A Lexical Approach", "Bipolar Disorders in Chinese Culture: From a Perspective of Harmony", and "Predicting Affective States of Bipolar disorder by the Chinese Adjective Descriptors of Personality"). In this chapter, we would like to discuss the relationship between Chinese family and more types of psychological disorders.

The family is made up of individuals, but it is also part of the larger society (Goode 1964). As one of the most momentous social institutions, family is regarded as the first institution of human beings. It is the basic primary group and the natural matrix of personality worldwide (Young 1939). There are several definitions of family given by different sociologists. MacIver and Page (1959) refer family to a group defined by a sex relationship sufficiently precise and enduring to provide for the procreation and upbringing of children. It is in essence a social unit comprised of two or more people who live together and are related by blood, marriage or adoption (Doob 1997). According to Akubue and Okolo (2008), family is a group of people who interact and communicate with others such as husband, wife and children.

H. Fan · W. Wang (✉)
Department of Clinical Psychology and Psychiatry/School of Public Health, Zhejiang University College of Medicine, Hangzhou, China
e-mail: drwangwei@zju.edu.cn

Y. Xu
Department of Sleep Medicine, the Seventh Hospital of Hangzhou, and Mental Health Center, Zhejiang University College of Medicine, Hangzhou, China

© Springer Nature Singapore Pte Ltd. 2019
W. Wang (ed.), *Chinese Perspectives on Cultural Psychiatry*,
https://doi.org/10.1007/978-981-13-3537-2_11

Meanwhile, as a complex, ever-changing system, family always changes its size and make-up, this affects its needs and customs (Skinner et al. 2000). Consequently, all these definitions suggest that the family, as a system of relationships existing between the members, always has an influence on every individual inside.

Family functions as a system, and its functions satisfy different needs of associated members. The fundamental functions of family include the reproduction of child birth, child rearing and child care, socialization of family members, personality development, educative roles, care of dependent adults, placement function (e.g., marriage in a family), economic sufficiency of family, health care, recreation (through celebration and festival, reunion of family members), wish fulfillment (through moral and emotional support, love, affection), and property transmission (Das 2016). Moreover, family, as a universal social institution, performs six social functions such as the regulation sexual behavior, reproduction, economic cooperation, education (or socialization), affection, protection, emotional support, and social status (Anastasiu 2012). It has also been acknowledged that family functions reflect social conditions and social rank differences (Duvall 1957).

From a clinical point of view, the McMaster Model of Family Functioning (Epstein et al. 1981) is a good example for conceptualization of family function. It helps to distinguish between healthy and unhealthy families by structural and organizational properties of the family group as well as the patterns of transactions among family members. Six dimensions of family functioning are identified in the model: (1) Problem Solving, defined as the family's ability to resolve effective problems threatening the integrity and functional capacity of the family; (2) Communication, referring to the exchange of information such as verbal messages, among family members; (3) Roles, whether the family has established outlines of behavior for dealing with a series of family functions including provision of resources, providing nurturance and support, supporting personal development, maintaining and managing the family systems and providing adult sexual gratification; (4) Affective Responsiveness, being concerned with the extent to which individual family members are able to experience appropriate affect such as welfare and emergency emotions over a range of stimuli; (5) Affective Involvement, assessing the extent to which family members are interested in and largely visible to each other's activities and concerns, and intermediate levels of involvement to be regarded as the healthiest, neither too little nor too much; and (6) Behavior Control, evaluating the approach to which a family expresses and maintains standards for the behavior of its members, in situations of different sorts such as dangerous, psychological and social. Hence, there has been a need for assessment tools and procedures designed to measure family functions, which could likewise provide therapists and researchers with reliable information about whether the family functioning properly or not, in a quite wide range of clinically relevant dimensions. A self-report questionnaire based on the McMaster Model of Family Functioning, the Family Assessment Device (Epstein and Bishop 1983; Miller et al. 1985; Mansfield et al. 2015) is a nice candidate. For example, using the questionnaire, investigators recognized connections between poor family functioning and clinical variables of severity in bipolar disorder patients (Reinares et al. 2016). It has shown that a worse family functioning is related to bipolar disorder patients with lifetime suicide attempt (Berutti et al. 2016).

Taking Chinese culture into account, Chinese family exhibits some distinguishing characteristics. For instance, the joint family plays a vital role in traditional culture, such that the family consists of a father, a mother and their married children and grandchildren living in the same household. The sort of group involves three or even four generations of near blood relatives, in distinction to the smaller family of parents and children called the marriage group. Levy (1949) systematically analyzed the family structure of traditional China under the five general categories of role differentiation, including allocation of solidarity, economic allocation, political allocation, and the allocation of integration and expression, and found that "modern industry is the first genuine threat" to the Chinese family, which is in turn one of the greatest obstacles to modern industry. Hence, the structure of the traditional Chinese family might be doomed in the industrial society. However, in consideration of the impact of traditional, social, political, and economic factors in Chinese family structure, it could be suggested that a rapid decrease in stem families is not likely drawing closer in the coming future, though the value and consumption patterns of nuclear family is changing and will eventually make it the dominant pattern (Tsui 1989). Even now in Chinese urban areas 50–70% of young children are mainly looked after by their grandparents (Lu 2004; Li 2005), which indicates the great influence on family members by three- or more-generation family.

Nevertheless, according to Maslow's (1970) Hierarchy of Needs Theory, once a family fails to satisfy the needs of any family member, psychological problems appear. With regard to family affected by Chinese culture, it functions under the influence of Chinese culture values from different aspects, such as *Li* (see Chapter "Hierarchical Needs and Psychological Disorders in China"), *Guanxi* (see Chapter "Societal Culture from Late Imperial to Contemporary China: As Indirectly Reflected in A Dream of Red Mansions"), and so forth. Although the culture provides Chinese family with help for functioning smoothly, it cannot satisfy all the needs of the members, and it is the time when psychological problem occurs. However, the relationship between functions of Chinese family and psychological disorders is still unclear.

2   Regulation of Sexual Behavior

Sex is essential for the human beings. Family came into being to allowing institutionalized sex relationship between couples, aiming at satisfying the sexual needs, instincts of the wife and husband. Family regulates sex behavior of the members through the mechanism of marriage.

The most negative performance in this function of Chinese family is the attitude to sex. Many scholars considered sexual attitudes in the Chinese culture suppressive. There are some images/pictures portrayed by some psychiatrists, transculturalists, anthropologists, and psychologists, who are mostly Chinese (Suen

1983; Tseng and Hsu 1970), and who experience and understand Chinese culture quite deeply. In their opinions, the whole matter comes down to the Chinese reverence for *Li* (Chapters "Hierarchical Needs and Psychological Disorders in China" and "Societal Culture from Late Imperial to Contemporary China: As Indirectly Reflected in A Dream of Red Mansions") with its strict moral and social codes, ruled by Confucianism, leading to the suppression of sexual needs and expression.

The fact is that, the Chinese are in general more conservative than people from other cultures in expectation. A study compared the sex role attitude in Chinese and American, indicating that the Chinese hold more conservative views, although in both cultures, females were found to be significantly more liberal (Chia et al. 1994). Another study about Chinese and English persons' attitudes toward marriage and sexual behaviors concluded similarly that traditional values in mate-selection preferences persisted more in China, which indicated a relatively conservative sexual culture that existed in China up to present; yet traditional morality and attitudes prevail, especially among women (Higgins et al. 2002). Meston et al. (1996) revealed that Asian students were significantly more conservative than non-Asian students on interpersonal sexual behavior and sociosexual restrictiveness.

For the Chinese, the inherent conservatism of the Confucian doctrine defines "traditional views" in their cultures. Chia et al. (1994) found some possible explanations for the finding that women prefer masculine, dominant males to a lesser degree than do American women. The reason might be that Chinese men are socialized in the Confucian tradition that *Junzi* (see Chapters "Hierarchical Needs and Psychological Disorders in China" and "Societal Culture from Late Imperial to Contemporary China: As Indirectly Reflected in A Dream of Red Mansions") has to be well-versed in *Shi Shu Li Yue* (诗书礼乐, Poetry, Books, Rituals, and Music), it is likely that the ideal man in Chinese society has never been the "macho type" as in USA. According to Confucian philosophy, both man and woman should be cultivated for the virtue of *Rén* (see Chapter "Hierarchical Needs and Psychological Disorders in China"), selflessness, kindness, and reciprocity (Hsu 1985); moderation is highly valued (Chia et al. 1997), and one is always encouraged to control their desire. For the Chinese, love should be kept within one's heart, rather than expressed overtly through affectionate behaviors such as hugging, kissing, and cuddling (So and Cheung 2005).

Unfortunately, the Confucian conservative concept results in contrary to expectation. The forced suppression of desire may provide some short-term relief, but the suppression may often backfire, leading to so-called ironic rebound effects. Thus, the phrnomenon calls for attention to the desire content the individual tries to suppress (Wegner 1994). The generally maladaptive effect of suppression makes it possible that some people may suffer less (or more) from the ironic rebound effects (Hofmann et al. 2015). According to Maslow's Hierarchy of Needs Theory, the need of sex is one of the basic distincts of an individual. Therefore for sex, the suppression of the desire results in psychological problems.

On the other hand, due to the need of sex, sex workers have existed for a longtime despite whoring behavior is illegal in current Chinese society. Hong and Li (2008) reviewed behavioral studies in English on female sex workers in China from 1990 to

2006, indicating that female sex workers in China are young, mobile, and some of them are engaged in drug abuse or the HIV-related sexual risk behaviors. Excessive suppression of sex not only dissatisfies the basic needs, but causes illegal sexual transaction and then negative consequences of mental health.

3   Education (or Socialization)

Family is the primary agent of education, which is equated to the socialization of children (Murdock 1949). The discipline that is learnt and followed in the family is the foundation of control. Socialization provided by the family plays a fundamental role naturally in the use of a certain language, learning a set of values, beliefs, skills, etc.

China is the cradle of Confucian culture, but there are also many other cultural values which are contradicted each other. Individuals are educated to practice as the values set all the time. Faure and Fang (2008) selected eight pairs of paradoxical Chinese values that coexist in today's China: (1) *Guanxi* vs. Professionalism; (2) Importance of face vs. Self-expression and directness; (3) Thrift vs. Materialism and ostentatious consumption; (4) Family and group orientation (Collectivism) vs. Individuation (Individualism); (5) Aversion to law vs. Respect for legal practices; (6) Respect for etiquette, age and hierarchy vs. Respect for simplicity, creativity and competence; (7) Long-term orientation vs. Short-term orientation; and (8) Traditional creeds vs. Modern approaches. When meeting troubles, the Chinese would make their choices between these values with their own morality. The Confucianism also forms the foundation of Chinese cultural tradition and fosters the bases of Chinese interpersonal behaviors (Pye 1972). Confucius defined *Wu Lun* (see Chapter "Hierarchical Needs and Psychological Disorders in China"), i.e., *Zhong, Xiao, Rěn* (忍), *Ti, Xin*, as five basic human relations and their principles.

Family members meet all these contradictory value orientations in the process of socialization under the background of this culture. In family, individuals are also educated to behave as these principles set by human relations, to ensure a harmonious society, so that relationships are structured to deliver optimal benefits for both parties. The Confucian moral notion, instead of law, makes China, with its loose legal framework and lax enforcement possible to be an integrated society. Thus, it is the rule by man, rather than rule by law (Hao 1999; Jenco 2010). Hence, individuals are faced with confusion caused by contradictions all the time, trying to keep balance by their own conscientiousness, where psychological disorders are developed easily. It is obvious that when a person in a dilemma that trust and filial piety are incompatible, there are no statutes to apply, whichever side chosen to stand on, the person must harm the interests of the other side, and the family relationship will be destructed. Then, the feeling of guilt, strongly affected by the manipulation of moral beliefs (Smith et al. 2002), will appear, becoming the source of psychological disorders. Feeling of guilt is one important reason of depression (Hamilton 1960; Barraclough et al. 1974; Alexander et al. 1999), further leading to suicide (Hamilton 1960; Kim et al. 2011). It can be imagined that ubiquitous moral decisions in the context of Chinese culture produce an overall feeling of guilt, to serve as the breeding ground of depression.

In spite of all the evidence, investigators have focused on the dimensional structures of Collectivism compared with those of Individualism (Gao 2001). Collectivism emphasizes interdependence, interpersonal harmony, co-operation, and the subordination of personal goals to in-group goals (Triandis et al. 1988). Specifically in family, Collectivism may encourage greater responsiveness to family members as a means of fostering harmony and mutual obligation (Lebra 1976; Markus and Kitayama 1991; Heine 2001). The obsession with preserving harmony in society and family systems eventually leads to the excessive power distance and rigid rules, at the expense of flexibility and professionalism (Chan et al. 2001). The obsession is remarkably correlated with responsibility and guilt, which involves a range of phenomena including anger and guilt, control of thoughts, the fusion of thoughts and action, resistance to additional responsibility, procrastination and unfinished tasks, hypochondriasis, and brief holidays (Rachman 1993). In light of these facts, it becomes clear that Chinese values may give rise to guilt as well as to the obsession and depression of psychological disorders.

4 Affection, Protection and Emotional Support

On the other aspect, the family functions to provide affection, protection, and emotion support for associated members within the system. Family satisfies psychological needs, such as the love, affection, sense of belonging, self-confidence, and intimate relationship and concern, which are working together as a fuel to run the family. The absence of the above needs causes many psychological problems with an individual.

Supportive characteristics of the family and kin systems are functioning effectively as modulators of stress, such as a haven for rest and recuperation, a source and validator of identity, and a contributor to emotional mastery (Caplan 1976). From this point of view, family prominently satisfies the love/belonging needs of its members. Nevertheless, Chinese parents need to improve their behaviors by correction of their recognition. Due to traditional values in Chinese culture, Chinese parents highly expect of their children be accomplished in four categories of attributes: the family-related attributes, academic-related, conduct-related, and other attributes (Shek and Chan 1999), by incorporating elements of authoritarian parenting (high control and set standard of conduct) with high involvement and concern for the child (Chao 1994). Most parents show enough affection for their children, however in China, the parental affection (warmth) is still expressed in a limited way. Existing studies suggest that in collectivistic cultures, intimacy needs of romantic partners are primarily satisfied through interdependent family relationships rather than through romantic relationships (Hsu 1985; Dion and Dion 1993). For example, the emphasis on verbal, explicit, direct, and expressive communication styles in individualistic settings (Gudykunst and Matsumoto 1996), affords more open self-disclosure than the indirect, nonverbal, ambiguous, contextual, and less expressive communication styles that dominate in collectivistic settings (Argyle et al. 1986). Consistent with these explanations, some research has found that Chinese, who are typically more collectivist, tend to be less self-disclosing within close relationships than are people from Western cultures, who are typically individualist (Goodwin and Lee 1994; Chen 1995).

The affection of parents could moderate the stressful life events during adolescence (Wagner et al. 1996), which is very essential to children. Investigators have examined the associations between the two key parenting dimensions of warmth and control on child outcomes in original and immigrant Chinese families, they have reported that warmth is associated with positive child outcomes (Lim and Lim 2004). In another study, the suicidal ideation was significantly associated with perceived authoritarian parenting, low parental warmth, high maternal overcontrol, negative child-rearing practices, and a negative family climate (Lai and McBride-Chang 2001). Chen et al. (2000) showed the gender differences in parents, which maternal warmth had significant contributions to the prediction of emotional adjustment, paternal warmth significantly predicted later social and school achievement. Parental warmth was found related to a decrease in depression in a sample of immigrant Chinese adolescents (Skinner and Crane 1999), and associated with fewer symptoms of depression and fewer conduct problems (Wagner et al. 1996). High warmth was reported associated with enhanced emotional well-being and self-esteem (Scott and Scott 1989), which is supported by the study that warmth was observed to have the strongest negative association with measures of adolescent distress (Chiu et al. 1992). On the other hand, the high expectation from parents tends to value group cohesion over individualization and independence, and the indifference factor of the Parental Bonding Instrument (Parker et al. 1979), a widely used assessment tool for measuring parental characteristics that affect parent-child bonds, may reflect aspects of parenting specific to Chinese culture (Liu et al. 2011). Offsprings from divorced families are more prone to development of personality disorder that those from intact families (Xu et al. 2016). Inappropriate parental bonding or chronic traumatic attachment styles also have respective relationships with the functional and emotional disturbances experienced by patients with primary dysmenorrhea (Xu et al. 2016).

Consequently, based on similar affective dimension of parenting, Chinese parents express less affection to children than Western parents do, producing more risks of psychological disorders for children. The process to turn around could be explained from the cognitive-behavioral perspective (Kendall and Ingram 1989; Kendall 2011): parents might change the expression of their love to their children against the culture context, and the children might feel positive emotion and affection, therefore their cognition might encourage them behave better.

5 Other Functions

Social status is an important function of family as well, because family is the basic unit of social organization as stated before. Individuals define themselves directly in terms of roles they play within the family. The social class is defined when a family member is born, and the status is always permanent, and difficult to change later.

Traditional Chinese families are authoritarian and hierarchical, with the dominance of elders and men (Lang 1946; Ho 1987). The hierarchy in the family is often backed by legal and moral rules, such as the social hierarchy system. The five basic human relations and their principles, the *Wu Lun* (see Chapter "Hierarchical Needs and Psychological Disorders in China"), defined by Confucius evidently show the level of class. All family members are framed into the hierarchy system. More often than not, roles of men and their behaviors tend to be greater in status and agency than those of women (Eagly and Wood 1999). Confucian social ethics shaped the traditional ideology, for example, one of *Wu Lun* is that wives are subordinate to husbands (Bond and Hwang 1986). Consistently, Chinese women in the mainland (Zuo 2003) and Hong Kong of China (Tang and Tang 2001) are more likely to assume domestic roles while their husbands are more likely to join the paid workforce, always called the backbone or the head of a family. The desire to have higher social status is one of a vital need in Maslow's Hierarchy of Needs Theory (i.e., the need of esteem), which has been suppressed by Confucianism similarly to what has been done with the need of sex.

For instance, a study on 1132 Chinese wives showed that 67.2% of the surveyed women reported at least one incidence of verbal or sexual abuse, and 10% experienced at least one incidence of physical abuse by their husbands during the surveyed year, and this just because the husbands thought their wives had failed to live up to their prescribed roles and trespassed cultural rules that required them to remain submissive and dependent (Tang 1999). The violence of husbands indicates that the national desire for keeping benevolence and kindness leading to the ironic rebound effect, which Chinese men have brought tyranny so much under the past to women that their masculine, dominant type are strongly harmful to women (Chia et al. 1994). The disappointing consequences are similar to those family dysfunctions influenced by the cultural factors mentioned above.

Another function that fulfils the acquirement of family members is the recreation or leisure, i.e., family provides entertainment to its members by entertaining them in various ways (Holman and Epperson 1984; Mancoske 2014). Activities such as spending time with others in leisure and recreation reduce stress and provide relaxation for the people involved. In such an environment, family performs the role of a modern club. In ancient period family was the only center of recreation, where all the members together reunite family members, organize family feasts, visit family relations, organize family picnics, etc. However, in China, drinking is an essential link in the party, which is also a socially acceptable habit.

6 Conclusion

Generally speaking, family refers to the group comprising parents and children. In some cases, it may also refer to a group of relatives and their dependents forming one household. Sharing common residence, family members are usually born there in family, grow in it, work for it, die in it, and also develop emotional attachment to it. They have reciprocal rights and duties towards each other. Family is known as the first school of social man, where the parental care-giver imparts to children the first lesson regarding social responsibility and acceptance of self-discipline. Obviously, family plays a central role in the society, acts as the backbone of the social structure.

The culture and society are connected and influence one another. This is still the case in contemporary China, where the traditional culture, especially Confucianism, still holds a crucial position in value and influences the structure and functions of a family. Empirical evidence demonstrated the pros and cons of Chinese culture in a convincing way. Nevertheless, the traditional values about moderation (suppression of normal desire), Collectivism, the authoritarian and hierarchy lead to a large number of problems for mental health. It should be on the alert that once the negative aspect of traditional Chinese culture is neglected, there will be long-lasting psychological effects on individuals.

In line with Maslow's Hierarchy of Needs Theory, the functions of family can satisfy the essential desires of individuals. However, when the needs are dissatisfied, individual's desire would be suppressed, which conversely might lead to ironic rebound effects, then the recognition transform, and finally the psychological disorders. Cultural and cross-cultural studies have recognized the influence on some respects of family functions, such as parental bonding styles, while other respects of family can be studied further.

References

Akubue, F. N., & Okolo, A. N. (2008). *Sociology of education*. Nsukka: Great A. P. Express Publishers.

Alexander, B., Brewin, C. R., Vearnals, S., Wolff, G., & Leff, J. (1999). An investigation of shame and guilt in a depressed sample. *British Journal of Medical Psychology, 72*, 323–338.

Anastasiu, I. (2012). The social functions of the family. *Euromentor Journal – Studies About Education, 3*, 133–139.

Argyle, M., Henderson, M., Bond, M., Iizuka, Y., & Contarello, A. (1986). Cross-cultural variation in relationship rules. *International Journal of Psychology, 21*, 287–315.

Barraclough, B., Bunch, J., Nelson, B., & Sainsbury, P. (1974). A hundred cases of suicide: Clinical aspects. *British Journal of Psychiatry, 125*, 355–373.

Berutti, M., Dias, R. S., Pereira, V. A., Lafer, B., & Nery, F. G. (2016). Association between history of suicide attempts and family functioning in bipolar disorder. *Journal of Affective Disorders, 192*, 28–33.

Bond, M. H., & Hwang, K. (1986). The social psychology of Chinese people. *International Journal of Intercultural Relations, 11*, 212–214.

Caplan, G. (1976). The family as a social support system. In G. Caplan, M. Killilea, & R. B. Abrahams (Eds.), *Social systems and mutual help: Multidisciplinary explorations*. New York: Grune and Stratton.

Chan, K. H., Lew, A. Y., & Tong, M. Y. J. W. (2001). Accounting and management controls in the classical Chinese novel: A Dream of the Red Mansions. *International Journal of Accounting, 36*, 311–327.

Chao, R. K. (1994). Beyond parental control and authoritarian parenting style: Understanding Chinese parenting through the cultural notion of training. *Child Development, 65*, 1111–1119.

Chen, G. M. (1995). Differences in self-disclosure patterns among Americans versus Chinese: A comparative study. *Journal of Cross-Cultural Psychology, 26*, 84–91.

Chen, X., Liu, M., & Li, D. (2000). Parental warmth, control, and indulgence and their relations to adjustment in Chinese children: A longitudinal study. *Journal of Family Psychology, 14*, 401–419.

Chia, R. C., Moore, J. L., Lam, K. N., Chuang, C. J., & Cheng, B. S. (1994). Cultural differences in gender role attitudes between Chinese and American students. *Sex Roles, 31*, 23–30.

Chia, R. C., Allred, L. J., & Jerzak, P. A. (1997). Attitudes toward women in Taiwan and China. *Psychology of Women Quarterly, 21*, 137–150.

Chiu, M. L., Feldman, S. S., & Rosenthal, D. A. (1992). The influence of immigration on parental behavior and adolescent distress in Chinese families residing in two Western nations. *Journal of Research on Adolescence, 2*, 205–239.

Das, S. (2016). *Introduction to community nutrition. Textbook of community nutrition* (Rev. 2nd ed., pp. 1–8). Kolkata: Academic Publishers.

Dion, K. K., & Dion, K. L. (1993). Individualistic and collectivistic perspectives on gender and the cultural context of love and intimacy. *Journal of Social Issues, 49*, 53–69.

Doob, C. B. (1997). *Sociology: An introduction* (5th ed.). New York: The Harcourt Press.

Duvall, E. M. (1957). *Family development*. Oxford: Lippincott.

Eagly, A. H., & Wood, W. (1999). The origins of sex differences in human behavior: Evolved dispositions versus social roles. *American Psychologist, 54*, 408–423.

Epstein, N. B., & Bishop, D. S. (1983). McMaster family assessment device. *Journal of Family Therapy, 9*, 171–180.

Epstein, N. B., Bishop, D. S., & Baldwin, L. M. (1981). McMaster Model of Family Functioning: A view of the normal family. In F. Walsh (Ed.), *Normal family processes*. New York: Guilford.

Faure, G. O., & Fang, T. (2008). Changing Chinese values: Keeping up with paradoxes. *International Business Review, 17*, 194–207.

Gao, G. (2001). Intimacy, passion, and commitment in Chinese and US American romantic relationships. *International Journal of Intercultural Relations, 25*, 329–342.

Goode, W. J. (1964). *The family* (p. 2). New Jersey: Prentice Hall.

Goodwin, R., & Lee, I. (1994). Taboo topics among Chinese and English friends. *Journal of Cross-Cultural Psychology, 25*, 325–328.

Gudykunst, W. B., & Matsumoto, Y. (1996). Cross-cultural variability of communication in personal relationships. In W. B. Gudykunst, S. Ting-Toomey, & T. Nishida (Eds.), *Communication in personal relationships across cultures* (pp. 19–56). Thousand Oaks: SAGE.

Hamilton, M. (1960). A rating scale for depression. *Journal of Neurology, Neurosurgery and Psychiatry, 23*, 56–62.

Hao, Y. (1999). From rule of man to rule of law: An unintended consequence of corruption in China in the 1990s. *Journal of Contemporary China, 8*, 405–423.

Heine, S. J. (2001). Self as cultural product: An examination of East Asian and North American selves. *Journal of Personality, 69*, 881–906.

Higgins, L. T., Zheng, M., Liu, Y., & Sun, C. H. (2002). Attitudes to marriage and sexual behaviors: A survey of gender and culture differences in China and United Kingdom. *Sex Roles, 46*, 75–89.

Ho, D. Y. F. (1987). Fatherhood in Chinese culture. In M. E. Lamb (Ed.), *The father's role: Cross-cultural perspectives* (pp. 227–245). Hillsdale: Erlbaum.

Hofmann, W., Kotabe, H. P., Vohs, K. D., & Baumeister, R. F. (2015). Desire and desire regulation. In W. Hofmann & L. F. Nordgren (Eds.), *The psychology of desire (Chap. 3)* (pp. 61–81). New York: Guilford.

Holman, T. B., & Epperson, A. (1984). Family and leisure: A review of the literature with research recommendations. *Journal of Leisure Research, 16*, 277–294.

Hong, Y., & Li, X. (2008). Behavioral studies of female sex workers in China: A literature review and recommendation for future research. *AIDS and Behavior, 12*, 623–636.

Hsu, F. L. K. (1985). The self in cross-cultural perspective. In A. J. Marsella, G. DeVos, & F. L. K. Hsu (Eds.), *Culture and self: Asian and western perspectives* (pp. 24–55). London: Tavistock.

Jenco, L. K. (2010). "Rule by man" and "rule by law" in early Republican China: Contributions to a theoretical debate. *Journal of Asian Studies, 69*, 181–203.

Kendall, P. C. (2011). Guiding theory for therapy with children and adolescents. In P. C. Kendall (Ed.), *Child and adolescent therapy: Cognitive-behavioral procedures* (4th ed., pp. 3–24). New York: Guilford.

Kendall, P. C., & Ingram, R. E. (1989). Cognitive-behavioural perspectives: Theory and research on depression and anxiety. In P. C. Kendall & D. Watson (Eds.), *Anxiety and depression: Distinctive and overlapping features (xviii)* (pp. 27–53). San Diego: Academic Press.

Kim, S., Thibodeau, R., & Jorgensen, R. S. (2011). Shame, guilt, and depressive symptoms: A meta-analytic review. *Psychological Bulletin, 137*, 68–96.

Lai, K. W., & McBride-Chang, C. (2001). Suicidal ideation, parenting style, and family climate among Hong Kong adolescents. *International Journal of Psychology, 36*, 81–87.

Lang, O. (1946). *Chinese family and society*. New Haven: Yale University Press.

Lebra, T. S. (1976). *Japanese patterns of behavior*. Honolulu: University of Hawaii Press.

Levy, M. J., Jr. (1949). *The family revolution in modern China*. Oxford: Harvard University Press.

Li, H. (2005). How grandparents educated children in three-generation family. *Preschool Research, 6*, 28–30 (in Chinese).

Lim, S. L., & Lim, B. K. (2004). Parenting style and child outcomes in Chinese and immigrant Chinese families-current findings and cross-cultural considerations in conceptualization and research. *Marriage and Family Review, 35*, 21–43.

Liu, J., Li, L., & Fang, F. (2011). Psychometric properties of the Chinese version of the Parental Bonding Instrument. *International Journal of Nursing Studies, 48*, 582–589.

Lu, L. (2004). Advantage and disadvantage for grandparents caring Child. *Family Education (China), 10*, 6–8 (in Chinese).

MacIver, R. M., & Page, C. H. (1959). The family. In *Society: An introductory analysis* (pp. 238–280). London: MacMillan.

Mancoske, R. J. (2014). The changing family and family policy. *Journal of Sociology and Social Welfare, 8*, 174–193.

Mansfield, A. K., Keitner, G. I., & Dealy, J. (2015). The family assessment device: An update. *Family Process, 54*, 82–93.

Markus, H. R., & Kitayama, S. (1991). Culture and the self: Implications for cognition, emotion, and motivation. *Psychological Review, 98*, 224–253.

Maslow, A. H. (1970). *Motivation and personality*. New York: Harper and Row.

Meston, C. M., Trapnell, P. D., & Gorzalka, B. B. (1996). Ethnic and gender differences in sexuality: Variations in sexual behavior between Asian and non-Asian university students. *Archives of Sexual Behavior, 25*, 33–72.

Miller, I. W., Epstein, N. B., Bishop, D. S., & Keitner, G. I. (1985). The McMaster family assessment device: Reliability and validity. *Journal of Marital and Family Therapy, 11*, 345–356.

Murdock, G. P. (1949). *Social structure*. New York: MacMillan.

Parker, G., Tupling, H., & Brown, L. B. (1979). A parental bonding instrument. *British Journal of Medical Psychology, 52*, 1–10.

Pye, L. W. (1972). *China: An introduction* (2nd ed.). Boston: Little Brown.

Rachman, S. (1993). Obsessions, responsibility and guilt. *Behaviour Research and Therapy, 31*, 149–154.

Reinares, M., Bonnín, C. M., Hidalgo-Mazzei, D., Colom, F., Solé, B., Jiménez, E., Torrent, C., Comes, M., Martínez-Arán, A., Sánchez-Moreno, J., & Vieta, E. (2016). Family functioning in bipolar disorder: Characteristics, congruity between patients and relatives, and clinical correlates. *Psychiatry Research, 245*, 66–73.

Scott, W. A., & Scott, R. (1989). *Adaptation of immigrants: Individual differences and determinants*. Oxford: Pergamon.

Shek, D. T., & Chan, L. K. (1999). Hong Kong Chinese parents' perceptions of the ideal child. *Journal of Psychology, 133*, 291–302.

Skinner, K. B., & Crane, D. R. (1999). *Associations between parenting, acculturation, and adolescent functioning among Chinese in North America*. Poster session presented at the 61st annual conference of the National Council on Family Relations, Irvine; November 12–15, 1999.

Skinner, H., Steinhauer, P., & Sitarenios, G. (2000). Family Assessment Measure (FAM) and process model of family functioning. *Journal of Family Therapy, 22*, 190–210.

Smith, R. H., Webster, J. M., Parrott, W. G., & Eyre, H. L. (2002). The role of public exposure in moral and nonmoral shame and guilt. *Journal of Personality and Social Psychology, 83*, 138–159.

So, H. W., & Cheung, F. M. (2005). Review of Chinese sex attitudes and applicability of sex therapy for Chinese couples with sexual dysfunction. *Journal of Sex Research, 42*, 93–101.

Suen, L. C. (1983). *The underlying structure of Chinese civilization* [Zhong-guo-wen-hua-di-shen-ceng-jie-gou]. Hong Kong: Yi Shan Publication (in Chinese).

Tang, C. S. K. (1999). Wife abuse in Hong Kong Chinese families: A community survey. *Journal of Family Violence, 14*, 173–191.

Tang, T. N., & Tang, C. S. (2001). Gender role internalization, multiple roles, and Chinese women's mental health. *Psychology of Women Quarterly, 25*, 181–196.

Triandis, H. C., Bontempo, R., Villareal, M. J., Asai, M., & Lucca, N. (1988). Individualism and collectivism: Cross-cultural perspectives on self-ingroup relationships. *Journal of Personality and Social Psychology, 54*, 323–338.

Tseng, W. S., & Hsu, J. (1970). Chinese culture, personality formation and mental illness. *International Journal of Social Psychiatry, 16*, 5–14.

Tsui, M. (1989). Changes in Chinese urban family structure. *Journal of Marriage and the Family, 51*, 737–747.

Wagner, B. M., Cohen, P., & Brook, J. S. (1996). Parent/adolescent relationships: Moderators of the effects of stressful life events. *Journal of Adolescent Research, 11*, 347–374.

Wegner, D. M. (1994). Ironic processes of mental control. *Psychological Review, 101*, 34–52.

Xu, K., Chen, L., Fu, L., Xu, S., Fan, H., Gao, Q., Xu, Y., & Wang, W. (2016). Stressful parental-bonding exaggerates the functional and emotional disturbances of primary dysmenorrhea. *International Journal of Behavioral Medicine, 23*, 458–463.

Young, K. (1939). *The family and its institutions. An introductory sociology* (Rev. Ed., xxv, pp. 215–230). New York: American Book Company.

Zuo, J. (2003). From revolutionary comrades to gendered partners: Marital construction of breadwinning in post-Mao urban China. *Journal of Family Issues, 24*, 314–337.

A Theoretical Framework Explaining Chinese Cultural Contributions to Psychological Disorders

Hongying Fan, Guorong Ma, and Wei Wang

1 The Framework

The most fundamental factor of the Chinese culture is the Confucianism. This book covers many studies on the relationship between Chinese culture and psychological disorders, and has demonstrated the unfortunate fact that Chinese culture also provides a perfect hotbed for the development of psychological disorders.

In previous chapters, we have discussed the characteristics of late imperial and contemporary Chinese societies, and the relationship between the Chinese culture/ family and psychological disorders, using Maslow's Hierarchy of Need Theory. At the societal level, Chinese culture is unable to meet all levels of human needs. The dissatisfaction with human's basic and developmental needs then impacts prominently on Chinese family and Chinese people. When deliberating the normal and abnormal personality traits of Chinese people, the famous novel DRM has provided us a rich source for studying individual characteristics in societal and family environments. Indeed, individuals' personality structure is shaped by Chinese culture in a way analogous to but distinct from Western culture. Meanwhile, individual's cognition, behavior, and emotion suffer constant damages from a variety of surrounding sources. When scrutinized on basic structures, each personality disorder has its core beliefs or behavioral features, an excellent example of which is the antisocial personality disorder. While for affective fluctuations, the bipolar disorder exemplifies the influence of Chinese culture on the emotional recognition and control. After these documentation, we have accomplished a theoretical frame for the relationship between Chinese culture and psychologic disorders (Fig. 1).

Much evidence point to the core value of Chinese culture, the "harmony", in the link, which is also appreciated all over the world. However, we have to highlight the

H. Fan · G. Ma · W. Wang (✉)
Department of Clinical Psychology and Psychiatry/School of Public Health, Zhejiang University College of Medicine, Hangzhou, China
e-mail: drwangwei@zju.edu.cn

© Springer Nature Singapore Pte Ltd. 2019
W. Wang (ed.), *Chinese Perspectives on Cultural Psychiatry*,
https://doi.org/10.1007/978-981-13-3537-2_12

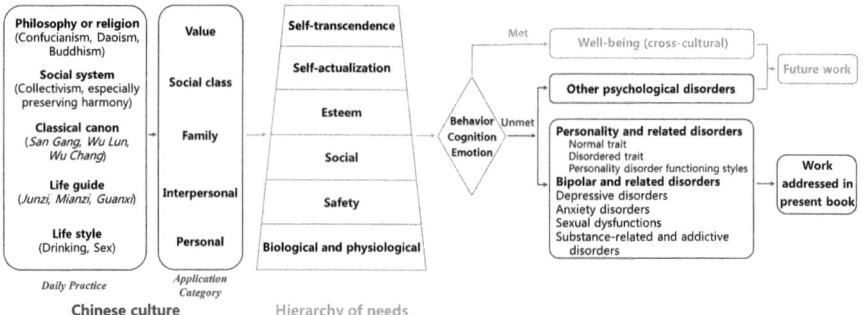

Fig. 1 The relationships between Chinese culture, individual's hierarchical needs, and psychological disorders. The daily practice of life style, guide, classical canon, social system, and philosophy or religion, are stratified into the personal, interpersonal, family, social class and value categories, which affect individuals' psychological processes (behavior, cognition and emotion) through their hierarchical needs. Most people have their needs satisfied and thus remain well-being, other people have their needs unmet and thus develop sorts of psychological disorders

question, why our harmony culture eventually leads to disharmony (disease)? Our results have implicated that all ideas, theories, thoughts and disciplines originating from the core values are not in harmony with individual's basic needs. For instance, the idea of *Zhong Yong* tells people "when the wood is in the forest, the wind will destroy it (木秀于林, 风必摧之)", therefore an individual should keep his weakness as well as strongpoint unexposed, otherwise he would be injured by external environment. Following the teachings, the creativities of people are restrained naturally. For instance, the Chinese people do appreciate intelligence very much, as illustrated by narrations in DRM (Chapter "Personality Traits Characterized by the Adjectives in A Dream of Red Mansions") and the first descriptions of personality trait (Chapter "Personality Traits in Contemporary China: A Lexical Approach"). The literature, the reflection and sublimation of life, also evidence the pitfalls of Chinese culture, such as the Romance of the Three Kingdoms (三国演义), a classic military novel of China, with plenty of war descriptions which advocating that a tricky way makes victory. Along the history line, Chinese people use tricks to break rules of every kinds, thus creating much anxiousness and disoharmony among colleagues, they also use tricks to solve an interpersonal problem and sometimes they tell lies to satifisy bosses or officials, or for a social desirability. Indeed, it is much terrible that people's basic needs are threatened due to a harmful culture, for instance, the issue of food safety is the first to bear the brunt (Lam et al. 2013; Lu et al. 2015). Social events such as the "poisonous" vaccine (Griffiths 2018) and melamine milk powder (Wen et al. 2016), making food by gutter oil (Lu and Wu 2014), and so forth, have brought health risks and insecurity, which are hot-topics these years. People may therefore question the reasons for these events, and begin to realize that it might be due the selfishness and the lie which are rooted deeply in the human dark side.

2 Future Work

Bearing in mind some limitations regarding the relationship between Chinese culture and psychological disorders proposed in the book, a reader can easily fix his eyes on the openings for future work along this line. Although many typical cultural elements, such as the drink custom, sexual attitude, moral rules, harmony seeking, Collectivism, hierarchical society, legal and moral systems, and others, are reported as risk factors in sorts of psychological disorders, still many other elements might have been neglected. First, regarding the present series of research, we have only mentioned bipolar disorders, depressive disorder, anxiety disorder, sexual dysfunction, personality disorder, and substance-related and addictive disorders, there are still many other psychological disorders which deserve to be studied, such as schizophrenia and sleep-wake disorders. Second, the sample sizes of our designs were small and not equally distributed in age and education. A more expanded recruitment of patients would make the current relationship clearer. Third, we only have concentrated on Chinese culture and Chinese people, without including cultures or people from other parts of the world. Comparative studies including Chinese and overseas (Western and neighboring) people would help elucidate the related concepts. Fourth, we only have de-briefed the personality disorder into trait-structures for antisocial personality disorder, the infrastructures of other personality disorders and their connections with Chinese culture might offer more poofs for the proposed theoretical framework. Fifth, in consideration of our research purpose – looking for the relationship between Chinese culture and psychological disorders, the positive influence of the Chinese culture on the psychological well-being has been less emphasized.

3 General Conclusions

Cultural issues have been mentioned in the DSM and ICD diagnostic systems to ellucudate the etiopathology, treatment and prevention of psychiatric/psychological disorders, and studies regarding the influence of Chinese culture on these disorders are increasing these years. We have found some evidence to support the theoretical framework illustrated in Fig. 1, especially the Chinese factors derived from Confucianism, Buddhism and Doism. Although the structures and the measurement scales of psychological disorders in China might be similar to those in other countries, the cultural contributions to these disorders are unique to the Chinese society. Therefore, considering that Chinese culture has expanded its impact on hundreds of millions of people all over the world, we believe that the framework offers some hints for the understanding, prevention and treatment of psychological disorders in both China and other parts of the world.

References

Griffiths, J. (2018, July 24). *Vaccine scandal exposes the contradictions at the heart of the "Chinese dream"*. Retrieved October 12, 2018, from https://edition.cnn.com/2018/07/24/asia/china-vaccine-scandal-intl/index.html

Lam, H. M., Remais, J., Fung, M. C., Xu, L., & Sun, S. S. M. (2013). Food supply and food safety issues in China. *Lancet, 381*, 2044–2053.

Lu, F., & Wu, X. (2014). China food safety hits the "gutter". *Food Control, 41*, 134–138.

Lu, Y., Song, S., Wang, R., Liu, Z., Meng, J., Sweetman, A. J., Jenkins, A., Ferrier, R. C., Li, H., Luo, W., & Wang, T. (2015). Impacts of soil and water pollution on food safety and health risks in China. *Environment International, 77*, 5–15.

Wen, J. G., Liu, X. J., Wang, Z. M., Li, T. F., & Wahlqvist, M. L. (2016). Melamine-contaminated milk formula and its impact on children. *Asia Pacific Journal of Clinical Nutrition, 25*, 697–705.

Appendix

© Springer Nature Singapore Pte Ltd. 2019
W. Wang (ed.), *Chinese Perspectives on Cultural Psychiatry*,
https://doi.org/10.1007/978-981-13-3537-2

Table A.1 Personality-descriptive terms (adjectives)/phrases and sentences/paragraphs, their respective DRM chapter number indices (following Chinese expressions), and their corresponding DSM-5 Section III criteria in each DRM character

Character name	Description in DRM (English – Chinese)		DSM-5 Section III
	Terms or phrases	Sentences or paragraphs	Personality functioning or facets trait
Jia Baoyu (贾宝玉)		A1.1 "What do you mean?" asked Xiren. "This is the beginning of a new year when all the ladies and girls are enjoying themselves. Why carry on like this?" "I don't care whether they're enjoying themselves or not." "If they are so obliging to each other, shouldn't you be obliging too? Wouldn't that be pleasanter for everyone?" "For everyone? Let them oblige each other while 'naked I go without impediment.'" Tears ran down his cheeks… (袭人见这话不是往日的口吻,因又笑道: "这是怎么说? 好好的大正月里, 娘儿们姊妹们都喜欢欢的, 你又怎么这个形景了?" 宝玉冷笑道. "他们姊妹们次不次欢喜, 也与我干干." 袭人笑道: "他们既随和, 你也随和, 岂不大家彼去无事, 彼此有趣?" 宝玉道: "什么是 '大家彼此'!他们有 '大家彼此', 我是 '赤条条来去无牵挂' "该及此句,不觉泪下, 22).	(Schizotypal) Identity: Emotional expression often not congruent with context.
	B1 Losing patience with all conventions (不喜务正, 19); B2 Highly-spirited and wilful (淘气憨顽, 19)	B1.1 His wild ways, aversion to study and delight in playing about in the women's apartments. (顽劣异常, 极恶读书, 最喜在内帏厮混, 3). B1.2 His father's departure left Baoyu free to do as he pleased in the Garden, and he frittered away whole months in idleness. ((贾政出门去后) 宝玉每日在园中任意纵性的逛荡, 真把光阴虚度, 岁月空添, 37). B1.3 Big as he is, he's unique in never having had any proper schooling. (他长了这么大, 独他没有上过正经学堂, 66). B1.4 He never studies books or practises military arts. (每日也不习文, 也不学武, 66). B1.5 Baoyu instantly felt as distraught as Monkey King on hearing the incantation to tighten th magic band around his head. Staggered, he racked his brains but could think of no way out except to cram in readiness for a test the following day. He fancied that if he could give correct answers from his books, other lapses would be overlooked and he might muddle through. Throwing a jacket round his shoulders he got up to study,	(Schizotypal) Self-direction: No clear set of internal standards.

thinking remorsefully, "I was sure he wouldn't test me these first few days, so I let things slide and got rusty. If I'd known, I'd have done some revising every day." (这里宝玉听了，便如孙大圣听见了紧箍咒一般，登时四肢五内一齐都不自在起来。想来想去，别无他法，且理熟了书，预备明儿盘考。只能书won事，也可搪塞一半。想罢，忙披衣起来要读书。心中又自后悔，这些日子只说不提了，偏又丢生，早知该天天好歹温习些的，73).		
C1.1 He's handsome and is taken for an intelligent boy, but for all he looks so smart he's actually muddle-headed, with nothing to say for himself in company. (外头人人看着好清俊的模样儿，心里自然是聪明的，谁知是外清而内浊，见了人，一句话也没有，66). C1.2 …he doesn't like meeting strangers, instead he just loves to fool about with the maids (又怕见人，只爱在丫头里闹，66).		(Schizotypal) Intimacy: Marked impairments in developing close relationships, associated with mistrust and anxiety.
D1.1 …he had come to the conclusion that while human beings were the highest form of creation, the finest essences of Nature were embodied in girls, men being nothing but the dregs and scum. To him, therefore, all men were filthy clods who might just as well not have existed. Only deference to Confucius, the greatest sage of all time who taught that fathers, uncles and brothers should be respected, made him keep on a fairly good footing with his brothers and boy cousins. It never entered his head that he as a man should set the younger boys a good example. (他便料定，原来天生人为万物之灵，凡山川日月之精秀，只钟于女儿，须眉男子不过是些渣滓浊沫而已，因有这个念在心，把一切男子都看成混沌浊物，可有可无。只是父亲叔伯兄弟中因孔子是第一人说下的，不可忤慢，只得要听他这句话，所以，弟兄之间不过尽其大概的情理罢了，并不想自己是丈夫，须要为子弟之表率，20). D1.2 Xiren knew all his foibles. Whereas hypocritical compliments disgusted him, true sentiments of this kind distressed him too. Regretting her tactlessness she hastily turned to subjects more to his taste. (袭人深知宝玉性情古怪，听见奉承吉利话又厌虚而不实，听了这些尽情实话又生悲感，便悔自己说冒撞了，连忙笑着用话截开，只拣那宝玉素昔喜谈者问之，36).	D1 Tco headstrong (性情乖僻, 3); D2 Very absurd and willful (愚拙偏僻, 5); D3 Headstrong and eccentric (禀性乖张, 性情乖诡, 5); D4 Really and truly fool (又傻又呆, 71)	(Schizotypal) Cognitive and perceptual dysregulation (an aspect of Psychoticism): Odd or unusual thought processes.

(continued)

Table A.1 (continued)

Character name	Description in DRM (English – Chinese)		DSM-5 Section III
	Terms or phrases	Sentences or paragraphs	Personality functioning or facets trait
E1 Foolhardy and eccentric (行为偏僻 性乖张, 3)		E1.1 (Jia Baoyu says:) "Girls are made of water, men of mud, I feel clean and refreshed when I'm with girls but find men dirty and stinking." (他 (贾宝玉) 说: "女儿是水作的 骨肉, 男人是泥作的骨肉. 我见了女儿, 我便清爽; 见了男子, 便觉浊臭逼人.", 2). E1.2 As for Xiren, these years had shown her that Baoyu was no ordinary youth but more high-spirited and willful than other boys, with some indescribably perverse streaks in his character. Of late he had been so indulged by his grandmother that his parents were unable to control him strictly and he had now become so reckless and headstrong that he was losing patience with all conventions. (如今日说袭人, 自幼见宝玉性格异 常, 其淘气憨顽自是出于众小儿之外, 更有几件千奇百怪口不能言的毛病儿. 近来仆 着他母每溺爱, 父祖亦不能十分严紧拘管, 更觉放荡弛纵, 任性恣情, 最不喜务正, 19). E1.3 "You must stop abusing Buddhist monks and Daoist priests and playing about with girls' cosmetics and powder. Most important of all, you must stop kissing the rouge on girls' lips and running after everything in red." (袭人道: "再不许毁僧谤道, 调脂弄粉. 还有更要紧的一件, 再不许吃人嘴上擦的胭脂了, 与那爱红的毛病儿", 19). E1.4 Now Baoyu had always been deplorably eccentric. (原来那宝玉自幼生成有一种 下流痴病, 29). E1.5 As soon as they were alone, the old women started talking as they ambled along. One of them said with a laugh, "No wonder Baoyu's called a handsome fool. Handsome is as handsome does, and anyone can see he's a bit touched. He scalds his own hand and asks someone else if it hurts—what could be more stupid than that?" "The last time I came here," the other rejoined, "I heard several of those girls say he's downright cracked. He got drenched himself in the rain and advised someone else to take shelter. Don't you call that soft? When there's no one about he laughs and cries to himself. When he sees a swallow he talks to the swallow, when he sees a fish in the stream he talks to the fish. He sighs or mumbles to the moon and stars, and has so little spirit he even puts up with the tantrums of those pert girls. When he's in a saving mood he	(Schizotypal) Eccentricity (an aspect of Psychoticism): Odd, unusual, or bizarre behavior; saying unusual or inappropriate things.

(continued)

treasures the least scrap of thread, but at other times he doesn't mind squandering millions". (那两个婆子见没人了，一行走，一行谈论。这一个笑道："怪道有人说，他家宝玉是外相好，里头糊涂，中看不中吃的。果然有些呆气。他自己烫了手，倒问人疼不疼，这可不是呆子？"那一个又笑道："我前一回来，听见他家许多人抱怨，千真万真的有些呆气。大雨淋的水鸡似的，他反告诉别人：'下雨了，快避雨去罢。'你说可笑不可笑？时常没人在跟前，就自哭自笑的；看见燕子，就和燕子说话；河里看见了鱼，就和鱼说话；见了星星月亮，不是长吁短叹，就是咭咭哝哝的。且连一点刚性也没有，连那些毛丫头的气都受的。爱惜东西，连个线头儿都是好的，糟蹋起来，那怕值千值万的都不管了。"；35).

E1.6 Baoyu had an inveterate dislike of entertaining literati or men in general. He hated putting on ceremonial dress to pay calls, return visits or offer congratulations or condolences. Delighted by his grandmother's decision, he not only stopped seeing most relatives and friends but even grew lax about asking after the health of his seniors each morning and evening. After paying his respects early in the morning to his grandmother and mother he spent the rest of the day amusing himself in the Garden, often glad to idle away his time by offering his services to the maids. When Baochai or any of the others advised against this it only angered him. "Imagine a pure, innocent girl joining the ranks of time-servers and place-seekers, who set such store by reputation!" he would fume. "This is all the fault of the ancients who had nothing better to do than coin maxims and codes to control stupid, uncouth men. It's too bad that in our time even those in refined ladies' chambers have been contaminated. This is an offence against Heaven and Earth which endowed them with the finest qualities." Going further in his anger against the ancients, he burned all the Confucian classics in his possession except the *Four Books*. His wild ways discouraged people from talking to him about serious matters. And the only person he really admired was Daiyu, precisely because she alone had never urged him to seek an official career or frame for himself. (那宝玉本就懒与士大夫诸男人接谈，又最厌峨冠礼服贺吊往还等事，近日愈发得了意，不但将亲戚朋友一概杜绝了，而且连家庭中晨昏定省亦都随他的便了。日日只在园中游卧，不过每日一清早到贾母、王夫人处走走就回来了，却每每甘心为诸丫鬟充役，竟也得十分闲消日月。或如宝钗辈有时见机导劝，反生起气来，只说："好好的一个清净洁白女儿，也学的钓名沽誉，入了国贼禄鬼之流。这总是前人无故生事，

Table A.1 (continued)

Character name	Description in DRM (English – Chinese)		DSM-5 Section III
	Terms or phrases	Sentences or paragraphs	Personality functioning or facets trait
		立言竖辞，原为导后世的须眉浊物。不想因此祸延古人，除四书外，竟将别的书焚了。我生不幸，亦且琼闺绣阁中亦染此风，真真有负天地钟灵毓秀之德！"众人见他如此疯癫，也都不向他说这些正经话了。独有林黛玉自幼不曾劝他去立身扬名等语，所以深敬黛玉，36）。	
		E1.7 (Jia Baoyu said:) "In my own case, if I had any luck I should die now with all of you around me; still better if your tears for me were to become a great stream and float my corpse away to some quiet spot deserted even by crows or any other birds, to vanish with the wind, never again to be born as a human being. That's how I should like to die." To cut short such wild talk Xiren said she was tired and gave up answering him. ((宝玉道:) "比如我此时若果有造化，该死于此时的，趁你们在，我就死了，再能够你们哭我的眼泪流成大河，把我的尸首漂起来，送到那鸦雀不到的幽僻之处，随风化了，自此再不要托生为人，就是我死的时了"。袭人忽见说出这些疯话来，忙说困了，不理他，36）。	
		E1.8 Baoyu carries on the whole time like a lunatic, talking in a way that no one understands, and what he gets up to goodness only knows (成天家疯疯癫癫的，说的话人也不懂，干的事人也不知，66）。	
		E1.9 The others hastily stopped him. "He's raving again," they said. "We mustn't talk to him. If we do, he talks like a fool or a lunatic." (众人不等说完，便说: "可是又疯了？别和他说话才好，若和他说话，不是呆话，就是疯话" 71）。	
		E1.10 (Jia Baoyu) shook a finger at them and swore: " How strange! How is it that once girls marry they get contaminated by men and become so obnoxious—even worse than men!" The matrons on duty at the gate burst out laughing. "Whatever is Master Bao talking about?" they cried. "Goodness knows where he gets hold of such good and all married women bad?" "That's right." Baoyu nodded. "Of course." ((贾宝玉) 指着 (那几个媳妇) 恨道: "奇怪，奇怪，怎么这些人只一嫁了汉子，染了男人的气味，就这样混账起来，比男人更可杀了！" 守园门的婆子听了，也不禁好笑起来，因问道: "这样说，凡女儿个个是好的了，女人各个是坏的了？" 宝玉点头道: "不错，不错！" 77）。	

	(Schizotypal) Unusual beliefs and experiences (an aspect of Psychoticism): Unusual experiences of reality.
F1.1 Five devils invoked by sorcery take possession of Baoyu and Xifeng (Concubine Zhao and Priestess Ma did something in secret). (The next moment he let out a piercing cry. "I'm dying!" He leapt several feet into the air, babbling and raving. By now Baoyu had turned the whole place upside down in search of a sword or stick to kill himself with. Baoyu and Xifeng had fallen into a coma. They lay on their beds burning with fever and babbling deliriously.). (魔魔法姊弟逢五鬼. (宝玉大叫一声: "我要死了!" 将身一纵, 离地跳有三四尺高, 口内乱嚷乱叫, 说起胡话来了. 宝玉亦拿刀弄杖, 寻死觅活的, 闹得天翻地覆. 他叔嫂二人越发糊涂, 不省人事, 睡在床上浑身火炭一般, 口内无般不说.), 25).	
F1.2 (Zijuan said) "Your cousin—back to Suzhou."…Baoyu was thunderstruck.… Qingwen noticed Baoyu's distraught look, the hectic flush on his cheeks and the sweat on his forehead. She at once let him by the hand to Happy Red Court…A fever was not too alarming, but his eyes were fixed and staring, saliva was trickling from the corners of his lips, and he seemed in a state of stupefaction. He would liedown if a pillow was put for him, would sit up if pulled, and drink tea if it was brought…Nanny Li, arriving presently, examined Baoyu carefully. When he made no answer to any of her questions she felt his pulse, then pinched his upper lip so hard that her fingers left deep imprints— yet he felt no pain…At sight of Zijuan the old lady's eyes flashed. "You bitch!" she stormed. "What did you say to him?" "Nothing, madam. Nothing but a few words in fun." At the sight of her Baoyu cried out and burst into tears, to the relief of everybody present. The Lady Dowager caught Zijuan's arm, thinking she had offended him, and urged him to beat her. But Baoyu seized hold of her and would not let go. "If you go," he shouted, "you must take me with you!" No one could understand this till Zijuan, when questioned explained her threat made in fun of going back to Suzhou. "Is that all?" exclaimed the Lady Dowager, the tears running down her cheeks. "So it because of a joke." She scolded Zijuan, "You're such a sensible girl normally, how could you tease him like that when you know how credulous he is?"…Just then it was announced that the wives of Lin Zhixiao and Shan Daliang had come to inquire after the young master. "Show them in," said the old lady. "It's thoughtful of them." But on hearing the name Lin, Baoyu grew frantic again. "No, no!" he shouted from his bed. "The Lins have come to fetch her. Drive them away!" Hastily chiming in, "Drive them away!" his grandmother assured him, "They're not from the Lin family. All those Lins are dead.	

(continued)

Table A.1 (continued)

Character name	Description in DRM (English – Chinese)		DSM-5 Section III
	Terms or phrases	Sentences or paragraphs	Personality functioning or facets trait
		Nobody will ever come to fetch her. Don't you worry." "Never mind who they are," stormed Baoyu tearfully. "No one but Cousin Daiyu should have the mane Lin." ... Baoyu's eye now fell on a golden boat with an engine, a toy from the West, which was on his cabinet. "Isn't that the boat coming to fetch them?" he shouted, pointing at it. "It's mooring there." The Lady Dowager ordered its instant removal, and when Baoyu reached out for it Xiren gave it to him. He tucked it under his bedding. "Now they won't be able to sail away," he laughed. Seizing tight hold of Zijuan he refused to let her go... Whenever he slept he had nightmares, and would wake up crying that Daiyu had gone or that people had come to fetch her ...By now Xiangyun was better, and she came every day to see Baoyu. Finding that he had recovered his faculties she mimicked his crazy behavior during his illness until, lying on his pillow, he had to laugh. Having no idea himself of what had passed, he could hardly believe what was told him. (紫鹃道："妹妹回苏州家去。"宝玉听了，便如头顶上响了一个焦雷一般...晴雯见他只是呆呆，一头热汗，满脸紫胀，忙拉他的手，一直到怡红院中...无奈宝玉发热事亦小可，更觉两个眼珠儿直直的起来，口角边津液流出，皆不知觉，给他个枕头，他便睡下，话也无回答，用手向他脉门摸了茶来，他便吃茶...一时李嬷嬷来了，看了半日，掐的指印如许来深，竟也不觉疼...贾母一见了紫鹃，不过说几句顽话...紫鹃忙道："并没说什么，不过说几句顽话。"谁知宝玉见了紫鹃，方"嗳哟"了一声，哭出来了。众人一见，方都放下心来。贾母便拉住紫鹃，只当他得罪了宝玉，所以拉紫鹃命他打。细问起来，方知宝玉一把拉住紫玉，死也不放，说："要去连我也带了去。"众人不解，细问紫玉，方知紫娟说"要回苏州去"又向紫鹃道："你这孩子素日是个伶俐聪敏的，你又知道他有个呆根子，平白的哄他作什么？"...正说着，人回林之孝家的，单大良家的都来瞧他，贾母流泪道："我当有什么要紧大事，原来是这句话。"贾母道："了不得了，林家的人接他们来了，快打出去罢。"又忙安慰说："那不是林家的人，林家之孝家的，快打出去罢。"又忙安慰说："那不是林家的人，林家的人都死绝了，没人来接他的，你只放心罢。"宝玉哭道："凭他是谁，除了林妹妹，都不许姓林的！"...一时宝玉又一眼	

	看见了十锦槅子上陈设的一只金西洋自行船，便指着乱叫，说："那不是接他们来的船来了？湾在那里呢！"贾母忙命拿下来。袭人忙拿下来，袭人递过去，宝玉便掖在被中，笑道："可去不成了！"一面说，一面死拉着紫鹃不放……有时宝玉睡去，必从梦中惊醒，不是哭了说黛玉已去，便是有人来接……因此时湘云之症已愈，天天过来他看。见宝玉明白了，便将他病中狂态形容了与他瞧，引的宝玉自己伏枕而笑。原来他起先那样竟是不知的，如今听人说还不信。	
	F1.3 A whole series of misfortunes "Baoyu's loss of his friend Liu Xianglian, the suicides of Third Sister You and Second Sister You, and Liu Wuer's illness brought on by mortification" had reduced Baoyu to such a state of dejection that he appeared dazed and often raved like a madman. (宝玉因听见了柳湘莲，剑刎了尤小妹，金逝了尤二姐，病了柳五儿，连连接着闲愁胡恨，一重不了一重添，弄得精色若痴，语言常乱，似染怔忡之疾，70).	(Schizotypal) Withdrawal (an aspect of Detachment): Reticence in social situations; avoidance of social contacts and activity; lack of initiation of social contact.
G1 Afraid of meeting strangers (怕见人, 66)	B1.5	
	H1.1 "For everyone? Let them oblige each other while 'naked I go without impediment.'" Tears ran down his cheeks… (宝玉道："什么是'大家彼此'!他们有'大家彼此'，我是'赤条条来去无牵挂'," 谈及此句，不觉泪下，22).	(Borderline) Identity: Chronic feelings of emptiness; dissociative states under stress.
	H1.2 "Who can compare with you, with not a care in the world?" asked Madam You. "All you do is play around with your girl cousins, eating when you're hungry, sleeping when you're tired and going on like this year after year, taking no thought at all for the future." "Every day I spend with my cousins is all to the good," he answered. "When I die that'll be the end. Who cares about the future?" … "A man's fate is uncertain," Baoyu quipped. "Who knows when he will die? If I died today or tomorrow, this year or next, I'd die content." (尤氏道："谁都像你？真是'一心无挂碍'，只知道和姊妹们顽笑，饿了吃，困了睡，再过几年，不过还是这样，一点后事也不想。"宝玉笑道："我能够和姊妹们过一日是一日，死了就完了。什么后事不后事!"……宝玉笑道："人事莫定，知道谁死谁活？倘或我在今日明日今年明年死了，也就算是遂心一辈子了"，71).	

(continued)

Table A.1 (continued)

Character name	Description in DRM (English – Chinese)		DSM-5 Section III
	Terms or phrases	Sentences or paragraphs	Personality functioning or facets trait
		I1.1 Now Baoyu had always been deplorably eccentric. Since childhood, moreover, he had been intimate with Daiyu, finding her a kindred spirit. Thus now that he knew a little more and had read some improper books, he felt none of the fine girls he had seen in the families of relatives and friends fit to hold a candle to here. He had long since set his heart on having her, but could not admit as much. So whether happy or angry, he used every means to test her secretly. And Daiyu, being rather eccentric too, would disguise her feelings to test him in return. Thus each concealed his or her real sentiments to sound the other out. The proverb says, "When false meets false, the truth will out." So inevitably, in the process, they kept quarrelling over trifles. (原来那宝玉自幼生成有一种下流痴病，况从幼时和黛玉耳鬓厮磨，心情相对；及如今稍明时事，又看了那些邪书僻传，凡远来近友之家所见的那些闺英闱秀，皆未有稍及黛玉者。所以早存了一段心事，只不好说出来，故每每或喜或怒，变尽法子暗中试探。那林黛玉偏生也是个多心病的，也每用假情试探。因你也将真心真意瞒了起来，只用假意，如此两假相逢，终有一真。其间瓑头假体逢，难保不有口舌之争，29)。	(Borderline) Intimacy: Intense, unstable, and conflicted close relationships, marked by mistrust neediness, and anxious preoccupation with real or imagined abandonment.
		J1.1 If the girls ignore him he keeps fairly quiet though he feels bored. He can always work off his temper by scolding some of his pages. But if the girls give him the least encouragement, he's so elated he gets up to all kinds of mischief; one moment he's all honey-sweet; the next, he's rude and recalcitrant; and in another minute he's raving like a lunatic. (姊妹们有日不理他，他倒还安静些。纵然他没趣，不过出了二门，背地里拿着他两个小么儿出气，咕唧一会子就完了。若这一日姊妹们和他多说一句话，他心里一乐，便生出多少事来。他嘴里一时甜言蜜语，一时有天无日，一时又疯疯傻傻。3)。 J1.2 Absurdly he courts care and melancholy/And raves like any madman in his folly (无故寻愁觅恨，有时似傻如狂。3)。 J1.3 This instantly threw Baoyu into one of his frenzies. Tearing off the jade he flung it on the ground. "What's rare about it?" he stormed. "It can't even tell good people from bad. What spiritual understanding has it got? I don't want this nuisance either." (宝玉听了，登时发作起痴狂病来，摘下那玉，就狠命摔去，骂道："什么罕物，连人之高低不择，还说'通灵'不'通灵'呢！我也不要这劳什子了！" 3)。	(Borderline) Emotional lability (an aspect of Negative Affectivity): Emotions that are easily aroused, intense, and/or out of proportion to events and circumstances.

	J1.4 When he sees the girls, if he's in the mood he'll play around with them quite forgetting his station; if he's not in the mood he'll go off by himself, ignoring everyone else. (有时见了我们, 喜欢时没上没下, 大家玩成一块; 不喜欢欢各自走了, 他也不理人, 66).	(Borderline) Separation insecurity (an aspect of Negative Affectivity): Fears of rejection by – and/or separation from – significant others, associated with fears of excessive dependency and complete loss of autonomy.
K1 Naturally timid (天生性怯, 79)	K1.1 Baoyu, on the other hand, wished that parties need never break up, flowers never fade; and although he could neither stop a feast from ending nor flowers from withering, he grieved every time this happened (那宝玉的情性只愿常聚, 生怕一时散了添悲; 那花只愿常开, 生怕一时谢了没趣; 只到筵散花谢, 虽有万种悲伤, 也就无可如何了, 31). K1.2 "If you both sleep on that clothes-warmer, I'll be all alone out here.' objected Baoyu. 'I'd be too scared to get a wink of sleep.'" (宝玉笑道: "这个话, 你们两个都在那上头睡了, 我这外边没个人, 我怪怕的, 一夜也睡不着". 51). F1.2 K1.3 However, he often woke up in the night and being very timid would always call for someone (宝玉夜间常醒, 又极胆小, 每醒必唤人. 77).	
L1 Flinging down wretchedly (恟倒, 28); L2 Heart-broken (心碎肠断, 28)	L1.1 "I only beseech you all to stay and watch over me until the day that I turn into floating ashes—no, not ashes. Ashes have a trace of form and consciousness. Stay until I've turned into a puff of smoke and been scattered by the wind. Then you'll no longer be able to watch over me, and I shall no longer be able to care about you – you can let me go, and I'll have to let you go wherever you please as well." ("…只求你们同看着我, 守着我, 等我有一日化成了灰,—灰还有形有迹, 还有知识, 等我化成一股轻烟, 风一吹便散了的时候, 你们也管不得我, 我也顾不得你们了…", 19). L1.2 He wished he were some insensible, stupid object, able to escape all earthly entanglements and be free from such wretchedness… (真不知此时此际欲为何等蠢物, 杳无所知, 逃大造, 出尘网, 始可解释这段悲伤, 28). E1.7 L1.3 "I only wish I could die this very minute and tear out my heart to show you. Then all the rest of me, skin and bones, could be turned into ashes—no, ashes still have form—better be turned into smoke. But smoke still congeals and can be seen by men—it would have to be scattered in a flash, by a great wind, to the four quarters. That would be a good death." ("我只愿这会子立刻我死了, 把心进出来你们瞧见了, 然后连皮带骨一概都化成一股灰,—灰还有形迹, 不如再化一股烟,—烟还可凝聚, 人还看见, 须得一阵大乱风吹吹散了, 这才好", 57). H1.2	(Borderline) Depressivity (an aspect of Negative Affectivity): Pessimism about the future.

(continued)

Table A.1 (continued)

Character name	Description in DRM (English – Chinese)		DSM-5 Section III
	Terms or phrases	Sentences or paragraphs	Personality functioning or facets trait
	M1 Reckless and headstrong (放荡弛纵, 任性恣情, 19); M2 Carrying away by all whims and fancies (任意任情的, 19)	J1.3 M1.1 Baoyu, in a foul temper, had decided to punish whoever opened the gate. Without waiting to see who it was, and assuming that this was one of the younger girls, he kicked Xiren so hard in the side that she let out a cry. "You low creatures!" he stormed. "I treat you so well that you've lost all sense of respect. Now you dare make fun of me!" (宝玉一肚子没好气, 满心里要把开门的踢几脚。及开了门, 并不看真是谁, 还只当是那些小丫头子们, 便抬腿踢在肋上。袭人"嗳哟"了一声, 宝玉还骂道: "下流东西们! 我素日担待你们得了意, 一点儿也不怕, 越发拿我取笑儿了", 30).	(Borderline) Impulsivity (an aspect of Disinhibition): Acting on the spur of the moment in response to immediate stimuli; difficulty establishing or following plans.
	N1 Doing things in unconventional way (随心所欲, 9); N2 Neglecting studies (荒疏学业, 33); N3 Free to do as pleased (任意纵性, 37)	B1.1 N1.1 He always followed his own bent regardless of what was due to his position (宝玉终是不安本分之人, 竟一味的随心所欲, 9). B1.4 B1.5	Distractibility (an aspect of Disinhibition): Difficulty concentrating and focusing on tasks; attention is easily diverted by extraneous stimuli; difficulty maintaining goalfocused behavior, including both planning and completing tasks.
Wang Xifeng (王熙凤)	O1 Regardless of anyone else (目若无人, 14); O2 Wantonly talkative (放诞, 3); N3 Pert (无礼, 3)	O1.1 Xifeng was thoroughly gratified by the authority she now wielded. (凤姐儿见自己威重令行, 心中十分得意, 14). O1.2 Mortified at being addressed like this in front of so many people, Xifeng flushed crimson, quite put out for a moment. (凤姐听了这话, 又当着许多人, 又羞又气, 一时抓寻不着头脑, 憋得脸紫涨, 71).	(Narcissistic) Identity: excessive reference to others for self-definition and self-esteem regulation; exaggerate self-appraisal inflated.

P1 Always having passion to shine (争强斗智, 55); P2 Likely to show smartness (多事逞才, 65).	P1.1 She looks down on everyone and just sucks up to the old lady and mistress. Whatever she says goes, and no one dares stop her. She tries to save up piles of silver so that Their Ladyships will praise her for being a good manager. (皆因他一时看的人都不及他，只一味哄着老太太、太太两个人喜欢。他说一是一，说二是二，没人敢拦他。又恨不得把银子省下来堆成山，好叫老太太、太太说他会过日子, 65).	(Narcissistic) Self-direction: Goal-setting based on gaining approval from others; personal standards unreasonably high in order to see oneself as exceptional; often unaware of own motivations.
	Q1.1 If she has a fault, it's that she's rather hard on those below her. (就只一件，待下人未免太严些个, 6). Q1.2 Xifeng scraped together less than an ounce of inferior scraps. (凤姐听了，只得将些渣末泡须凑了几钱，命人送去, 12). Q1.3 This flattery made Xifeng forget her exhaustion and start chatting more cheerfully. (一路奉承的凤姐越发受用，也不顾劳乏，更攀谈起来, 15). Q1.4 "Why hasn't she called to see Bao-yu?" She wondered. "Even if she's busy, you'd think she'd put in an appearance to please the Lady Dowager and Lady Wang. There must be some reason why she hasn't come." ((林黛玉)心里有事缠住了，他必定也是要来打个花胡哨，讨老太太和太太的好儿才是。今儿才是早晚不来，必有原故。, 35).	(Narcissistic) Empathy: Impaired ability to recognize or identify with the feelings and needs of others; excessively attuned to reactions of others, but only if perceived as relevant to self.
	Q1.4	(Narcissistic) Intimacy: Relationships largely superficial and exist to serve self-esteem regulation; mutuality constrained by little genuine interest in others' experiences and predominance of a need for personal gain.

(continued)

Table A.1 (continued)

Character name	Description in DRM (English – Chinese)		DSM-5 Section III
	Terms or phrases	Sentences or paragraphs	Personality functioning or facets trait
	R1 Overestimating (indulging) self-strength (自恃强壮, 55)	R1.1 She sat alone in her annex and not even joining the other young wives to greet lady guests. (独在抱厦内起坐, 不与众姊娌合群, 便有堂客来任, 也不与迎会, 14). R1.2 None of them could compare with Xifeng with her charm, ready tongue and elegance. Having no fear of anyone, she gave whatever orders she pleased and did as she liked, regardless of anyone else. (种种之类, 俱不及凤姐爷止舒徐, 言语慷慨, 珍贵宽大. 因此, 也不把众人放在眼里, 挥霍指示, 任其所为, 目若无人, 14).	(Narcissistic) Grandiosity (an aspect of Antagonism): Feelings of entitlement, either overt or covert.
	S1 Flattery and ceremonial (喜奉承尚排场, 24); S2 Tongue-clever (嘴乖, 35)	S1.1 Now Xifeng loved nothing better than displaying her administrative ability. (那凤姐素日最喜揽事办, 好卖弄才干, 13). P1.1 S1.2 If anything good happens, she rushes to take the credit before anyone else can report it. If anything bad happens, or if she herself makes some mistake, she ducks and shifts the blame on to other people, stirring up more trouble too on the side. (遇着有好事, 他就先抓尖儿; 或有了不好事或他自己错了, 他便一缩头推到别人身上来, 他还在旁劳边拨火儿, 65).	(Narcissistic) Attention seeking (an aspect of Antagonism): Excessive attempts to attract and be the focus of the attention of others; admiration seeking.
	T1 Crafty and vicious (心里歹毒, 65)	T1.1 Xifeng, though hating Qiutong, was eager to use her first to rid herself of Second Sister You by "killing with a borrowed sword" and "watching from a hilltop while two tigers fought." For once Qiutong had killed Second Sister You, she could do this new concubine in. (凤姐虽恨秋桐, 且喜借他先可发脱二姐, 自己且抽头, 用"借剑杀人"之法, 坐山观虎斗, 等秋桐杀了尤二姐, 自己再杀秋桐, 65).	(Antisocial) Self-direction: Absence of prosocial internal standards, association with failure to conform to lawful or culturally normative ethical behavior.
	U1 Haughty and hard-hearted (脸酸心硬, 14)	U1.1 (Xifeng abuses her power at Iron Threshold Temple) Thus the Zhang and Li families were unlucky enough to lose both girl and money. Only Xifeng was the gainer by three thousand taels…This emboldened her from that time on to undertake countless similar transactions. (王凤姐弄权铁槛寺, 结果, 张, 李两家受波拖, 真是人财两空. 这里凤姐却坐享了三千两…自此凤姐胆识愈壮, 便恣意的作为起来, 15–16).	(Antisocial) Empathy: Lack of concern for feelings, needs, or suffering of others; lack of remorse after hurting or mistreating another.

	U1.2 My plan is to fetch all the maids from the mistress' house here. No need to torture or beat them; we can just make them kneel in the sun on shards of porcelain with nothing to eat or drink. If they don't come clean, they'll have to kneel all day. Then even if they're made of iron, in a day they're bound to confess. (依我的主意，把太太屋里的丫头都拿来，虽不便擅加拷打，只叫他们垫着磁瓦子跪在太阳地下，茶饭也别给吃。一日不说跪一日，便是铁打的，一日也管招了，61).	(Antisocial) Manipulativeness (an aspect of Antagonism): Frequent use of subterfuge to influence or control others; use of ingratiation to achieve one's ends.
	V1.1 This put Xifeng on her mettle. "You know me," she replied. "I have never believed all that talk about Hell and retribution. I do what I please and am always as good as my word. Let them bring me three thousand taels and I will see to this for them." (凤姐听了这话，便发了兴头，说道："你是素日知道我的，从来不信什么是阴司地狱报应的，凭是什么事，我说要行就行。你叫他拿三千银子来，我就替他出这口气，"15). Q1.4 T1.1	
U1; T1	W1.1 Xifeng sets a vicious trap for a lover; Jia Rui looks into the wrong side of the precious mirror of love. (王熙凤毒设相思局，贾天祥正照风月鉴，12). U1.1 U1.2	(Antisocial) Callousness (an aspect of Antagonism): Lack of concern for feelings or problems of others; lack of guilt or remorse about the negative or harmful effects of one's actions on others; aggression.
X1 Showing of regard (假意殷勤, 12);	X1.1 Xifeng questions a page boy and hatches a plot (She then thought the whole business over carefully once more, and hit on a cunning plan to kill several birds with one stone, working out the sagest measures to achieve this. This done, instead of disclosing her plan to Pinger, she behaved as cheerfully as if nothing had happened, giving no sign of her fury and jealousy.). (讯家童凤姐着意阴谋（自己一个人将前事从头至尾细细的盘算了多时，得了一个"一击两鸣"一计害贤"的很主意出来。自己暗想："须得如此如此，方妥。"主意已定，也不告诉平儿，反外面作出欢笑自若无事的意思，并不露出恼恨妒嫉之意。), 67).	(Antisocial) Deceitfulness (an aspect of Antagonism): Dishonesty and fraudulence; embellishment or fabrication when relating events.

(continued)

Table A.1 (continued)

Character name	Description in DRM (English – Chinese)		DSM-5 Section III
	Terms or phrases	Sentences or paragraphs	Personality functioning or facets trait
	X2 Having shrew's honeyed talk and showing of being virtuous wife – but at heart crafty and cruel (花言巧语，外作贤良，内藏奸狡, 69)	X1.2 (Jia Lian) rewarded him (Jia Lian) with a new concubine—a seventeen-year-old maid of his named Qiutong. Jia Lian kowtowed his thanks and left in high spirits. Having paid his respect to the Lady Dowager and other members of the family he went home somewhat sheepishly to see Xifeng, but found her less stern than usual. She came out with Second Sister You to welcome him and ask after his health. Then Jia Lian, telling her of his father's gift, could not help looking pleased and proud. Xifeng immediately sent two servingwomen to fetch Qiutong by carriage. Before she had rid herself of one thorn in her side, here—out of the blue—was another! However, she had to watch her tongue and hide her anger by a show of complaisance, ordering a feast of welcome, then taking Qiutong to present her to the Lady Dowager and Lady Wang, much to her husband's amazement...Xifeng, though hating Qiutong, was eager to use her first to rid herself of Second Sister You by "killing with a borrowed sword" and "watching from a hilltop while two tiger fought."For once Qiutong had killed Second Sister You, she could do this new concubine in. ((贾赦) 将房中一个十七岁的丫鬟名唤秋桐者，赏他 (贾琏) 为妾. 贾琏即叩头领去，喜之不尽. 见了贾母和家中人，回来见凤姐. 未免脸上有些愧色. 谁知凤姐儿他反不似往日容颜，同尤二姐一同出迎，叙了寒温. 贾琏将秋桐之事说了，未免脸上有些得意之色. 凤姐听了，忙命两个媳妇坐车在那边接了来. 心中一剁未除，又凭空添了一剁，将好颜面换出来遮掩. 一面又命摆酒接风，一面带了秋桐来见可巧贾母先见贾琏回发脱二姐，自己且抽头，用"借剑杀人""之法，坐山观虎斗，等秋桐杀了尤二姐，自己再杀秋桐, 69).	
	T1;	Y1.1 "You can know a man's face but not his heart," she reflected, "I'll show the beast! If he tries anything like that with me, I'll sooner or later make him die at my hands, to let him know my ability." (凤姐儿故意的把脚步放送了些儿，见他去远了，心里暗付道: "这才是知人知面不知心呢，那里有这样禽兽的人呢!他如果如此，几时叫他死在我的手里，他才知道我的手段!", 11).	(Antisocial) Hostility (an aspect of Antagonism): mean, nasty or vengeful behavior.

(continued)

Y1 Sharp-, quick-tongued (口里尖快, 65)	Y1.2 As she did so, an acolyte of twelve or thirteen, holding a case of scissors for cutting the candle-wicks, came darting out to see the fun and ran into her. She boxed his ears so hard that he pitched to the ground. "Look out where you're going, little bastard!" she swore. (可巧有个十二三岁的小道士儿, 拿着剪筒, 照管剪各处蜡花, 正欲得便且藏出去, 不想一头撞在凤姐儿怀里. 凤姐便一扬手, 照脸一下, 把那小孩子打了一个筋斗, 骂道: "野牛肏的, 胡朝那里跑", 29).
	Y1.3 "That reminds me," said Lady Wang. "How much are the concubines Zhao and Zhou allowed a month?"... "Are they paid in full every month?" "Of course they are," declared Xifeng in surprise. "The other day I seem to have heard someone complaining that she was one string short. Why was that?" Xifeng replied readily, "The allowance for the concubines' maids used to be one string a month, but last year the gentlemen in the treasury decided to reduce it by half—to five hundred cash for each. As each of them has two maids, that makes one string less. They can't complain this was my doing. I'd like to give them the usual amount; but since the gentlemen cut it, how can I make good the cut? I'm only the intermediary, I've no say in the matter. I merely hand out what I'm given. Several times in fact I've suggested restoring their original pay, only to be told, 'This is the quota.' I can't do more. At least I pay them on the dot each month, whereas in the past those people in the treasury always kept them waiting. They were never paid so regularly before." A short silence followed....she (Wang Xifeng) remarked. "It's not my fault if I've been a long time. Her Ladyship has been raking up ancient history, and I had to answer her questions one by one." With a grim smile she added, "Well, from today on, I mean to show how ruthless I can be, and I don't care if they complain to Her Ladyship either. Tot those stupid, four-mouthed bitches! They'll come to no good end. How puffed up they are with their own consequence! But they'll lose the lot, and sooner than they think. Baming us, indeed, because either maids' pay is cut. Who do they think they are? Do they deserve maids?" Still pouring out abuse, she went off.... (王夫人问道: "正要问你, 如今赵姨娘, 周姨娘的月例多少?"...王夫人道: "可都按数给他们?" 凤姐见问的奇怪, 忙道: "怎么不按数给!" 王夫人道: "前儿我恍惚听见有人抱怨, 说短了一吊钱, 是什么原故?" 凤姐忙笑道: "姨娘们的丫头, 月例原是人各一吊. 从旧年他们外头商议的, 姨娘的丫头分例减半, 人各五百钱, 每位两个丫头, 所以短了一吊钱. 这也抱怨不着我, 我倒乐得给他们呢."... 王夫人听说, 也就罢了...

Table A.1 (continued)

Character name	Description in DRM (English – Chinese)		DSM-5 Section III
	Terms or phrases	Sentences or paragraphs	Personality functioning or facets trait
		(王熙凤) 又告诉众人道: "你们说我回了这半日的话, 太太把一百年的事都想 起来 问我, 难道我不说罢?" 又冷笑道: "我从今以后得好几样克毒罢了. 抱怨给太太听, 我也不怕. 糊涂油蒙了心, 烂了舌头不得好死的下作东西, 别作娘的春梦! 明儿一裹 脑子扣的日子还有呢. 如今裁了丫头的钱, 就抱怨了咱们. 也不想一想是奴儿? 也配 使两三个丫头了!"一面骂, 一面方走了. (第两次方走了, 36). Y1.4 She'll give you sweet talk when there's hatred in her heart, she's so double-faced and tricky. All the time she's smiling she tries to trip you up, making a show of great warmth while she stabs you in the back. That's the way she is. (嘴甜心苦, 两面三刀; 上 头一脸笑, 脚下便绊子; 明是一盆火, 暗是一把刀一都占全了, 65). Y1.5 Don't trust that shrew's (Wang Xifeng) honeyed talk and her show of being such a virtuous wife—at heart she's crafty and cruel. She's made up her mind to kill you (Second Sister You). (休信那妒妇花言巧语, 外作贤良, 内藏奸狡, 他发恨定要弄你一 死方罢, 69).	
		Z1.1 Xifeng sets a vicious trap for a lover (Wang Xifeng played with Jia Rui, who was made to stayed out for one night and almost froze to death; under Xifeng's instigation, Jia Qiang and Jia Rong forced Jia Rui to write and sign two I.O.U.s for each of fifty taels of silver which they pocketed: emptied a bucket of slops over Jia Rui's head in secret.). (王熙凤毒设相思局 (贾瑞被天一夜几乎不曾冻死; 贾蔷, 贾蓉逼贾瑞给二人 各写五十两次契; 将一净桶尿粪从上面直发下来泼了贾瑞一身一头), 12). U1.1 Z1.2 Xifeng, taken by surprise, gives way to jealousy (With that she struck Pinger again. Having no one to whom to complain of this injustice, Pinger holding back her tears nearly choked with rage…When Xifeng saw Pinger bent on suicide, she rammed her head against Jia Lian's chest and screamed, "You've all ganged up to do me in, and when I find out you all try to frighten me. Strangle me and have done with it!"). (发生不 测凤姐泼醋 (打的平儿有冤无处诉, 只气得干哭…平儿急了, 便跑出来找刀子要寻 死…这里凤姐见平儿寻死去, 便一头撞在贾琏怀里, 叫道: "你们一条藤儿害我, 被 我听见了, 倒都唬起我来. 你也勒死我!"), 44).	(Antisocial) Risk taking (an aspect of Disinhibition): Engagement in dangerous, risky, and potentially self-damaging activities, unnecessarily and without regard for consequences.

	X1.1	
	Z1.3 Craft Xifeng kills her rival by proxy, and Second Sister You swallows gold and dies. (弄小巧用借剑杀人, 觉大限吞生金自逝, 69).	
	AA1.1 And once seated there she asked her: "Why has no one received the allowance for this month yet?" "It'll be coming in a couple of days," Pinger whispered. "My mistress got this month's allowance some time ago but has loaned it out. She'll distribute it as soon as she's collected the interest. But mind you don't pass this on." "I can't believe she's put herself to all that trouble?" Pinger smiled. "These last few years she's been lending out this money for the monthly allowances together with her own. The interest she gets on these loans comes to more than a thousand taels of silver a year." "So the two of you, mistress and maid, have been using our money to get interest and kept us waiting like regular fools!" said Xiren with a smile. (袭人又叫任, 问道: "这个月的月钱, 连老太太和太太的还没放呢, 这是为什么?" 平儿见问, 忙转身至袭人跟前, 见方近无人, 才悄悄说道: "你快别问, 横竖再过几天就放了。" 袭人笑道: "这是为什么, 唬得你这样?" 平儿瞧瞧他道: "这个月的月钱, 我们奶奶早已支了, 放给人使呢。等别处的利钱收了来凑齐了, 才放呢。因为是你, 我才告诉你, 你可不许告诉一个人去。" 袭人笑道: "他难道还短钱使? 还没个足厌? 何苦还操这心。" 平儿笑道: "这几年拿着这一项银子, 翻出有几百来了。他的月例钱又使不着, 只他这梯己利钱, 一年不到, 上千的银子呢。" 袭人笑道: "拿着我们的钱, 你们主子奴才赚利钱, 哄的我们呆呆的等着.", 39).	(Antisocial) Irresponsibility (an aspect of Disinhibition): Disregard for—and failure to honor—financial and other obligations or commitments.
	AB1.1 "...She spies on me as if I were a thief. It's all right for her to talk to other men, but she won't let me say a word to another woman. If I do, she suspects the worst." ("他防我像防贼的, 只许他同男人说话, 不许我和女人略近些, 他就疑惑.", 21). AB1.2 If other women are jealous, she's a hundred times so. If the master happens to cast a second glance at any maid, she's liable to make a row then and there. (人家是醋罐子, 他是醋缸醋瓮. 凡丫头们二爷多看一眼, 他有本事当着爷打个烂羊头.", 21). AB1.3 Xifeng was convulsed with fury, convinced by their praise of Pinger that the latter must have been complaining about her behind her back too. (凤姐听了, 气的浑身乱战, 又听他俩都赞平儿, 便疑平儿素日背地里自然也有抱怨语了, 44).	Suspiciousness (an aspect of Detachment): Doubts about loyalty and fidelity of others; feelings of being mistreated, used, and/or persecuted by others.

(continued)

Table A.1 (continued)

Character name	Description in DRM (English – Chinese)		DSM-5 Section III Personality functioning or facets trait
	Terms or phrases	Sentences or paragraphs	
		AC1.1 Five devils invoked by sorcery take possession of Baoyu and Xifeng (Concubine Zhao and Priestess Ma did something in secret). (They were all in a great commotion and wondering what to do when in rushed Xifeng, brandishing a bright steel sword, with which she was trying to cut down all the chickens, dogs and people in her way…Baoyu and Xifeng had fallen into a coma. They lay on their beds burning with fever and babbling deliriously). (魔魇法姊弟逢五鬼，正没个主见，只见凤姐手持一把明晃晃钢刀砍进园来，见鸡杀鸡，见狗杀狗，见人就要杀人…他叔嫂二人愈发搧涂，不省人事，睡在床上洋身火炭一般，口内无般不说，25).	Unusual beliefs and experiences (an aspect of Psychoticism): unusual experiences of reality, including hallucination-like experiences.
Lin Daiyu (林黛玉)		AD1.1 "…That she'd lower and cheapen herself by joking with me? She's the daughter of a noble house, I'm a nobody. If she were to joke with me and I answered back, that would be degrading for her – was that the idea?…" ("…莫不是他和我顽，他就自轻自贱了，他原是公侯的小姐，我原是贫民的丫头，设若我回了口，岂不他自惹人轻贱呢…", 22). AD1.2 "In my case, they'd resent it even more. After all, I'm not a daughter of the house, I'm here because I've nowhere else to go. They resent me enough as it is. If I should push myself forward, they'd all start cursing me." ("况我又不是他们这里正经主子，原是无依无靠投奔了来的，他们已经多嫌着我了，如今我还不知进退，何苦叫他们咒我？", 45).	(Borderline) Identity: Unstable self-image, often associated with excessive self-criticism; chronic feelings of emptiness.
	AE1 Rather jealous and petty-minded (素习猜忌, 好弄小性儿, 27); AE2 Taking things to heart (心窄, 76)	AE1.1 She must watch her step in her new home, she decided, be on guard every moment and weigh every word, so as not to be laughed at for any foolish blunder. (因此步步留心，时时在意，不肯轻易多说一句话，多行一步路，惟恐被人耻笑了他去, 3); AE1.2 Daiyu smiled bitterly. "I wouldn't get mine till the others had taken their pick." (黛玉冷笑道："我就知道，别人不挑剩下的，也不给我", 7).	(Borderline) Empathy: Perceptions of others selectively biased toward negative attributes or vulnerabilities.

	AE1.3 "Mother always drags us in!" protested Baochai. Resting her head against her mother's breast she asked laughingly, "Shall we go now?" "Look at her," teased Daiyu. "Such a big girl, and when you're not around, aunt, she looks very dignified; but when she's with you she acts just like a baby." Caressing her daughter Aunt Xue told Daiyu, "This child means as much to me as Xifeng does to the old lady. When I've serious business, I consult her; when there's none, she amuses me. When I see her like this all my troubles melt away." Tears came into Daiyu's eyes. "She's doing this on purpose here, to wound me by reminding me that *I've* no mother." ...She (Aunt Xue) turned then to caress Daiyu as well. "Don't cry, there's a good child," she urged. "It upsets you to see how fond I am of your cousin, but I love you even more if you only knew it…" (宝钗道："惟有妈，说动话就拉上我们。"一面说，一面伏在他母亲怀里要个不走。黛玉笑道："你瞧，这么大了，离了姨妈他就是个样子的，见了姨妈他就撒娇儿。"薛姨妈用手搂着宝钗，叹道，没了事幸亏有他开我的心。我见了他这样，分明是气我没娘的人，故意来刺我的眼。"…(薛姨妈)摩挲黛玉，笑道："好孩子别哭。你见我疼你姐姐，你伤心了，不知我疼你心里更疼你呢…"，57).	(Borderline) Intimacy: Intense, unstable, and conflicted close relationships, marked by mistrust, neediness, and anxious preoccupation with real or imagined abandonment.
AF1 Sensitive and suspicious (多心, 22, 27)	AF1.1 Now her maid Xueyan brought in her little hand-stove. "Who told you to bring this?" demanded Daiyu. "Many thanks. Think I was freezing to death here?" "Zi juan was afraid you might be cold, miss, so she asked me to bring it over." Nursing the stove in her arms Daiyu retorted, "So you do whatever she asks, but let whatever I say go in one ear and out the other. You jump to ovey her instructions faster than if they were and Imperial edict." Although Baoyu knew these remarks were aimed at him, his only reply was to chuckle. And Baochai, aware that this was Daiyu's way, paid no attention either. (可巧，黛玉的小丫鬟雪雁走来，与黛玉送小手炉。黛玉因含笑问他："谁叫你送来的?亏你费心，那里就冷死了我。"雪雁道："紫鹃姐姐怕姑娘冷，使我送来的。"黛玉一面接了抱在怀中，笑道："也亏你倒听他的话。我平日和你说的，全当耳旁风，怎么他说了你就依，比圣旨还快呢?"宝玉听这话，知是黛玉借此奚落他，也无回复之词，只嘻嘻的笑两声罢了。宝钗素知黛玉是如此惯了的，也不去睬他，8). AF1.2 (Lin Daiyu said) "There's no need to swear. I know I have a place in your heart. But whenever you see her, you forget all about me." (Jia Baoyu said) "That's your imagination. I'm not like that." (林黛玉（对贾宝玉）道："你也不用说誓，我很知道你心里有妹妹，但只见了姐姐，就把妹妹忘了。"宝玉道："那是你多心，我再不的。"，28).	

(continued)

Table A.1 (continued)

Character name	Description in DRM (English – Chinese)		DSM-5 Section III
	Terms or phrases	Sentences or paragraphs	Personality functioning or facets trait
		I1.1	
		AF1.3 (Lin Daiyu said to Jia Baoyu) "How dense you are! You have jade, and someone else (Xue Baochai) has gold to match it. So don't you have a warm scent to match her cold scent?" ((林黛玉对贾宝玉道) "蠢才! 你有玉, 人家 (薛宝钗) 就有金配你; 人家有'冷香', 你就没有'暖香'去配?", 19). AF1.4 As for Daiyu, she was reflecting, "... Why get so worked up at the mention of gold (Xue Baochai) and jade (Jia Baoyu)? This shows you're thinking about them all the time. You're afraid I suspect this when I mention them, so you put on a show of being worked up – just to fool me." (那林黛玉心里想着: "...如何我只一提'金玉'的事, 你就着急? 可知你心里时时有'金玉', 见我一提, 你又怕我多心, 故意着急, 安心哄我", 29).	
	AG1 So sensitive (多心, 3); AG2 Feeling some twinges of jealousy (悒郁不忿, 5); AG3 Quick to take offence (爱恼的, 22); AG4 Too hasty (浮躁, 30);	AG1.1 The more she thought, the more distressed she felt. Oblivious of the cold dew on the green moss and the chill wind on the path, standing under the blossom by tile corner of the wall she gave way to sobs. (越想越伤感起来, 也不顾苍苔露冷, 花径风寒, 独立墙角边花阴之下, 悲悲戚戚呜咽起来, 26). AG1.2 She would often sit moodily frowning or sighing over nothing or, for no apparent reason, would give way to long spells of weeping. (无事闷坐, 不是愁眉便是长叹, 且好端端的不知为了什么, 常常的便自泪道不干的, 27). AG1.3 Daiyu enjoyed the general excitement too until it came home to her that she alone had no family but was all on her own, and at this thought she shed tears. (黛玉见了, 先是欢喜, 次后想起众人皆有亲眷, 独自己孤单, 无个亲眷, 不免又去垂泪, 49). AG1.4 Unable to suppress a laugh she (Lin Daiyu) replied... Then Daiyu spoke of Baoqin, and wept because she had no sister of her own. (黛玉听了, 禁不住也笑了起来, 因又笑道...黛玉因又说起宝琴来, 想起自己没有姊妹, 不免又哭了, 49).	(Borderline) Emotional lability (an aspect of Negative Affectivity): Unstable emotional experiences and frequent mood changes; emotions that are easily aroused, intense and/or out of proportion to events and circumstances.

AG5 Always crying (爱哭, 37, 64)	AG1.5 Gazing at them through tears she sighed: 'I come from south of the Yangzi, but my parents are dead and I'm all on my own, with no brothers; so I have to put up in my grandmother's house. My health is poor too, and though I'm well looked after by my grandmother, aunt and cousins, none of the Lin family ever calls to see me or brings me local products which I could gain face by distributing as presents. This shows how lonely it is, how utterly wretched, to have no family of one's own.' These reflections made her feel her heart would break. (惟有林黛玉，他见了江南家乡之物，反自触物伤情，因想起他的父母来了…想到这里，不觉就大伤起心来了，67). AG1.6 This big family reunion in the Jia mansion, which the Lady Dowager still complained was less lively than in the old days, as well as her reference to Baochai and Baoqin celebrating at home with their own family, had made Daiyu feel so disconsolate that she had slipped out to the corridor to shed tears. (只因黛玉见贾府中许多人赏月，贾母犹叹人少，不似当年热闹，又提宝钗姊妹家去，母女兄弟自去赏月等语，不觉对景感怀，自去俯栏垂泪，76).	(Borderline) Anxiousness (an aspect of Negative Affectivity): Intense feelings of nervousness, tenseness, or panic, often in reaction to interpersonal stresses; worry about the negative effects of past unpleasant experiences and future negative possibilities.
AH1 Worrying too much (忧虑过度, 67)	AE1.1 AH1.1 Rooted indignantly to the spot and tempted to let fly at her Daiyu reflected, "Although my aunt's house is a second home to me, I'm after all an outsider here. With both my parents dead, I've no one to turn to except this family. It would be foolish to start a real rumpus." As she thought thus, tears ran down her cheeks. (林黛玉听了，不觉气闷在心，自己回思一番："虽说是舅母家，如同自己家一样，到底是客边。如今父母双亡，无依无靠，现在他家依栖。如今认真淘气，也觉没趣。"一面想，一面又滚下泪珠来, 26).	
AH1	AI1.1 And Baoyu and Daiyu had drawn closer to each other than all the others. By day they strolled or sat together; at night they went to bed in the same apartment. On all matters, indeed, they were in complete accord. But now Baochai had suddenly appeared on the scene. Although only slightly older, she was such a proper young lady and so charming that most people considered Daiyu inferior to her. In the eyes of the world, of course, everyone has some merits. In the case of Daiyu and Baochai, one ws lovely as a flower, the other graceful as a willow, but each charming in her own way, according to	(Borderline) Separation insecurity (an aspect of Negative Affectivity): Fears of rejection by and/or separation from-significant others.

(continued)

Table A.1 (continued)

Character name	Description in DRM (English – Chinese)		DSM-5 Section III
	Terms or phrases	Sentences or paragraphs	Personality functioning or facets trait
		her distinctive temperament. Besides, Baochai's generous, tactful and accommodating ways contrasted strongly with Daiyu's stand-offish reserve and won the hearts of her subordinates, so that nearly all the maids liked to chat with her. Because of this, Daiyu began to feel some twinges of jealousy. (便是宝玉和黛玉二人之亲密友爱处, 亦自较别个不同一日则同行同坐, 夜则同息同止, 真是言和意顺, 略无参商. 不想如今来了一个薛宝钗, 年岁虽大不多, 然品格端方, 容貌丰美, 人多谓黛玉所不及. 而且宝钗行为豁达, 随分从时, 不比黛玉孤高自许, 目下无尘, 故比黛玉大得下人之心. 便是那些小丫头们, 亦多喜与宝钗去顽. 因此, 黛玉心中便有些怏怏不忿之意, 5).	
		AII.2 She was wondering whether or not to go back when the sound of talk and laughter inside – she distinguished the voices of Baoyu and Baochai – upset her even more. She thought back then to the events of the morning. "Baoyu must be angry with me, thinking I told on him," she reflected. "But I never did! You ought to investigate before flying into a temper like this. You can shut me out today, but shall we not see each other still tomorrow?" The more she thought, the more distressed she felt. Oblivious of the cold dew on the green moss and the chill wind on the path, standing under the blossom by the corner of the wall she gave way to sobs. (正是回去不是, 站着不是, 正没注意, 只听里面一阵笑语之声. 细听一听, 竟是宝玉, 宝钗二人. 林黛玉心中亦发动了气. 左思右想, 忽然想起了早起的事来: "必定是宝玉恼我告他的原故. 但只我何尝告你了, 越你也打听打听, 就恼我到这步田地. 你今儿不叫我进来, 难道明儿就不见面了?" 越想越伤感起来, 也不顾苍苔露冷, 花径风寒, 独立墙角边花阴之下, 悲悲戚戚呜咽起来, 26).	
		AII.3 "There's no need to swear. I know I have a place in your heart. But whenever you see her, you forget all about me." "That's your imagination. I'm not like that." (林黛玉道: "你也不用说誓, 我很知道你心里有妹妹, 但只见了姐姐, 就把妹妹忘了." 宝玉道: "那是你多心, 我再不的.", 28).	

		(Borderline) Depressivity (an aspect of Negative Affectivity): Frequent feelings of being down, miserable, and/or hopeless; difficulty recovering from such moods; pessimism about the future.
AJ1 In tears always (满眼抹泪, 3); AJ2 So upset (伤感, 3,); AJ3 Feeling distressed (伤感, 26); AJ4 Giving way to sobs (悲悲戚戚, 26); AJ5 Weeping (哭, 26, 27, 29, 30, 57); AJ6 Crying (哭, 32); AJ7 Giving way to own grief (伤感, 28, 57, 64, 76); AJ8 Sobbing even more bitterly (越发伤心大哭, 29);	AJ1.1 Zijuan and Xueyan knew their young mistress' ways. She would often sit moodily frowning or sighing over nothing or, for no apparent reason, would give way to long spells of weeping. At first they had tried to comfort her, imagining that she missed her parents and home or that someone had been unkind; but as time went by and they found this was her habit they paid little further attention. (紫鹃, 雪雁素日知道林黛玉的情性: 无事闷坐, 不是愁眉便是长叹; 且好端端的不知为了什么, 常常的便自泪道不干的. 先时还有人劝, 怕他思父母, 想家乡, 受了委屈, 只得用话宽慰解劝. 谁知后来一年一月的竟常常的如此, 把这个样儿看惯了, 也都不理论了, 27).

AJ1.2…he (Jia Baoyu) caught the sound of sobs on the other side. Someone (Lin Daiyu) was lamenting and weeping there in a heart-rending fashion. (只听山坡那边有鸣咽之声, 一行数落着, 哭的好不伤感, 27).

AJ1.3 Each year for three hundred and sixty days, The cutting wind and biting frost contend. How long can beauty flower fresh and fair? In a single day wind can whirl it to its end…Now you are dead I come to bury you; None has divined the day when I shall die; Men laugh at my folly in burying fallen flowers, But who will bury me when dead I lie? See, when spring draws to a close and flowers fall, This is the season when beauty must ebb and fade; The day that spring takes wing and beauty fades/Who will care for the fallen blossom or dead maid? (一年三百六十日, 风刀霜剑严相逼 明媚鲜妍能几时, 一朝飘泊难寻觅…尔今死去侬收葬, 未卜侬身何日丧? 侬今葬花人笑痴, 他年葬侬知是谁? 试看春残花渐落, 便是红颜老死时. 一朝春尽红颜老, 花落人亡两不知! 27).

AJ1.4 Daiyu nodded and tears ran down her cheeks as she reflected wistfully how good it was to have parents. (黛玉看了不觉点头, 想起有父母的人的好处来, 早又泪珠满面, 35). |

(continued)

Table A.1 (continued)

Character name	Description in DRM (English – Chinese)		DSM-5 Section III
	Terms or phrases	Sentences or paragraphs	Personality functioning or facets trait
	AJ9 Weeping and chocking (一行嗚哭、一行气喘, 29); AJ10 Being in tears (滚下泪来, 32); AJ11 Having habit of crying (每每好哭, 34); AJ12 Always crying (爱哭, 37); AJ13 Weeping again (哭哭啼啼, 67); AH1	AJ1.5 Then Daiyu spoke of Baoqin, and wept because she had no sister of her own. "There you go again, upsetting yourself for no reason," scolded Baoyu. "Just see, you're thinner this year than last, yet you won't look after yourself. Every day you work yourself up for no reason at all and aren't satisfied until you'be had a good cry." Wiping her tears she answered, "I've been feeling sick at hearts, but I don't seem to cry as much as before. Though my heart aches, I haven't many tears to shed." "You just imagine that because you're so used to crying," he objected. "How can anyone's tears dry up?" (黛玉因又说起宝琴来, 想起自己没有姊妹, 不免又哭了. 宝玉忙劝道: "你又寻烦恼了. 你瞧瞧, 今年比旧年越发瘦了, 你还不保养. 每天好好的, 你必是自寻烦恼, 哭一会子, 才算完了这一天的事." 黛玉拭泪道: "近来我只觉心酸, 眼泪却像比旧年少了些的. 心里只管酸痛, 眼泪却不多." 宝玉道: "这是你哭惯了, 心里疑认, 已有眼泪的了?", 49). AE1.3 AJ1.6 Baoyu knew just how narrow-minded and hyper-sensitive she (Lin Daiyu) was, how eager to outshine others in every way. When she saw that Baochai's brother had brought all these things from the south, from her old home, to give away as presents, she must have been painfully reminded of her own loss and other causes for grief. (宝玉深知黛玉之为人: 心细心窄, 而又多心要强, 不落人后, 因见了人家哥哥自江南带了东西来送人, 又系故乡之物, 勾起别的痛肠来, 是以伤感是实, 67).	
AG4	AK1.1 Going crossly back to her own room, she took her scissors and started cutting up the sachet she had been making for him at Baoyu's own request. (赌气回房, 将前日宝玉所烦他作的那个香袋儿—才做了一半—赌气拿过来就剪, 18). AK1.2 At this Daiyu forgot her nausea and rushed over to snatch the jade, seizing a pair of scissors to cut off the tassel. Xiren and Zijuan intervened too late to save it. (林黛玉听了, 也不顾病, 赶来夺过去, 顺手抓起一把剪子来要剪. 袭人、紫鹃刚要夺, 已经剪了几段, 29).	(Borderline) Impulsivity (an aspect of Disinhibition): Acting on the spur of the moment in response of outcomes.

AL1 Snorting (冷笑, 7, 8, 19, 20, 21, 22, 29, 31, 36); AG2; AE1; AL2 Narrow minded and making cutting-remarks (爱刻薄人, 心里又细, 27); AL3 Making cutting-remarks (不让人, 36)	AL1.1 "Why should I egg him on?" Daiyu gave a little snort. "I can't be bothered with offering him advice either. You're too pernickety, nanny. The old lady often gives him wine, so why shouldn't he have a drop more here with his aunt? Are you suggesting that antie's an outsider and he shouldn't behave like that here?" Amused yet vexed, Nanny Li expostulated, "Really, every word Miss Lin says cuts sharper than a knife. How can you suggest such a thing?" Even Baochai couldn't suppress a smile. She pinched Daiyu's cheek and cried, "What a tongue the girl has! One doesn't know whether to be cross or laugh." (林黛玉冷笑道: "我为什么助他? 我也犯不着劝他. 往常老太太又给他酒吃, 如今在姨妈这里多吃一口, 料也不妨事. 必定姨妈这里是外人, 不当在这里的, 也为可定." 李嬷嬷听了, 又是急, 又是笑, 说道: "真真这林姐儿说出一句话来, 比刀子还尖. 你这算了什么?" 宝钗也忍不住, 笑着把黛玉腮上一拧, 说道: "真真这个颦丫头的一张嘴, 叫人爱又不是, 喜欢又不是.", 8).	(Borderline) Hostility (an aspect of Antagonism): Persistent or frequent angry feelings; anger or irritability in response to minor slights and insults.
	AL1.2 "How do you do pick on one!" cried Xiangyun. "Always finding fault! Even if you are better than all the rest of us, there's no need to go making fun of everyone else. But I know someone you'd never dare find fault with. If you do, I'll really respect you." "Who's that?" Daiyu promptly asked." Dare you pick fault with Cousin Baochai? If so, good for you. I may not be up to you, but you've met your match in her." "Oh, her," Daiyu snorted. "I wondered whom you meant. How could I ever presume to find fault with her?" (史湘云道: "他再不放人一点儿, 专挑人的不好. 你自己便比世人好, 也不犯着见一个打趣一个. 指出一个人来, 你敢挑他, 我就挑你." 黛玉忙问是谁. 湘云道: "你敢挑宝姐姐的短处, 就算你是好的. 我靠不如你, 他怎么不及你呢?" 黛玉听了, 冷笑道: "我当是谁, 原来是他. 我那里敢挑他呢!", 20).	
	AL1.3 "If that's how you feel, you'd better hire a special company to play my favourite pieces instead of expecting me to cash in on someone else's birthday." (林黛玉冷笑道: "你既这样说, 你特叫一班戏来, 拣我爱听的唱给我看. 这合子犯不上跐着人借光儿问我.", 22).	
	AL1.4 "A fine question to ask!" Daiyu gave a short laugh. "I don't know. For you I'm a figure of fun, to be compared with an actress in order to raise a laugh." (林黛玉冷笑道: "问的我倒好, 我也不知为什么原故. 我原是给你们取笑的?一拿我比戏子取笑.", 22).	

(continued)

Table A.1 (continued)

Character name	Description in DRM (English – Chinese)		DSM-5 Section III
	Terms or phrases	Sentences or paragraphs	Personality functioning or facets trait
		AL1.5 "I wouldn't have minded so much if you hadn't made eyes at Xiangyun," Daiyu went on. "Just what did you mean by that? That she'd lower and cheapen herself by joking with me? She's the daughter of a noble house, I'm a nobody. If she were to joke with me and I answered back, that would be degrading for her – was that the idea? That was certainly kind on your part. Too bad she didn't appreciate your thoughtfulness, but flared up all the same. Then you tried to excuse yourself at my expense, calling me 'petty-minded and quick to take offence.' You were afraid she might offend me, were you? But what is it to you if I get angry with her? Or if she offends me?" (黛玉又道："这一节还想得。再你为什么又使眼色儿？这安的是什么心？莫不是他和我顽，他就自轻自贱了一他原是公侯的小姐，我原是贫民的丫头，他和我顽，设若我回了口，岂不他自惹人轻贱呢一是这主意不是？这却也是你的好心，只是那一个偏又不领你这好情，一般也恼了。你又拿我作情，倒说我小性儿，行动肯恼。你又怕他得罪了我，我恼他。我恼他与你何干？他得罪了我，又与你何干？", 22). AL1.6 Daiyu had been delighted to hear him make fun of Baochai. She would, indeed, have joined in if not for Baochai's retort regarding the fan. She decided, as it was, to change the subject. "What were the two operas you saw, cousin?" she asked. Daiyu's enjoyment of her discomfiture at Baoyu's remark had not escaped Baochai, who smiled at this question. (林黛玉听见宝玉奚落宝钗，心中着实得意，才要搭言也趁势儿取个笑，不想蔑儿因找扇子，宝钗又发了两句话，他便改口笑道：宝姐姐，你听两出什么戏？宝钗因见林黛玉面上有得意之态，一定是听了宝玉奚落之言，遂了他的心愿，30). AL1.7 "How good you (Xue Baochai) always are to others!" Daiyu exclaimed with a sigh. "I'm so touchy that I used to suspect your motives." (黛玉叹道："你(薛宝钗)素日待人，固然是极好的，然我最是个多心的人，只当你心里藏奸", 45).	

		Grandiosity (an aspect of Antagonism): Feelings of entitlement, either overt or covert; firmly holding to the belief that one is better than others; condescension toward others.
AM1 Being standoffishly reserved and winning hearts of subordinates (孤高自许，目无下尘，5)	AL1.2 AM1.1 "We should have started a club like this long ago," observed Baoyu. "Start one if you like, but don't count me in," said Daiyu. "I'm up to it." "If you're not, who is?" countered Yingchun with a smile. "This is a serious business," declared Baoyu. "We should encourage each other, not back out out of politeness. Let's all give our ides for general discussion." (宝玉笑道："可惜迟了，早该起个社。" 黛玉道："你们只管起社，可别算上我，我是不敢的。" 迎春笑道："你不敢谁还敢呢?" 宝玉道："这是一件正经大事，大家鼓舞起来，不要你谦我让的。各有主意自管说出来，大家平章。", 37).	
AG1	AN1.1 "How good you (Xue Baochai) always are to others!" Daiyu exclaimed with a sigh. "I'm so touchy that I used to suspect your motives...If I started demanding bird's-nest now, the old lady, Lady Wang and Xifeng wouldn't say anything, but those below would be bound to think me too pernickety. Look how jealous these people are and how much gossip there is here because the old lady favors Baoyu and Xifeng. In my case, they'd resent it even more. After all, I'm not a daughter of the house, I'm here because I've nowhere else to go. They resent me enough as it is. If I should push myself forward, they'd all start cursing me." (黛玉叹道："你(薛宝钗)素日待人，固然是极好的，然我最是个多心的人，只当你心里藏奸。...这会子我又兴出新文来熬什么燕窝粥，老太太，太太，凤姐姐这三个人便没话说，那些底下的婆子，丫头们，未免不嫌我太多事了。你看这里这些人，因见老太太多疼了宝玉和凤丫头两个，他们尚虎视眈眈，背地里言三语四的，何况于我?况我又不是他们这里正经主子，原是无依无靠投奔了来的，他们已经多嫌着我了。如今我还不知进退，何苦叫他们咒我?", 45). AN1.2 (Daiyu says:) "...I have nothing. Yet all I eat, wear and use, down to the least blade of grass or sheet of paper, is the same as their own girls get. Naturally those petty-minded people dislike me." (黛玉道："...我是一无所有，吃穿用度，一草一纸，皆是和他们家的姑娘一样，那起小人岂有不多嫌的。", 45). AE1.3	Suspicious (an aspect of Detachment): Expectations of–and sensitivity to–signs of interpersonal ill-intent or harm; doubts about loyalty and fidelity of others; feelings of being mistreated, used, and/or persecuted by others.

(continued)

Table A.1 (continued)

| Character name | Description in DRM (English – Chinese) | | DSM-5 Section III |
	Terms or phrases	Sentences or paragraphs	Personality functioning or facets trait
Xue Baochai (薛宝钗)	AI1.1 AE1.3 AL1.7		Antagonism (vs. Agreeableness): an exaggerated sense of self-importance, as well as a callous antipathy toward others, encompassing both unawareness of others' needs and feelings.
Qingwen (晴雯)		AO1.1 …she retorted with a snigger…sneered Qingwen… (Xiren said,) pushing Qingwen away. "We're the ones to blame." This "we", obviously meaning Baoyu and herself, made Qingwen even more jealous…she cried with a scornful laugh… "I'm too silly to be up to talking to you," snorted Qingwen. (…晴雯冷笑道…冷笑道…(袭人) 推晴雯道: "…原是我们的不是," 晴雯听他说 "我们" 两个字, 自然是他和宝玉了, 不觉又添了酸意, 冷笑几声…晴雯冷笑道: "我原是糊涂的人, 那里配和我说话呢!", 31). AO1.2 (Qingwen said:) "If that's so, get me a fan to tear up. I love ripping things apart." With a smile he (Jia Baoyu) handed her his own. Sure enough, she ripped it in two, then tore it to pieces.…Just then along came Sheyue. "What a wicked waste!" she cried. "Stop it." Baoyu's answer was to snatch her fan from her and give it to Qingwen, who promptly tore it up and joined in his loud laughter. (晴雯笑道: "既这么说, 你就拿了扇子来我撕. 我最喜欢撕的." 宝玉听了, 便笑着递与他. 晴雯果然接过来, 嗤的一声, 撕了两半, 接着嗤嗤又听几声…只见麝月走过来, 笑道: "少作些孽罢." 宝玉赶上来, 一把将他手里的扇子也夺了, 递与晴雯. 晴雯接了, 也撕了几下子, 二人都大笑, 31).	Empathy (moderate impairment): Is generally unaware of or unconcerned about effect of own behavior on others, or unrealistic appraisal of own effect.

AP1 Jealous (酸, 31)	AP1.1 "No wonder!" Qingwen snorted as they walked on. "Now that she's climbed to a higher branch of the tree, she won't pay any more attention to us. Our lady may have thrown her a word or two, without even knowing her name, and she's already eaten up with pride. What's so marvellous about running a little errand? We shall see if anything comes of it or not. If she's all that clever she'd better clear out of this Garden and stay perched on the top of the tree." (晴雯冷笑道："怪道呢，原来爬上高枝儿去了，把我们不放在眼里. 不知说了一句半句话，名儿姓儿知道了不曾呢？就把他兴得这样！这一遭半遭儿的算不得什么, 过了后儿还得听'咖', 有本事从今儿出了这园子，长长远远的在高枝儿上才算得.", 27). AO1.1	Intimacy (severe impairment): Has some desire to form relationships in community and personal life is present, but capacity for positive and enduring connections is significantly impaired.
AQ1 Sharp-tongued (口角锋芒, 77)	AQ1.1 She laughed mockingly at the sight of them. "Fancy! You haven't yet drunk the bridal cup but already you're doing her hair." (只见晴雯忙走进来取钱。一见了他两个, 便冷笑道："嗳, 交杯盏还没吃, 倒上头了！", 20). AQ1.2 It so happened that Qingwen was in a bad humour, having just quarreled with Bihen, and at Baochai's arrival she transferred her anger to the visitor; Now this fresh knocking on the gate only incensed her further. (谁知那晴雯和碧痕正拌了嘴，没好气, 忽见宝钗来了, 那晴雯正把气移在宝钗身上; 忽听又有人叫门, 晴雯越发动了气, 26). AP1.1 AO1.1 AO1.2 AQ1.3 'Don't be angry,' begged Baoyu, making her lie down again. "You (Qingwen) lose your temper far too easily, and of course being ill today makes you extra fractious." (宝玉忙按他, 笑道："别生气...你 (晴雯) 素习好生气, 如今肝火自然盛了.", 51). AQ1.4 I haven't told Qingwen because she's as hot-tempered as crackling charcoal. She'd be bound to flare up and start beating or cursing the girl. (晴雯那蹄子是块爆炭, 要告诉了他, 他是忍不住的。一时气了, 或打或骂, 51). AQ1.5 Qingwen, who was worried because the medicine had done her no good and now started abusing the doctor. "He's nothing but a swindler and quack," she complained. "His medicine's no use at all." (这里晴雯吃了药, 仍不见病退, 急的乱骂大夫, 说: "只会骗人的钱, 一剂好药也不给人吃.", 52).	Hostility (an aspect of Negative Affectivity and an aspect of Antagonism): Persistent or frequent angry feelings; anger or irritability in response to minor slights and insults.

(continued)

Table A.1 (continued)

Character name	Description in DRM (English – Chinese)		DSM-5 Section III
	Terms or phrases	Sentences or paragraphs	Personality functioning or facets trait
	AR1 Careless and thoughtless (顾前不顾后的, 31); AR2 Hasty and impatient (性急, 52)	AQ1.6 Zhuier had to come closer. Then Qingwen, lunging forward, grabbed one of her hands and began jabbing it with a hairpin from under her pillow. (坠儿只得前凑. 晴雯使冷不防欠身一把将他的手抓住, 向枕边取了一丈青, 向他手上乱戳, 52). AR1.1 Indeed, Qingwen's eyebrows had shot up and her eyes were round with rage. She wanted to summon Zhuier then and there. (晴雯听了, 果然气的蛾眉倒蹙凤眼圆睁, 即时就叫坠儿, 51). AR1.2 ...her (Qingwen's) hair loosely knotted. Crash! She flung the lid back and raised the case bottom upwards in both hands to empty all its contents on the floor. (只见晴雯挽着头发闯进来, 豁一声将箱子掀开, 两手捉着底子朝天, 往地下尽情一倒, 将所有之物尽都倒出, 74).	Impulsivity (an aspect of Disinhibition): Acting on the spur of the moment in response to immediate stimuli; acting on a momentary basis without a plan or consideration of outcomes.
Xue Pan (薛蟠)	AS1 Good for nothing (老大无成, 4); AS2 Having disgraceful behavior (横行霸道; AS3 Wild and lawless (恣心纵欲, 34); AS4 Fearing (defying) neither Heaven nor Earth (天不怕地不怕的, 34); AS5 Wild and headstrong (无法无天, 47)	AS1.1 Presuming on his powerful connections, he had had a man beaten to death and was now to be tried in the Yingtian prefectural court. (...殡表兄薛蟠, 仗财仗势打死人命, 现在应天府案下审理, 3). AS1.2 An auspicious day for departure had just been chosen when he met the kidnapper who was selling Yinglian and, struck by her good looks, promptly purchased her. When Feng Yuan demanded her back. Xue Pan relying on his powerful position ordered his bullies to beat the young man to death. Then entrusting the family affairs to some clansmen and old servants, he left with his mother and sister. To him a murder charge was just a trifle which could easily be settled with some filthy lucre. To him a murder charge was just a trifle which could easily be settled with some filthy lucre. (正择日一定起身, 不想偏遇见了拐子重卖英莲. 薛蟠见英莲生得不俗, 立意买他, 又遇冯家来夺人, 因恃强喝令手下豪奴将冯渊打死. 他便将家中事务一一的嘱托了族中人并几个老家人, 他竟带了母妹竟自起身长行去了. 人命官司一事, 他竟视为儿戏, 自为花上几个臭钱, 没有不了的, 4). AS1.3 He merely learned a few characters at school, spending all his time on cockfights, riding or pleasure trips. Although a Court Purveyor, he knew nothing of business or worldly affairs. (虽也上过学, 不过略识几字, 终日惟有斗鸡走马, 游山玩水而已. 虽是皇商, 一应经纪世事全然不知, 4).	(Antisocial) Self-direction: Goal setting based on personal gratification; absence of prosocial internal standards, associated with failure to conform to lawful or culturally normative ethical behavior.

	AS1.4 To his relief, after less than a month he found himself on familiar terms with half the Jia sons and nephews, and all the rich young men of fashion among them enjoyed his company. One day they would meet to drink, the next to look at flowers, and soon they included him in gambling parties or visits to the courtesans' quarters, with the result that Xue Pan rapidly became even ten times worse than before. (谁知在此住了不上一月的日期，贾宅族中凡有的子侄，俱已认熟了一半，凡是那些纵绔习气者，莫不喜与他来往。今日会酒，明日观花，甚至聚赌嫖娼，渐渐的薛蟠比当日更坏了十倍。)	(Antisocial) Empathy: Lack of concern for feelings, needs, or suffering of others; lack of remorse after hurting or mistreating another.
	AS1.5 But he was like the fisherman who fishes for three days and then suns his net for two. The fee he paid Jia Dairu was thrown away, for he had no intention of really studying, his sole aim being to find some 'sweet-hearts' there. (…因此也假来上学读书，不过是三日打鱼，两日晒网，白送些束修礼物与贾代儒，却不曾有一些儿进益，只图结交些契弟。)	
AT1 Showing insolent in speech (性情奢侈, 4; 言语傲慢, 4); AS2	AT1.1 Goaded by these taunts, Xue Pan grabbed hold of a doorbar and rushed to find Xiangling. Without giving her a chance to speak he started beating her, insisting that she was the one who had worked this witchcraft. (薛蟠更被这一席话激怒，顺手抓起一根门闩来，一径抢步找着香菱，不容分说，便劈头劈脸打起来，一口咬定是香菱所施, 80). AS1.2	(Antisocial) Manipulativeness (an aspect of Antagonism): Frequent use of subterfuge to influence or control others.
AU1 Doing evil with family's money and powerful backing (倚财仗势, 4)	AS1.2	
	AV1.1 Then young Xue, who will never give an inch to anyone, ordered his men to beat Feng Yuan into a pulp. Three days after being carried home he died. "Young Xue had already fixed on a day to set off for the capital. But happening to see this girl two days before leaving he decided to buy her and take her along, not knowing the trouble that would come of it. Then, having killed a man and carried off a girl, he set off with his household as if nothing had happened, leaving his clansmen and servants here to settle the business. A trifling matter like taking a man's life wouldn't frighten him away." He started a big fight and then dragged her off by force more dead than alive. (那薛家公子	(Antisocial) Callousness (an aspect of Antagonism): Lack of concern for feelings or problems of others; lack of guilt or remorse about the negative or harmful effects of one's actions on others; aggression.

(continued)

Table A.1 (continued)

Character name	Description in DRM (English – Chinese)		DSM-5 Section III
	Terms or phrases	Sentences or paragraphs	Personality functioning or facets trait
		岂是让人的! 便喝着手下人一打, 将冯公子打个稀烂, 抬回家去三日死了. 这薛公子原是早已择定日子上京去的, 头起身两日前, 就偶然遇见这丫头, 意欲买了就进京的, 谁知闹出这事来. 既打了冯公子, 夺了丫头, 他便没事人一般, 只管带了家眷走他的路, 他这里自有弟兄奴仆在此料理, 也并非为此些些小事值得他一逃走的, 4). AT1.1	
		AW1.1 …he (Xue Pan) reflected, "Since my beating I've been ashamed to show my face, wishing I could disappear for a year or so; but I have nowhere to hide. I can't go on shamming illness indefinitely. Besides, all these years I've never taken to books or soldiering, and although I'm in business I've never handled a balance or abacus and know nothing either about local customs and different parts of the country. I may as well take some capital and travel around with Zhang Dehui for a year. It doesn't matter whether I make money or not; I can at any rate hide my face for a while and enjoy some sight-seeing at the same time." …(Aunt Xue) withheld her consent…But Xue Pan, once his mind was made up, was stubborn. "You keep complaining every day of my lack of worldly wisdom, my ignorance and failure to learn," he protested. "Yet now that I've resolved to stop fooling around, come to grips with life and establish myself by learning to run the business, you won't let me. What do you expect me to do?" ((薛蟠) 心中村度: "我如今捱了打, 正难见人, 想着要像个一年半载, 又没处去躲. 天天装病, 也不是事. 况且我长了这么大, 文又不文, 武又不武, 虽说做买卖, 究竟联手算盘从没拿过, 地土风俗远近道路又不知道, 不如也打点后几个本钱, 和张德辉逛一二年来. 赚钱也罢, 不赚钱也罢, 且躲躲羞去. 二则逛逛山水也是好的." …(薛蟠妈) 不命他去…薛蟠主意已定, 哪里肯依, 只说: "天天又说我不知世事, 这个也不知, 那个也不学. 如今我发狠把那些要紧的都断了, 如今要成人立事, 学习做买卖, 又不准我了, 叫我怎么样呢?", 48).	(Antisocial) Deceitfulness (an aspect of Antagonism): Embellishment or fabrication when relating events.

AS2; AX1 Making trouble (生事招人, 47); AX2 So irascible (浮躁, 66)	AV1.1	(Antisocial) Hostility (an aspect of Antagonism): Persistent or frequent angry feelings; anger or irritability in response to minor slights and insults; mean, nasty, or vengeful behavior.
	AX1.1 Xue Pan was still raging at Liu Xiangliang from his *kang (a heatable brick bed)*, ordering his servants to go and pull down Liu's house, beat him to death, or take the case to court. (薛蟠睡在炕上，痛骂柳湘莲。又命小厮们去拆他的房子，打死他，和他打官司，47).	
	AX1.2 By now Jingui had told Baochan in confidence to spend the night with Xue Pan in Xiangling's room and become his concubine. When Xiangling ordered to sleep with her, demurred, she accused her of thinking her bed to dirty or of being too lazy to wait on his mistress at night. "He's grabbed my maid, yet doesn't send you to attend me. What's his idea? Is he trying to hound me to death?" Xue Pan, hearing this, reared he might be thwarted again and therefore joined in too. "You ungrateful bitch!" he roared at Xiangling. "Go on at once, or I'll beat you!" (彼时金桂已暗和宝蟾说明，今夜和薛蟠在香菱房中去成亲，命香菱过来陪自己先睡。尤是香菱不肯，那金桂说他嫌脏了，再必是图安逸，怕夜里劳动服侍，又骂说: "你那没见过世面的主子，见一个，爱一个，把我的人霸占了去，又不叫你来，到底是什么主意？想必是逼我死罢了。"薛蟠听了这话，又怕闹黄了宝蟾之事，忙又过来骂香菱: "不识抬举！再不去睡，便要打了！", 79).	
	AX1.3 Then Xue Pan looked for Baochan and, failing to find her, loosed off more abuse at Xiangling. After dinner that evening, befuddled with wine, he happened to scald his feet because the bath water was rather hot. Blaming this on Xiangling he ran out, stark naked as he was, to kick and beat her. (薛蟠再来找宝蟾，已无踪迹了，于是恨的只骂香菱。至晚饭后，已吃得醺醺然，洗澡时不防水略热了些，烫了脚，便说香菱有意害他，赤条精光的赶着香菱踢打了两下，79).	
AY1 Careless (不防头的, 34); AS4;	AY1.1 ...this young Xue, otherwise known as the Stupid Tyrant, is the most vicious ruffian alive, who throws money about like dirt. (这薛公子的混名人称 "呆霸王", 最是天下第一个弄性尚气的人，而且使钱如土，4).	(Antisocial) Risk taking (an aspect of Disinhibition): Engagement in dangerous, risky, and potentially self-damaging activities, unnecessarily and without regard for consequences.

(continued)

Table A.1 (continued)

Character name	Description in DRM (English – Chinese)		DSM-5 Section III
	Terms or phrases	Sentences or paragraphs	Personality functioning or facets trait
	AY2 Never behaving quietly (从不安分守己, 48, 79).	AY1.2 Blunt, outspoken Xue Pan could not stand such insinuations. Baochai's warning against ooling about outside and his mother's charge that his careless talk had caused Baoyu's logging made him stamp with rage and swear he must clear himself...he fumed. "...Well, I'm not afraid. I'll go and kill Baoyu then pay with my life—make a clean sweep!" He seized the door bar and started rushing out. Xue Pan's eyes nearly started from his head in fury...he bellowed. "...We'd better all die and be done with it." (薛蟠本是个心直口快的人，一生见不得这样藏头露尾的事，又见宝钗劝动他不要逛去，他母亲又说他犯舌，宝玉之才是他治的，早已急的乱跳，赌身发誓的分辩，又骂众人："...既拉上，我也不怕，越性进去把宝玉打死了，我替他偿了命，大家干净。"一面嚷，一面抓起一根门闩来就跑...薛蟠急的眼似铜铃一般，嚷道："...不如大家死了清净。", 34).	Personality functioning or facets trait
	AS3; AZ1 Thoughtless (顾前不顾后, 34); AZ2 Blurting out whatever happens to be in mind (心里有什么口里就说什么, 34).	AY1.2	Impulsivity (an aspect of Disinhibition): Acting on the spur of the moment in response to immediate stimuli; acting on a momentary basis without a plan or consideration of outcomes.
	BA1 Off with the old love and on with the new (得新弃旧, 9); BA2 Discarding the old as soon as having something new (怜新弃旧, 79)	BA1.1 "...but a profligate like Xue Pan is sure to have troops of maids and concubines and to be thoroughly debauched – he could never be as true to one girl as Feng Yuan." ("...想其为人，自然娇妾众多，淫佚无度，未必及冯渊定情于一人者", 4). BA1.2 Now Jia Rui was an unscrupulous, grasping scoundrel who used his position in the school to fleece the boys. In return for money and good meals from Xue Pan, he had not checked his disgraceful behavior but actually abetted him in order to curry favor. But Xue Pan was as fickle as water-weed which drifts east today, west tomorrow. Having recently acquired new friends he had dropped Sweetie and Lovely, to say	(Antisocial) Irresponsibility (an aspect of Disinhibition): Lack of respect for – and lack of follow – through on – agreements and promises.

	nothing of Jin Rong whom they had replaced…Jia Rui had nobody to put in a good word for him. Instead of blaming Xue Pan's fickleness, he bore his favourites a grudge for this. And because he, Jin Rong and the rest all had this grievance against the two boys, when Jin Rong and Sweetie came in with their complaint it only increased his annoyance. Not daring to reprove Qin Zhong he made a scapegoat of Sweetie, abusing him roundly for being a trouble-maker. (原来这贾瑞最是个图便宜没行止的人, 每在学中以公报私, 勒索子弟们请他. 后又附助着薛蟠, 反助纣为虐讨好儿. 偏那薛蟠本是浮萍心性, 今日爱东, 明日爱西, 近来又有了新朋友, 把香, 玉二人丢开一边. 故贾瑞也无了提携帮补他, 因此贾瑞, 金荣等一干人也正在醋妒他两个. 今见香, 玉二人不在薛蟠前提携帮补他, 贾瑞心中便更不自在起来. 虽不好呵叱秦钟, 却拿着香怜作法, 反说他多事, 着实抢白了几句, 9).	
	BA1.3 Now Xue Pan was a living example of the saying "*To covet the land of Shu after getting the region of Long (covet Sichuan after capturing Gansu – have insatiable desires)*." After marrying Jingui, he was struck by her maid Baochan's charms. As she seemed approachable as well as alluring, he often flirted with her when asking her to fetch him tea or water. (只因薛蟠天性是 "得陇望蜀" 的, 如今得娶了金桂, 又见金桂的丫鬟宝蟾有三分姿色, 举止轻浮可爱, 便时常要茶要水的故意撩逗他, 79).	
Jia Yucun (贾雨村)	BB1.1 But although a capable administrator Yucun wa grasping and ruthless, while his arrogance and insolence to his superiors mad them view him with disfavor. ((贾雨村) 虽才干优长, 未免有些贪酷之弊, 且又恃才侮上, 那些官员皆侧目而视, 2).	(Antisocial) Identity: Egocentrism; self-esteem derived from personal gain, power, or pleasure.
	BC1.1 Ingrained duplicity, tampering with the rites and, under a show of probity, conspiring with his ferocious underlings to foment trouble in his district and make life intolerable for the local people. (生性狡猾, 擅篡礼仪, 且沽清正之名, 而暗结虎狼之属, 致使地方多事, 民命不堪, 2).	(Antisocial) Self-direction: Absence of prosocial internal standards, associated with failure to conform to lawful or culturally normative ethical behavior.

(continued)

Table A.1 (continued)

Character name	Description in DRM (English – Chinese)		DSM-5 Section III
	Terms or phrases	Sentences or paragraphs	Personality functioning or facets trait
		BD1.1 There was also a confidential letter for Feng Su asking him to persuade Mrs. Zhen to let the prefect have Jiaoxing as his (Jia Yucun's) secondary wife. Feng Su could hardly contain himself for joy. Eager to please the prefect, he prevailed on his daughter to agree and that very same night put Jiaoxing in a small sedan-chair and escorted her to the yamen. We need not dwell on Yucun's satisfaction. He gave Feng Su a hundred pieces of silver and sent Mrs. Zhen many gifts, urging her to take good care of her health while he ascertained her daughter's whereabouts. ((贾雨村)又寄一封密书与封肃, 转托问甄家娘子要那娇杏作二房. 封肃喜的屁滚尿流, 巴不得去奉承, 便在女儿前一力撺掇成了, 乘夜只用一乘小轿, 便把娇杏送进去了. 雨村欢喜, 自不必说, 乃封百金赠封肃, 外谢甄家娘子许多物事, 令其好生养赡, 以待寻访女儿下落, 2).	(Antisocial) Intimacy: Incapacity for mutually intimate relationships, as exploitation is a primary means of relating to others; use of dominance or intimidation to control others.
		BE1.1 All this was due to the attendant who had been a novice in Gourd Temple, but Yucun, dismayed by the thought that this man might disclose certain facts about the days when he was poor and humble, later found some fault with him and had him exiled to a distant region. (此事皆由葫芦庙内之沙弥新门子所出, 雨村又恐他对人说出当日贫贱时的事来, 因此心中大不乐业, 后来到底寻了个不是, 远远的充发了, 4). BE1.2 Then that black-hearted scoundrel Jia Yucun heard about it and hatched a scheme. He had the idiot taken to his yamen on a charge of owing the government some money, and ordered the default to be made good by the sale of his property. So the fans were seized, paid for at the official price and brought to our house. As for that Stone Idiot, who knows whether he's alive or dead? …It's nothing to boast of, if somebody is willing to ruin a family for such a trifling reason. (谁知雨村那没天理的听见了, 便设了个法子, 讹他拖欠了官银, 拿他到衙门里去, 说所欠官银, 变卖家产赔补, 把这扇子抄了来, 作了官价送了来. 那石呆子如今不知是死是活……为这点子小事, 弄得人坑家败业, 48).	(Antisocial) Manipulativeness (an aspect of Antagonism): Frequent use of subterfuge to influence or control others.
		BE1.2	(Antisocial) Callousness (an aspect of Antagonism): Lack of concern for feelings or problems of others.

Appendix

Character	Traits	Text	Definition
		BF1.1 But Yucun, although mortified and enraged, betrayed no indignation and went about looking as cheerful as before. (那雨村心中虽十分惭恨,却面上全无一点怨色,仍是嘻笑自若, 2).	(Antisocial) Deceitfulness (an aspect of Antagonism): Dishonesty and fraudulence; embellishment or fabrication when relating events.
		BE1.2	(Antisocial) Hostility (an aspect of Antagonism): Mean behavior.
		BE1.2	(Antisocial) Risk taking (an aspect of Disinhibition): Engagement in dangerous and risky activities, unnecessarily and without regard for consequences.
		BG1.1 "But do you know who the girl is?" "How could I know?" "She's by way of being Your Honor's benefactress." The attendant sniggered. "She's Yingju, the daughter of Mr. Zhen who lived next to Gourd Temple."…So Yucun twisted the law to suit his own purpose and passed arbitrary judgement (Let the kidnapper and buyer go and conceal the trace of Yingju). ("这日别说, 老爷, 你当被卖之丫头是谁?" 雨村道: "我如何得知?" 门子冷笑道: "这人算来还是老爷的大恩人呢! 他就是葫芦庙旁住的甄老爷的小姐, 名唤英菊的."…雨村便徇情枉法, 胡乱判断了此案.	(Antisocial) Irresponsibility (an aspect of Disinhibition): Disregard for financial and other obligations or commitments.
Jia Huan (贾环)	BH1 Lack of self-respect (不尊重, 20); BH2 Having vulgar, common appearance (人物委琐, 举止荒疏, 23); BH3 Being a spiteful brat (黑心不知道理下流种子, 25)	BH1.1 (Jia Huan) had always hated Baoyu. At the sight of him teasing Cai Xia, he felt ready to explode with jealousy. He dared not protest outright, but he had mulled over a plan and now that they were so close he saw his chance to put it into action. He would blind Baoyu with burning candle-wax! Deliberately knocking over the candlestick, he splashed the hot melted wax on his half-brother's face. ((贾环)素日原恨宝玉, 如今又见他和彩霞闹, 心中越发按不下这口毒气. 虽他不敢明言, 却每每暗中算计, 只是不得下手. 今见相离甚近, 便要用热油烫瞎他的眼睛, 因而故意装作失手, 把那一盏油汪汪的蜡灯往宝玉脸上只一推, 25).	(Antisocial) Self-direction: Absence of prosocial internal standards, associated with failure to conform to lawful or culturally normative ethical behavior.

(continued)

Table A.1 (continued)

Character name	Description in DRM (English – Chinese)		DSM-5 Section III
	Terms or phrases	Sentences or paragraphs	Personality functioning or facets trait
		BI1.1 The unfairness of this made Ying'er fume, but she dared not answer back. As she slapped down some cash she muttered under her breath: "Fancy a young gentleman cheating! Even I wouldn't make such a fuss over a few cash. Last time we played with Baoyu he lost a whole packet, yet he didn't mind…"… "How can I compare with Baoyu?" whined Jia Huan. "You keep in with him because you're afraid of him, but you bully me because I'm a concubine's son."…(Jia Huan said to his mother—Concubine Zhao:) "I was playing with Cousin Baochai. Ying'er was mean to me and cheated me…" (Xifeng said to Jia Huan:) "…But instead of doing as I say, you let other people warp your mind and teach you these sneaky ways. You've no self-respect but will lower yourself. You behave spitefully yourself and then complain that everybody else is unfair!" (莺儿满心委屈, 见宝钗说, 不敢则声, 只得放下钱来. 口内嘟囔说: "一个作爷的, 还赖我们这几个钱, 连我也不在眼里. 前儿我和宝二爷顽, 他输了那些, 也没着急…"…贾环便说: "我拿什么比宝玉呢? 你们怕他, 都和他好, 都欺负我是太太养的."…贾环便说: "同宝姐姐顽的, 莺儿欺负我, 赖我的钱,"…凤姐向贾环道: "…你不听我的话, 反叫这些人教的歪心邪意, 狐媚子霸道的. 自己不尊重, 要往下流走, 安着坏心, 还只管怨人家偏心…", 20).	(Antisocial) Empathy: Lack of concern for feelings, needs, or suffering of others; lack of remorse after hurting or mistreating another.
		BJ1.1 It only made Jia Huan more suspicious, however. He fetched out all Caiyun's secret gifts to him and threw them at her face. "Sneaky double-crosser!" he swore. "I don't want this trash of yours. If you weren't on good terms with Baoyu, why should he cover up for you? If you had any guts, you wouldn't have let a single person know you'd given me these things. Now that you've blabbed about it I'd lose face if I kept them." Caiyun frantically assured him that she was not on friendly terms with Baoyu, nor had she told anyone. Sobbingly she tried in all sorts of ways to convince him, but Jia Huan stubbornly refused to believe her. "If not for our past friendship," he cried, "I'd go and tell sister-in-law Xifeng that you stole these things and offered them to me, but I dared not take them. Just think what would happen then!" With that he stormed out. (谁知贾环听如此说, 便起了疑心, 便将彩云凡私赠之物都拿了出来, 照着贾彩云的脸摔了去, 说: "这两面三刀的东西! 我不和宝玉好, 他如何肯替你应. 你既有担当给了我,	(Antisocial) Intimacy: marked impairments in developing close relationships, associated with mistrust and anxiety.

		(Antisocial) Callousness (an aspect of Antagonism): Lack of concern for feelings or problems of others; lack of guilt or remorse about the negative or harmful effects of one's actions on others; aggression.
原该不与一个人知道, 如今你既然告诉他, 如今我再要这个, 也没趣儿." 彩云见如此, 急的赌身发誓, 至于哭了, 百般解说, 贾环执意不信, 说: "不看你素日之情, 去告诉一声去, 就说你偷来给我, 我不敢要, 你细想去." 说毕, 撺手出去了 (62).	BH1.1	
		(Antisocial) Deceitfulness (an aspect of Antagonism): Dishonesty and fraudulence.
BK1.1 At that Baoyu pressed closer and took her hand. "I'll ask your mistress for you tomorrow," he said softly. "Then we can be together." Jinchuan made no reply. "Or rather I'll ask her as soon as she wakes." The girl opened her eyes then and pushed him away. "What's the hurry? 'A cold pin may fall into the well, but if it's yours it remains yours.' Can't you understand that proverb? I'll tell you something amusing to do. Go to the small east courtyard and see what your brother Huan and Caiyun are up to." "I don't care what they're up to. It's you I'm interested in." At this point Lady Wang sat up and slapped Jinchuan's face. "Shameless slut!" she scolded. "It's low creatures like you who lead the young maters astray." Baoyu had vanished like smoke as soon as his mother sat up. (宝玉上来便拉着手, 悄悄的笑道: "我明日和太太讨你, 咱们在一处罢." 金钏儿不答. 宝玉又道: "不然, 等太太醒了我就讨." 金钏儿睁开眼, 将宝玉一推, 笑道: "你忙什么! 金簪子掉在井里头, 有你的只是有你的, 连这句话难道也不明白? 我倒告诉你个巧宗儿, 你往东小院子里拿环哥儿同彩云去." 宝玉笑道: "凭他怎么去罢, 我只守着你." 只见王夫人翻身起来, 照金钏儿脸上就打了个嘴巴子, 指着骂道: "下作小娼妇, 好好的爷们, 都叫你教坏了." 宝玉见王夫人起来, 早一溜烟去了, 30). BK1.2 "My mother told me," Jia Huan went on in a whisper, "that the other day Brother Baoyu grabbed hold of Jinchuan in my lady's room and tried to rape her. When she wouldn't let him, he beat her. That's why she drowned herself in a fit of passion." (贾环便悄悄说道: "我母亲告诉我说, 宝玉哥哥前日在太太屋里, 拉着太太的丫头金钏儿强奸不遂, 打了一顿, 那金钏儿便赌气投井死了." 33).		

(continued)

Table A.1 (continued)

Character name	Description in DRM (English – Chinese)		DSM-5 Section III
	Terms or phrases	Sentences or paragraphs	Personality functioning or facets trait
	BL1 Spineless (没气性的, 20); BL2 Shameless/ mean and sneaky (下流, 20); BH1; BL3 Having sneaky ways (歪心邪意, 20)	BL1.1 But Jia Huan so resented the sight of Baoyu sharing the same cushion with his aunt, who was fonding him and making much of him, that before long he signalled to Jia Lan that they should leave. (贾环见宝玉同那夫人坐在一个坐褥上,那夫人又百般摩挲抚弄他,早已心中不自在了,坐不多时,便和贾兰使眼色儿要走. 24). BH1.1	(Antisocial) Hostility (an aspect of Antagonism): Persistent or frequent angry feelings; mean, nasty, or vengeful behavior.
		BH1.1	(Antisocial) Risk taking (an aspect of Disinhibition): Engagement in dangerous, risky, and potentially self-damaging activities, unnecessarily and without regard for consequences.
		BH1.1	(Antisocial) Impulsivity (an aspect of Disinhibition): Acting on the spur of the moment in response to immediate stimuli; acting on a momentary basis without a plan or consideration of outcomes.
		BM1.1 Finally, however, the dice came to rest at one. In exasperation he snatched up both dice and grabbed the stakes, insisting that he had thrown six. "Fancy a young gentleman cheating!" (那骰子偏生转出幺来. 贾环急了,伸手便抓起骰子来,然后就拿钱,说是个六点... "一个作爷的,还赖我们这几个钱", 20).	(Antisocial) Irresponsibility (an aspect of Disinhibition): Disregard for—and failure to honor financial and other obligations or commitments.

Concubine Zhao (赵姨娘)		
	BN1.1 Sensing something behind this, the concubine brightened up. "In secret? Do explain how," she cried. "I've thought of that, but there's no one capable of doing it. If you'll show me some way, I'll make it well worth your while." (赵姨娘闻听这话里有道理，心内暗暗的欢喜，便说道："怎么暗里算计？我倒有这个意思，只是没这样的能干人。你若教给我这法子，我大大的谢你。", 25). BN1.2 The rest don't matter, but if Concubine Zhao and that lot saw things from here they'd try some mean trick to break them, and the mistress wouldn't pay too much attention. (别人还可以，赵姨奶奶一伙的人见了这是这屋里的东西，又该使黑心弄坏了才罢, 37).	(Antisocial) Self-direction: Absence of prosocial internal standards, associated with failure to conform to lawful or culturally normative ethical behavior.
BO1 Being the limit (昏愦的不像了, 27)	BO1.1 (Five devils invoked by sorcery take possession of Baoyu and Xifeng. Concubine Zhao and Priestess Ma did something in secret) By the third day the patients were lying at death's door and the whole household despaired. Then, as all hope was relinquished, preparations were started for the funeral. The Lady Dowager, Lady Wang, Jia Lian, Pinger and Xiren wept even more bitterly than the rest, unable to take food or sleep. Only the Concubine Zhao and Jia Huan were secretly exulting. ((魔法姊弟逢五鬼) 看看三日光阴，那凤姐和宝玉躺在床上，亦发连进气都将没了. 合家人口无不慌，贾母、王夫人、贾琏、平儿、袭人这几个人，更比诸人哭的忘餐废寝，寻死觅活. 赵姨娘，贾环等自是称愿, 25). BO1.2 Her (Jia Tanchun, Concubine Zhao's daughter) distress reminded Li Wan and the others of all the instances of Concubine Zhao's outrageous behavior, which had involved Tanchun, making her embarrassed to face Lady Wang. (李纨等见他 (贾探春，赵姨娘的女儿) 说的恳切，又想他素日赵姨娘每生诽谤，在王夫人眼前亦为赵姨娘所累, 56).	(Antisocial) Empathy: Lack of concern for feelings, needs, or suffering of others.
	BP1.1 "You can talk, but you don't dare go either," he muttered. "You just want me to go and have a row with them. If they report me to our school and I get a beating, of course you won't feel the pain. Each time you've egged me on and trouble came of it so that I got beaten or cursed, you've always kept quiet. Now you're egging me on again to quarrel with those servantgirls…" ((贾环) 说道："你这么会说，你又不敢去，指使了我去闹. 倘或往学里告了去打，你敢自不疼呢? 遭遭调唆了我闹去，闹出了事来，我挨了打骂，你一般也低了头. 这会子又调唆了我和毛丫头们去闹…", 60).	(Antisocial) Intimacy: Use of dominance or intimidation to control others.

(continued)

Table A.1 (continued)

Character name	Description in DRM (English – Chinese)		DSM-5 Section III
	Terms or phrases	Sentences or paragraphs	Personality functioning or facets trait
		BQ1.1 It was Concubine Zhao who kept begging me to filch things, and I gave some of them to Master Huan—that's the truth. Even when the mistress is at home, we often take this or that to give to friends. (偷东西原是赵姨奶奶央告我 (彩云) 再三, 我拿了些与环哥哥是情真. 连太太在家我们还拿过, 各人去送人, 也是常事, 61). BQ1.2 As for Concubine Zhao, because Caiyun had given her so many things on the sly and Yuchuan had raised such a fuss, she was afraid others would find out the truth… Caiyun, weeping her eyes out, looked quite heart-broken no matter how the concubine tried to comfort her. "Good child, how ungrateful he is. Let me put these things away, and in a couple of days he'll come to his senses again." She wanted to take things. (赵姨娘正因原彩云赠了许多东西, 玉钏儿吵出, 生恐查诘出来….气的彩云哭个泪干肠断. 赵姨娘百般的安慰他: "好孩子, 他辜负了你的心, 我看的真. 让我收起来. 过两日他自然回转过来了." 说着, 便要收东西, 62).	(Antisocial) Manipulativeness (an aspect of Antagonism): Frequent use of subterfuge to influence or control others.
		BO1.1	(Antisocial) Callousness (an aspect of Antagonism): Lack of concern for feelings or problems of others.
	BR1 Having sly, low, dirty mind (阴微卑贱的见识, 27)	BR1.1 As for Concubine Zhao, because Caiyun had given her so many things on the sly and Yuchuan had raised such a fuss, this kept her in a constant cold sweat as she waited to hear the upshot. (赵姨娘正因因彩云私赠了许多东西, 玉钏儿吵出, 生恐查诘出来, 每日里一把汗打听信儿, 62).	(Antisocial) Deceitfulness (an aspect of Antagonism): Dishonesty and fraudulence.
		BS1.1 Although the concubine was eaten up by jealousy of Xifeng and Baoyu, she dared not show it either. (那赵姨娘素日里虽然常怀嫉妒之心, 不忿凤姐, 宝玉两个, 也不敢露出来, 25). BO1.1 BN1.2	(Antisocial) Hostility (an aspect of Antagonism): Persistent or frequent angry feelings; mean or vengeful behavior.

BS1.2 "How could she give you anything good?" sneered Concubine Zhao at this point. "Who told you to go there begging? No wonder they made a fool of you. If I were you, I'd take it back and throw it in her face. Now's the time, while some have gone to the funeral and others are ill in bed, to raise a rumpus and let no one have any peace. This way we can get our own back…." (赵姨娘便说:"有好的给你!谁叫你要去了,怎怨他们!依我,拿了去照脸给他去,趁着这回子撞尸的撞尸去了,挺床的便挺床,吵一出子,大家别心净,也算是报仇…", 60). BS1.3 "Why stir up more trouble?" put in Caiyun quickly. "Whatever happens, we'd better put up with it." "Don't you barge in," retorted Concubine Zhao. "This has nothing to do with you. Better seize this chance, while we've got a good excuse, to bawl out those dirty bitches." (彩云忙说:"这又何苦生事,不管怎样,忍耐些罢了了"。赵姨娘道:"你快休管,横竖与你无干。乘着抓住了理,骂给那些浪淫妇们一顿,也是好的。", 60).	
BO1.1	(Antisocial) Risk taking (an aspect of Disinhibition): Engagement in dangerous, risky, and potentially self-damaging activities, unnecessarily and without regard for consequences.
BT1.1 Emboldened by this, Concubine Zhao made her way confidently to Happy Red Court…Instead of answering, she stepped forward and threw the powder in Fangguan's face. "You trollop!" she swore, pointing a finger at her. "We bought you with our money to train as an actress. You're nothing but a painted whore. Even the lowest slave in our house ranks higher than you, yet you make up to some people and look down on others…"…The concubine was so angry that she darted forward and slapped Fangguan on both cheeks. (赵姨娘听了,越友得了意,仗着胆子便一径到了怡红院中…赵姨娘也不答话,走上来便将粉照着芳官脸上撒来,指着芳官骂道:"小淫妇!你是银子钱买来学戏的,不过娼妇粉头之流!我家里下三等奴才也比你高贵些的,你都会看人下菜碟儿…"…赵姨娘气的便上来打了(芳官)两个耳刮子, 60).	(Antisocial) Impulsivity (an aspect of Disinhibition): Acting on the spur of the moment in response to immediate stimuli.

(continued)

Table A.1 (continued)

Character name	Description in DRM (English – Chinese)		DSM-5 Section III
	Terms or phrases	Sentences or paragraphs	Personality functioning or facets trait
Jia Xichun (贾惜春)		BU1.1…Xichun laughing and chatting with Zhineng, a young nun from the Water Moon Convent… "I was just telling Zhineng that I'd shave my head some day and become a nun too, and now you turn up with flowers." Xichun smiled. "Where shall I wear them if my head is shaved?" (只见惜春正同水月庵的小姑子智能儿一处顽笑, …惜春笑道: "我这里正和智能儿说, 我明儿也剃了头同他作姑子去呢, 可巧又送了花儿来, 若剃了头, 可把这花儿戴在那里呢?" 7).	Self-direction (extreme impairment): Has poor differentiation of thoughts from actions, so goal-setting ability is severely compromised, with unrealistic or incoherent goals.
	BV1 Eccentric and upright (孤介, 75)	BV1.1 But Xichun although young had a will of her own and was most uncompromising and eccentric. However hard they pleaded, she was adamant as she felt the maid had disgraced her. "I don't want Ruhua," she insisted. (谁知惜春虽然年幼, 却天生成一种百折不回的廉介孤独解性, 任人怎说, 他只以为丢了他的体面, 咬定牙断乎不肯, 不要入画, 74).	Intimacy (moderate impairment): Intimate relationships are predominantly based on meeting self-regulatory and self-esteem needs.
	BW1 Heartless and cold (心冷口冷, 74)	BV1.1	Callousness (an aspect of Antagonism): Lack of concern for the feelings or problems of others.
Jia Rui (贾瑞)		BA1.2 BX1.1 Jia Rui meets and lusts after Xifeng (Jia Rui's sister-in-law). (见熙凤 (贾瑞的嫂子) 贾瑞起淫心, 11). Y1.1	(Antisocial) Self-direction: Goal setting based on personality gratification; absence of prosocial internal standards, associated with failure to conform to lawful or culturally normative ethical behavior.

BA1.2		(Antisocial) Intimacy: Incapacity for mutually intimate relationships, as exploitation is a primary means of relating to others.
BA1.2		(Antisocial) Manipulativeness (an aspect of Antagonism): Frequent use of subterfuge to influence or control others; use of ingratiation to achieve one's ends.
BA1.2		(Antisocial) Callousness (an aspect of Antagonism): Lack of concern for feelings or problems of others.
BY1.1	Xifeng sets a vicious trap for a lover (Wang Xifeng played with Jia Rui, who was made to stayed out for one night and almost froze to death)…In a cold sweat with fright, Jia Rui tried to lie his way out. "I went to my uncle's house, and because it was late he kept me for the night." ((王熙凤毒设相思局 (贾瑞被关一夜,几乎不曾冻死)…贾瑞也捻着一把汗, 少不得回来撒谎, 只说: "往舅舅家去了, 天黑了, 留我住了一夜.", 12).	
BA1.2		(Antisocial) Hostility (an aspect of Antagonism): Anger or irritability in response to minor slights and insults.

(continued)

Table A.1 (continued)

Character name	Description in DRM (English – Chinese)		DSM-5 Section III
	Terms or phrases	Sentences or paragraphs	Personality functioning or facets trait
		BX1.1 BZ1.1 The lame Daoist priest took from his wallet a mirror…he told Jia Rui. "But you must only look into the back of the mirror. On no account look into the front – remember that!" (Jia Rui) picked it up and look into the back…He turned the mirror over and there inside stood Xifeng, beckoning to him. In raptures he was wafted as if by magic into the mirror, where he indulged with his beloved in the sport of cloud and rain, after which she saw him out…the young man was not satisfied. He turned the mirror over again, Xifeng beckoned to him as before, and in he went. But after this had happened four times and he was about to leave her for the fourth time…The attendants had simply observed him look into the mirror, let it fall and then open his eyes and pick it up again. This time, however, when the mirror fell he did not stir. They pressed round and saw that he had breathed his last. (跛足道人) 从褡裢中取出一面镜子来…遂与贾瑞道: "千万不可照正面, 只照他的背面, 要紧, 要紧!"…贾瑞收了镜子来…向 反面一照…又将正面一照, 只见凤姐站在里面招手叫他. 贾瑞心中一喜, 荡悠悠的觉得进了镜子, 与凤姐云雨一番, 凤姐仍送他出来…(贾瑞) 心中到底不足, 又翻过正面来, 只见凤姐还招手叫他, 他又进去. 如此三四次. …旁边伏待贾瑞的众人, 只见他先还拿着镜子照, 落下来, 未后镜子落下来, 便不动了. 众人上来看, 已没了气, 12).	(Antisocial) Risk taking (an aspect of Disinhibition): Engagement in dangerous, risky, and potentially self-damaging activities, unnecessarily and without regard for consequences.
		BX1.1 BZ1.1	(Antisocial) Impulsivity (an aspect of Disinhibition): Acting on a momentary basis without a plan or consideration of outcomes.

Xia Jingui (夏金桂)		
	CA1.1 She (Xia Jingui) had as high an opinion of herself as if she were a goddess, and treated others like dirt…Now that she was married, she felt it incumbent on her to behave as the mistress of the house, not with the gentle shyness befitting a girl—she must show her authority to keep others under her thumb. (爱自己尊若菩萨，视他人秽如粪土…今日出了阁，自为要作当家的奶奶，比不得作女儿时腼腆温柔，须要拿出这威风来，才钤压得住人，79). CA1.2 One day after drinking he (Xue Pan) consulted her (Jingui) on something he wished to do and, when she would not hear of it, losing his temper he made an angry retort then went ahead and did it. Then Jingui…pretended to be ill.… Seeing that her husband was lowering his colors and her mother-in-law was good-natured, Jingui pressed her attack by degrees. At first she simply kept Xue Pan under her thumb; later she tried artfully to control Aunt Xue as well, and Baochai too. (一日薛蟠酒后，不知要行何事，先与金桂商议，金桂执意不从。薛蟠忍不住便发了几句话，赌气自行了．这金桂便…装起病来．那金桂见丈夫藏躲渐回，婆婆良善，也就渐渐的持戈试马起来。先时不过挟制薛蟠，后来以狡诈骗媚，将及薛姨妈，后渐至薛宝钗，79).	(Antisocial) Self-direction: Goal setting based on personal gratification.
	CB1.1 At home she had vented her temper on her maids, forever cursing them or beating them. (在家中时常就和丫鬟们使性弄气，轻骂重打的，79). CB1.2 As her family owned so many osmanthus trees, she had been given the pet name Jingui—Golden Osmanthus; so she forebade the whole household to use these two words. Any maid careless enough to slip up and do so was severely beaten and punished. Then, realizing the impossibility of banning any reference to osmanthus, she decided to give the flower a new name; and recalling the story of the osmanthus and the Moon Goddess, she changed the name of the flower to "moon-goddess flower" to add to her own dignity in this way. (因他家多桂花，他小名就做金桂。他在家时，不许人口中带出"金桂"二字来，凡有不留心误道一字者，他便定要苦打重罚才罢．他因想桂花一字是禁止不住的，须另换一名，因想桂花曾有广寒嫦娥之说，便将桂花改为嫦娥花，又寓自己身份如此，79).	(Antisocial) Empathy: Lack of concern for feelings, needs, or suffering of others.

(continued)

Table A.1 (continued)

Character name	Description in DRM (English – Chinese)		DSM-5 Section III
	Terms or phrases	Sentences or paragraphs	Personality functioning or facets trait
		CC1.1 "It's Xiangling I want to trap, but I can't find any pretext," she reflected. "As he's keen on Baochan now, I may as well let him have her and he's bound to lose interest in Xiangling. Then I can settle her hash. Since Baochan is my maid, she'll be easy to handle later." (金桂亦颇觉察其意, 想着: "正要摆布香菱, 无处寻隙, 如今他既看上了宝蟾, 如今且合出宝蟾去与他, 他一定就和香菱疏远了, 我且乘他疏远之时, 便摆布了香菱. 那时宝蟾原是我的人, 也就好处了.", 80). CC1.2 When this had happened several times, Jingui became even more over-bearing and Xue Pan even more spineless. (如今习惯成自然, 反使金桂越发长了威风, 薛蟠越发软了气骨, 79).	(Antisocial) Intimacy: Incapacity for mutually intimate relationships, as exploitation is a primary means of relating to others, including by deceit and coercion.
CD1 Trying artfully to control others, (尚娇诈媚, 79)		CA1.1 CA1.2	(Antisocial) Manipulativeness (an aspect of Antagonism): Frequent use of subterfuge to influence or control others.
		CB1.1 CE1.1 Xiangling had no choice but to carry her bedding over. And when Jingui ordered her to sleep on the floor, again she had to comply. But no sooner had she lain down than Jingui called for tea, then presently told her to massage her legs, rousing her seven or eight times altogether, so that there was no sleep for Xiangling that night. (金桂命他在地下铺睡. 香菱无奈, 只得依命. 刚睡下, 便叫倒茶, 一时又叫捶腿, 如是一夜七八次. 总不使其安逸稳卧片时, 79).	(Antisocial) Callousness (an aspect of Antagonism): Lack of concern for feelings or problems of others.
CD1		CF1.1 Baochai had long recognized her impropriety and knew how to cope with it, giving her hints not to over-reach herself. When Jingui saw that she was not to be bullied, she tried to pick fault with her in various ways; but being unable to find any chinks in her armour, she finally had to come to terms with her. (宝钗久察其不轨之心, 每随机应变, 暗以言语弹压其志. 金桂知其可乘, 又无隙可乘, 只得曲意俯就,79).	(Antisocial) Deceitfulness (an aspect of Antagonism): Dishonesty and fraudulence.

	CF1.2 Meanwhile, hiding her resentment, she went on tormenting Xiangling. After a fortnight she suddenly shammed ill, complaining of an unbearable pain in her heart and the loss of the use of her limbs. Then one day, from Jingui's pillow-case there fell out a paper effigy inscribed with the date of her birth and her horoscope. Five needles had been thrust through it: one through the heart and one through each of the limbs. (一面隐忍，一面设计摆布香菱. 半月光景，忽又装起病来，只说心疼难忍，四肢不能转动. 闹了两日，忽又从金桂的枕头内抖出纸人来，上面写着金桂的年庚八字，有五根针钉在心窝并四肢骨节等处，79).	
CB1.1 CE1.1		(Antisocial) Hostility (an aspect of Antagonism): Persistent or frequent angry feelings; mean behavior.
CB1.1 CE1.1 CF1.2		(Antisocial) Risk taking (an aspect of Disinhibition): Engagement in dangerous, risky, and potentially self-damaging activities, unnecessarily and without regard for consequences.
	CG1.1 When Jingui happened to be in a good mood, she would gather a party together to play cards, dice and make merry. All her life she had loved gnawing bones, so she had chickens or ducks killed every day and the meat given to others while she herself chewed the fried bones to go with her wine. When she tired of this, or when anything offended her, she would flare up and begin scolding again. (金桂不发作性气，有时欢喜，便纠聚人来斗纸牌、掷骰子作乐. 又生平最喜啃骨头，每日务要杀鸡鸭，将肉赏人吃，只单以油炸焦骨头下酒. 吃的不奈烦或动了气，便肆行海骂，说："有别的忘八粉头乐的，我为什么不乐!"，80).	(Antisocial) Impulsivity (an aspect of Disinhibition): Acting on the spur of the moment in response to immediate stimuli.
CB1.1 CB1.2		(Narcissistic) Empathy: Impaired ability to recognize or identify with the feelings and needs of others.

(continued)

Table A.1 (continued)

| Character name | Description in DRM (English – Chinese) | | DSM-5 Section III |
	Terms or phrases	Sentences or paragraphs	Personality functioning or facets trait
		CA1.1	(Narcissistic) Intimacy: Relationships largely superficial and exist to serve self-esteem regulation;
		CA1.1 CB1.2	(Narcissistic) Grandiosity (an aspect of Antagonism): Believing that one is superior to others and deserves special treatment; self-centeredness; feelings of entitlement; condescension toward others.
		CA1.1 CA1.2	(Narcissistic) Attention seeking (an aspect of Antagonism): Admiration seeking.
		CG1.1	Emotional lability (an aspect of Negative affectivity): Instability of emotional experiences and mood; emotions that are easily aroused, intense, and/ or out of proportion to events and circumstances.

Miaoyu (妙玉)	CH1 Very unconventional (不合时宜, 63)	CH1.1 She came to the capital with her tutor last year. She's been living in the Sakyamuni Convent outside the West Gate. Her tutor…passed away last winter. "In that case, why not ask her here?" put in Lady Wang. "She'd refuse," objected Lin Zhixiao's wife. "She'd be afraid of being looked down on in a noble household." ((妙玉) 去岁随了师父上来, 现在西门外牟尼院住着。他师父…于去冬圆寂了…王夫人不等回完, 便说: "既这样, 我们何不接了他来。" 林之孝家的回道: "请他, 他说 '侯门公府, 必以贵势压人, 我再不去的。'", 18). CH1.2 She's so aloof and unconventional that she looks down on everybody. (他为人孤僻, 不合时宜, 万人不入他目, 63).	(Obsessive-Compulsive) Empathy: Difficulty understanding and appreciating the ideas, feelings, or behaviors of others.
	CI1 Very aloof (为人孤僻, 63)	CI1.1 (Jia Baoyu) said, "After we've gone, shall I send a few pages with some buckets of water from the stream to wash your floors?" "That's a good idea." She (Miaoyu) smiled. "Only make them leave the buckets by the wall outside the gate. They mustn't come in."…By this time the Lady Dowager was ready to leave, and Miaoyu did not press her hard to stay but saw them out and closed the gate behind them. ((贾宝玉) 道: "等我们出去了, 我叫几个小么儿来河里打几桶水来洗地如何?" 妙玉笑道: "这更好了, 只是你嘱咐他们, 抬了水只搁在山门外头墙根下, 别进门来。"…贾母已经出来, 要回去。妙玉亦不甚留, 送出山门, 回身便将门闭了, 41). CI1.2	(Obsessive-Compulsive) Intimacy: Rigidity and stubbornness negatively affect relationships with others.
		CJ1.1 "Don't put away that Cheng Hua bowl (a bowl made in the Cheng Hua period (1465-1487))," cried Miaoyu hastily. "Leave it outside." Baoyu knew that because Granny Liu had used it, she thought it too dirty to keep. (妙玉忙命: "将那成窑的茶杯别收了, 搁在外头去罢。" 宝玉会意, 知为刘姥姥吃了, 他嫌脏不要了, 41). CJ1.2 "All right," she said. "It's a good thing I'd never drunk out of it, or I'd have smashed it. But I can't give it to her myself. If you want to give it to her, I've no objection. Go ahead and take it." (妙玉听了, 想了一想, 点头说道: "这也罢了。幸而那杯子我没吃过的, 若我使过, 我就砸碎了也不能给他。你要给他, 我也不管你, 只交给你, 快拿去罢。" 41). CJ1.1	(Obsessive-Compulsive) Rigid perfectionism (an aspect of Disinhibition): Rigid insistence on everything being flawless, perfect, and without errors or faults, including one's own and others' performance; difficulty changing ideas and/or viewpoint.

(continued)

Table A.1 (continued)

Character name	Description in DRM (English – Chinese)		DSM-5 Section III
	Terms or phrases	Sentences or paragraphs	Personality functioning or facets trait
		CK1.1 Daiyu, knowing her eccentricity, did not like to say too much or stay too long. After finishing her tea she signaled to Baochai and the two girls left. (黛玉知他天性怪僻，不好多话，亦不好多坐，吃过茶，便约着宝钗走了出来，41). CI1.1	(Obsessive-Compulsive) Intimacy avoidance (an aspect of Detachment): Avoidance of close relationships and interpersonal attachments.
	CL1 Smiling disdainfully (冷笑, 41)	CL1.1 "To have a chat with Miaoyu," was the (Xing Xiuyan's) answer. In surprise he (Jia Baoyu) remarked, "She's so aloof and unconventional that she looks down on everybody. If she thinks so highly of you, this show you're not vulgar like the rest of us." "She may not really think highly of me," replied Xiuyan with a smile, "but we were next-door neighbors for ten years...in a house." (岫烟笑道："我找妙玉说话." 宝玉听了诧异，说道："他为人孤僻，不合时宜，万人不入他目。原来他推重姐姐，竟知姐姐不是我们一流的俗人?" 岫烟笑道："他也未必身心重我，但我和他做过十年的邻居，只一墙之隔...住了十年.", 63).	(Obsessive-Compulsive) Restricted affectivity (an aspect of Detachment): indifference or coldness.
CH1.1	CM1 Eccentric (天性怪僻, 41); CM2 Headstrong and eccentric (放诞诡僻, 63)	CH1.1 CM1.1 She'd offended certain powerful people by her eccentric ways. (不合时宜, 权势 不容, 63).	Withdrawal (an aspect of Disinhibition): Preference for being alone to being with others; reticence in social situations; avoidance of social contacts and activity; lack of initiation of social contact.

Character	Code	Quote	Trait
		CN1.1 Miaoyu smiled disdainfully, "Can you really be so vulgar as not even to tell the difference? This is snow I gathered from plum-blossom five years ago while staying in Curly Fragrance Nunnery on Mount Xuanmu. I managed to fill that whole dark blue porcelain pot, but it seemed too precious to use so I've kept it buried in the earth all these years, not opening it till this summer. Today is only the second time I've used it. Surely you can taste the difference? How could last year's rain-water be as light and pure as this?" (妙玉冷笑道，"你这么个人，竟是大俗人，连水也尝不出来。这是五年前我在玄墓蟠香寺住着，收的梅花上的雪，共得了那一鬼脸青的花瓮一瓮，总舍不得吃，埋在地下，今年夏天才开了。我只吃过一回，这是第二回了。你怎么尝不出来？隔年蠲的雨水那有这样轻浮，如何吃得。" 41).	Hostility (an aspect of Negative Affectivity and an aspect of Antagonism): Persistent or frequent angry feelings; anger or irritability in response to minor slights and insults.
	CO1 Proud (骄傲, 18)	CH1.2	Grandiosity (an aspect of Antagonism): Believing that one is superior to others and deserves special treatment; condescension toward others.
Jia Jing (贾敬)	CP1 Expecting to attain immortality shortly (自为早晚就要飞升, 13)	CP1.1 Jia Jing alone was untouched by the death of his eldest grandson's wife. Expecting to attain immortality shortly himself, how could he go home to be soiled by mundane dust and squander all the merit he had acquired? So he left all the funeral arrangements to his son. (那贾敬闻得长孙媳妇死了，因自为早晚就要飞升，如何肯又回家染了红尘，将前功尽弃呢？因此并不在意，全凭贾珍料理, 13).	(Schizotypal) Identity: Distorted self-concept.
	CQ1 Wearing out with senseless and striving for immortality (枉作虚为, 63)	CQ1.1 But he's so wrapped up in Daoism that he takes no interest in anything but distilling elixirs; give all his mind to become an immortal. (如今一味好道，只爱烧丹炼汞，余者一概不在心上....心想作神仙, 2).	(Schizotypal) Self-direction: Unrealistic goals.

(continued)

Table A.1 (continued)

Character name	Description in DRM (English – Chinese)		DSM-5 Section III
	Terms or phrases	Sentences or paragraphs	Personality functioning or facets trait
		CQ1.1 CR1.1 They knew, however, that for years he had been practising absurd Daoist breathing exercises. As for his yoga, worship of the stars, keeping vigil on certain nights, taking sulphide of mercury and wearing himself out with his senseless striving for immortality—these were what had carried him off. (素知贾敬导气之术总属虚诞，更至参星礼斗，守庚申，服灵砂，妄作虚为，过于劳神费力，反因此伤了性命的，63).	(Schizotypal) Cognitive and perceptual dysregulation (an aspect of Psychoticism): Odd or unusual thought processes.
		CP1.1 CR1.1	(Schizotypal) Unusual beliefs and experiences (an aspect of Psychoticism): Thought content and views of reality that are viewed by others as bizarre or idiosyncratic.
CS1 Distilling elixirs every day (天天修炼, 63)		CS1.1 His Lordship (Jia Jing) had just concocted a new elixir with some secret formula, and that was his undoing. We'd warned him not to take such things, before achieving a certain potency; but last night, during his vigil, unknown to us he took some and became an immortal. (原是老爷秘法新制的丹砂吃坏事，小道们也曾劝说："功行未到，且服不得." 不承望老爷于今夜守庚申时，悄悄的服了下去，便升仙了，63).	(Schizotypal) Eccentricity (an aspect of Psychoticism): Odd, unusual, or bizarre behavior.
		CP1.1	(Schizotypal) Restricted affectivity (an aspect of Detachment): Indifference or coldness.

		(Schizotypal) Withdrawal (an aspect of Detachment): Avoidance of social contact and activity.
CT1.1 "I'm used to a peaceful life and don't want to be disturbed by all the commotion in your house. Of course, you're inviting me to go and have everyone kowtow to me because it's my birthday, but it would be a hundred times more to my liking if you had my annotated *Rewards and Punishments* (A Daoist tract on divine retribution) neatly copied out and printed. Suppose you entertain the two families for me at home the day after tomorrow instead of having them come here. Don't send me any presents either. In fact, there's no need for you to come yourself the day after tomorrow. You can kowtow to me now, if that will make you feel better. If you bring a great crowd to disturb me on my birthday, I shall be very displeased." ("我是清净惯了的，我不愿意往你们那里去场中去闹去。你们必定说是我的生日，要叫我去受众人些头，莫过你把我从前注的阴骘文给令人好好的写出来罢。比叫我花好好的款待他们就是了。也不必给我送什么东西来，这两日一家子要来，你就在家里好好的写出来罢。倘或后日有些不乐意，莫过你把我从前注的阴骘文给令人好好的写出来。连你后日也不必来，你要心中不安，你今日就给我磕了头去。倘或后日你要来，又跟随多少人来闹我，我必和你不依"，10).		
CT1.2 The only one not invited was Jia Jing, who abstained from both wine and meat. After the ancestral sacrifice on the seventeenth he moved back outside the city to live in seclusion; but even during his stay at home he remained quietly in his room, ignoring all the festivities around him. (贾敬素不茹酒，也不去请他，于后十七日祖祀已完，他便仍出城去修养。便这几日在家内，亦是静室默处，一概无听无闻，不在话下，53).		

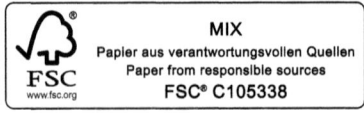

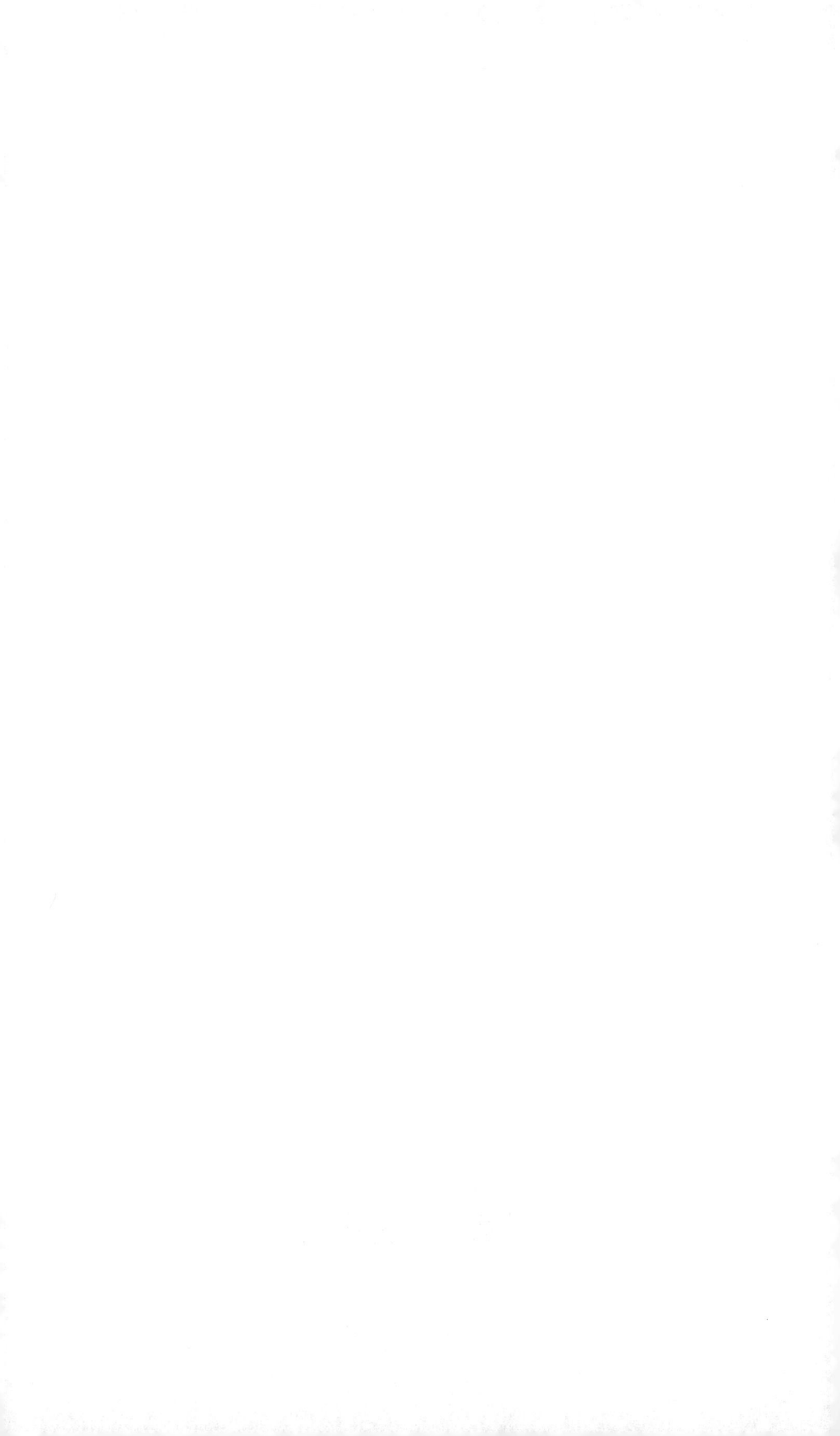